T0317571

Quality in Laboratory Hemostasis and Thrombosis

Quality in Laboratory Hemostasis and Thrombosis

Second Edition

Edited by

Steve Kitchen, PhD

Clinical Scientist
Sheffield Hemophilia and Thrombosis Centre
Royal Hallamshire Hospital
Sheffield; and
Scientific Director, UK National External Quality Assessment Scheme (NEQAS)
for Blood Coagulation
Scientific Director, WHO and WFH International External Quality Assessment
Programs for Blood Coagulation
Sheffield, UK

John D. Olson, MD, PhD

Professor and Vice Chair for Clinical Affairs
Department of Pathology
University of Texas Health Science Center; and
Director of Clinical Laboratories
University Health System
San Antonio, TX, USA

F. Eric Preston, MD, FRCPath, FRCP

Emeritus Professor of Hematology
University of Sheffield
Sheffield; and
Director, WHO and WFH International External Quality Assessment Programs
for Blood Coagulation
Sheffield, UK

Foreword by Professor Dr Frits R. Rosendaal

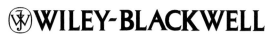

WILEY-BLACKWELL

A John Wiley & Sons, Ltd., Publication

Registered office: John Wiley & Sons, Ltd, The Atrium, Southern Gate, Chichester, West Sussex, PO19 8SQ, UK

Editorial offices: 9600 Garsington Road, Oxford, OX4 2DQ, UK
The Atrium, Southern Gate, Chichester, West Sussex, PO19 8SQ, UK
111 River Street, Hoboken, NJ 07030-5774, USA

For details of our global editorial offices, for customer services and for information about how to apply for permission to reuse the copyright material in this book please see our website at www.wiley.com/wiley-blackwell

Library of Congress Cataloging-in-Publication Data

Quality in laboratory hemostasis and thrombosis / edited by Steve Kitchen, John D. Olson, F. Eric Preston ; foreword by Frits R. Rosendaal. – 2nd ed.
    p. ; cm.
    Includes bibliographical references and index.
    ISBN 978-0-470-67119-1 (hardback : alk. paper)
    I. Kitchen, Steve, Dr. II. Olson, John David, 1944- III. Preston, F. E.
    [DNLM: 1. Hemostatic Techniques.   2. Anticoagulants.   3. Blood Coagulation Disorders, Inherited–diagnosis.   4. Blood Coagulation Factors.   5. Clinical Laboratory Techniques. 6. Thrombophilia–diagnosis. WH 310]

    616.1′57075–dc23

                                                                2012044510

A catalogue record for this book is available from the British Library.

1 2013

Contents

Contributors

Trevor W. Barrowcliffe MA, PhD
Formerly National Institute for Biological Standards
    and Control (NIBSC)
Potters Bar, Hertfordshire, UK

Mary E. Bauman RN, MN, NP
Stollery Childen's Hospital
University of Alberta
Edmonton, AB, Canada

Anthony K.C. Chan MBBS, FRCPC, FRCPath
McMaster Children's Hospital/Hamilton Health
    Sciences Foundation
Chair in Pediatric Thrombosis and Hemostasis
Department of Pediatrics, McMaster University
Hamilton, ON, Canada

Vanessa Chan BSc, MLT
Department of Paediatric Laboratory Medicine
The Hospital for Sick Children
Toronto, ON, Canada

Wayne L. Chandler MD
Coagulation Laboratory
Department of Pathology and Genomic Medicine
The Methodist Hospital Physician Organization
Houston, TX, USA

Myriam Dardikh MSc
Department of Laboratory Medicine
Laboratory of Haematology
Radboud University Nijmegen Medical Centre
Nijmegen, The Netherlands

Philippe de Moerloose MD
Haemostasis Unit
Department of Internal Medicine
University Hospital and Faculty of Medicine
Geneva, Switzerland

Morten Dunø MD, PhD
Department of Clinical Genetics
Copenhagen University Hospital (Rigshospitalet)
Copenhagen, Denmark

Emmanuel J. Favaloro PhD, FFSc (RCPA)
Department of Hematology
ICPMR, Westmead Hospital
Westmead, NSW, Australia

Dorothy (Adcock) Funk MD
Colorado Coagulation
a business unit of Esoterix, Inc., Englewood, CO,
    USA

Chris Gardiner PhD
Haematology Department
University College London Hospitals NHS Trust; and
Nuffield Department of Obstetrics and Gynaecology
John Radcliffe Hospital
Oxford, UK

Anne C. Goodeve PhD
Sheffield Haemostasis Research Group
Department of Cardiovascular Science
University of Sheffield
Sheffield; and
Sheffield Diagnostic Genetics Service
Sheffield Children's NHS Foundation Trust
Sheffield, UK

Elaine Gray PhD
National Institute for Biological Standards and
    Control
Potters Bar, Hertfordshire, UK

Michael Greaves MD FRCP FRCPath
Aberdeen Royal Infirmary
Head of College of Life Sciences and Medicine,
University of Aberdeen, Scotland, UK

Anthony R. Hubbard PhD
National Institute for Biological Standards and
    Control
Hertfordshire, UK

Martine Jandrot-Perrus MD, PhD
INSERM U698 and Paris 7 University
Paris, France

Ian Jennings PhD
UK NEQAS for Blood Coagulation
Sheffield, UK

Marilyn Johnston MLT, ART
Hemostasis Reference Laboratory
Hamilton, ON, Canada

Dianne Kitchen FIBMS
UK NEQAS Blood Coagulation
Sheffield, UK

Steve Kitchen PhD
Sheffield Hemophilia and Thrombosis
    Centre
Royal Hallamshire Hospital
Sheffield; and
UK National External Quality Assessment Scheme
    (NEQAS) for Blood Coagulation
WHO and WFH International External
    Quality Assessment Programs for Blood
    Coagulation
Sheffield, UK

Britta Laros-van Gorkom MD, PhD
Department of Haematology
Radboud University Nijmegen Medical
    Centre
Nijmegen, The Netherlands

Stefan Lethagen MD, PhD
Copenhagen University
Copenhagen; and
Medical and Science
Haemophilia R&D
Novo Nordisk A/S, Denmark

Giuseppe Lippi MD
Clinical Chemistry and Haematology Laboratory
Department of Pathology and Laboratory Medicine
Academic Hospital of Parma
Parma, Italy

Samuel Machin MB ChB, FRCP, FRCPath
Haematology Department
University College London Hospitals NHS Trust; and
Haemostasis Research Unit, Haematology Department
University College London
London, UK

Ian Mackie PhD, FRCPath
Haematology Department
University College London Hospitals NHS Trust
Haemostasis Research Unit
Haematology Department
University College London
London, UK

Richard A. Marlar PhD
Pathology and Laboratory Medicine
Oklahoma City VA Medical Center; and
Department of Pathology
University of Oklahoma Health Sciences Center
Oklahoma City, OK, USA

M. Patricia Massicotte MD, MHSc
Stollery Childen's Hospital
University of Alberta
Edmonton, AB, Canada

Jane C. Moore ART, BSc
Departments of Pathology and Molecular Medicine,
    and Medicine
Michael G. DeGroote School of Medicine, McMaster
    University
Hamilton Regional Laboratory Medicine Program
Hamilton, ON, Canada

Lars Bo Nielsen MD, PhD
Department of Clinical Biochemistry
Rigshospitalet and Department of Biomedical
    Sciences; and
University of Copenhagen
Copenhagen University Hospital (Rigshospitalet)
Copenhagen, Denmark

Alan Nurden PhD
Centre de Référence des Pathologies Plaquettaires
Plateforme Technologique d'Innovation Biomédicale
Hôpital Xavier Arnozan
Pessac, France

Paquita Nurden MD, PhD
Centre de Référence des Pathologies Plaquettaires
Plateforme Technologique d'Innovation Biomédicale
Hôpital Xavier Arnozan
Pessac, France

John D. Olson MD, PhD
Department of Pathology
University of Texas Health Science Center
San Antonio, TX, USA

Ian R. Peake PhD
Sheffield Haemostasis Research Group
Department of Cardiovascular Science
University of Sheffield
Sheffield, UK

F. Eric Preston MD, FRCPath, FRCP
University of Sheffield
Sheffield; and
WHO and WFH International External Quality
    Assessment Programs for Blood Coagulation
Sheffield, UK

Guido Reber PhD
Haemostasis Unit
Department of Internal Medicine
University Hospital and Faculty of Medicine
Geneva, Switzerland

Alok Srivastava MD, FRACP, FRCPA, FRCP
Department of Hematology
Christian Medical School
Vellore, India

Armando Tripodi PhD
Angelo Bianchi Bonomi Hemophilia and Thrombosis
    Center
Department of Internal Medicine
University School of Medicine and IRCCS Cà
    Granda Maggiore Hospital Foundation
Milan, Italy

Bert Verbruggen PhD
Laboratory of Clinical Chemistry and Haematology
Jeroen Bosch Hospital's-Hertogenbosch,
The Netherlands

Isobel D. Walker MD MPhil (Medical Law),
FRCPath
University of Glasgow, Glasgow; and
NEQAS for Blood Coagulation
Sheffield, UK

Theodore (Ted) E. Warkentin MD
Departments of Pathology and Molecular Medicine,
    and Medicine
Michael G. DeGroote School of Medicine
McMaster University
Transfusion Medicine
Hamilton Regional Laboratory Medicine Program
Hamilton, ON, Canada

Foreword

Thou art always figuring diseases in me, but thou art full of error: I am sound

(William Shakespeare. Measure for measure (1604); Act I, Scene II)

A correct diagnosis is the cornerstone of medicine. Without it, no remedy can be prescribed, or prognosis given. Although laboratory tests are only a part of the diagnostic arsenal, together with history taking, clinical examination, and imaging techniques, few diagnoses are arrived at without some form of laboratory test. Inadequate tests may lead to either false reassurance or false alarm. They may lead to the erroneous choice not to give treatment when treatment would be beneficial, or even to prescribe the wrong treatment, which is likely to be harmful. It is therefore of the utmost importance that whenever laboratory tests are performed, the results are reliable.

Laboratory tests in the field of thrombosis and hemostasis are notoriously difficult, which is related to the large variety in techniques that are used, and the sensitivity of many assays to small preanalytical and analytical variation. Therefore, quality assurance is crucial, and no hemostasis laboratory can afford not to invest in internal and external quality control. The book, Quality in Laboratory Hemostasis and Thrombosis, edited and written by authorities in the field, since its first edition in 2008, has become a indispensable help for those who wish to set up a hemostasis laboratory, as well as those who already work in such a place. For, to quote from the first chapter: "Process is never optimized; it can always be improved."

The book has two parts: the first eight chapters give a scholarly overview of the concepts that underlie quality assurance, explaining the various aspects of test validation, with its components, of which accuracy and precision are the most important: does a test measure what it is supposed to measure, and does it do so with acceptable reproducibility. Subsequent chapters in this first part explain in detail how internal quality control deals with precision and external quality control with accuracy. The development of international standards is an important and ongoing

development in improving accuracy and comparability of hemostasis laboratory tests. Here, the Scientific and Standardization Committee of the International Society on Thrombosis and Haemostasis, working together with the World Health Organization, has played a major role. Over the years we have witnessed the emergence of large external quality assurance programs, in which samples are sometimes sent to more than a thousand participating laboratories. Such programs not only allow laboratories to evaluate their performance, but also to group results by reagent or instrument, which leads to valuable insights, and further quality improvement. Newly added chapters to the second edition deal with the causes of laboratory error, the understanding of which is indispensable in optimizing laboratory performance, and the performance and interpretation of hemostatic tests in children.

In the second part of the book, Chapters 9 through 23, a detailed description is given of all major assays in hemostasis, grouped in a series of chapters on coagulation factor assays, on primary hemostasis (platelets and von Willebrand factor), and on thrombophilia testing and anticoagulant treatment monitoring. These chapters give the reader invaluable information on the performance and interpretation of these tests. A newly added chapter that was much missed in the first edition deals with heparin-induced thrombocytopenia.

The ultimate test for a laboratory test is whether it improves medical care, that is, reduces morbidity and mortality, which depends on the effect a negative or positive test result has on the treatment of a patient. A test that does not affect clinical management is a waste of resources. Both at the beginning and the end of laboratory tests there is usually a clinician, who first makes the decision to order a test, and subsequently has to interpret the test result. Although these clinical decisions and interpretation are not part of the content of this book, which would have made it unwieldy to say the least, these are of obvious importance, and one of the tasks of the individuals working in hemostasis laboratories is to educate clinicians about the clinical value of the various assays. I am quite confident that in the field of hemostasis and thrombosis more useless than useful testing is done, and that in medicine as a whole the greatest waste of money is on redundant diagnostics. The practice of medicine knows a wide variety of tests, which generally serve three purposes, either to diagnose a disease, or to test for a risk factor for disease, or to screen for either of these. This distinction is rarely sharply made, while it seems that clinically one type (diagnosing a disease) is almost always indicated and useful, and another type (testing for risk factors) only rarely is. While it is logical to find out which disease a patient with complaints has, it is not so logical to try and identify the causes of that disease, or even to try and identify those risk factors in nondiseased individuals, such as relatives of individuals with thrombosis. The reason the distinction between diagnosing a disease and identifying a risk factor is not always sharply made, is possibly because in some diseases in the field, notably bleeding disorders, there is an almost one-to-one relationship between the cause of the disease and the disease itself. While excessive bleeding is the disease and the clotting factor level a cause, individuals with no factor VIII or IX will invariably have the clinical disease of hemophilia, and therefore, measuring the clotting factor level has become synonymous to diagnosing hemophilia. This is quite different for thrombosis. Thrombosis (deep vein thrombosis or pulmonary embolism) is a disease, whereas thrombophilia is not. Given the multicausal nature of the etiology of thrombosis, in which multiple risk factors need to be present to lead to disease, it is far from self-evident that testing for thrombophilic abnormalities has any clinical value. So far, there are no clinical studies that show a benefit of such testing, although it is performed on a broad scale. Whenever you order a test or are requested to perform a test, question whether the result could possibly change anything. If not, or if the only benefit is to satisfy the doctor's curiosity, the test should not be done.

The reliability of a particular assay should be viewed in the context in which the test is ordered. Suppose one would order a test for high factor VIII as a prothrombotic risk factor, the above mentioned notwithstanding, an error of five IU/dL would be irrelevant, since the purpose is to discriminate between levels of over 150 or 200 IU/dL versus plasma concentrations around 100 IU/dL. The same error in a factor VIII assay to diagnose hemophilia A could be disastrous.

A clinician, when ordering a test, will have to deal with so-called prior probabilities, which is of particular relevance in screening tests. A slightly prolonged aPTT has a vastly different meaning when found in a healthy woman who had four uneventful deliveries who has come to the hospital for a tubal ligation, than in an 18-month-old boy who needs to undergo a duodenoscopy with possible biopsies. She is unlikely to have a bleeding tendency, even when the aPTT is prolonged, while the young boy may suffer from hemophilia. Screening tests affect the likelihood of disease, which, according to Bayes' theorem, is also a function of the prior probability of disease. Virtually, all tests that use reference ranges based on statistical cutoff values, such as the population mean plus or minus two standard deviations, are screening tests, that do neither establish a risk factor or a disease, but only, when abnormal, affect the likelihood of that state. Nature does not use standard deviations, and using a cutoff of two standard deviations by definition finds 2.5% of the population below, or over, such a cutoff. In reality, diseases and risk factors may have prevalences that exceed, or, more usual, lie far below this figure. Tests using "normal ranges" therefore can never establish an abnormality, and should be followed by more specific tests, such as clotting factor assays or genetic tests.

Over the last decades, major progress has been made in quality assurance of hemostatic laboratory assays. In this new edition of Quality in Laboratory Hemostasis and Thrombosis, all chapters have been updated and several new chapters have been added. This book will remain an indispensable part of every hemostasis laboratory, where, given its hands-on nature, it will rarely sit to get dusty on the shelves.

Frits R. Rosendaal
Former Chairman ISTH Council, President XXIV ISTH Congress, Former Chairman Netherlands Society of Thrombosis & Haemostasis, Leiden University Medical Centre, The Netherlands

Preface

In the past two to three decades, few disciplines, if any, in laboratory medicine have seen the growth in the number and complexity of testing as that experienced in the discipline of hemostasis and thrombosis. These rapid changes have presented challenges for laboratories as they develop quality programs for the oversight of this testing. The quality issues extend across all levels of testing and all sizes of laboratories. The field of laboratory medicine continues to evolve and there have been important advances since the first edition of this text was published. We, therefore, accepted the invitation to bring this text up to date in the second edition.

In our original discussions about a title for the first edition, we had an interesting discussion regarding possibilities of " … the Hemostasis and Thrombosis Laboratory" and " … Laboratory Hemostasis and Thrombosis." The distinction is subtle but relevant, the former being a place and the latter a discipline. Quality issues in this discipline extend well beyond the walls of the laboratory. In this second edition, we have retained contributions from all the original recognized experts which have been updated, and added a few new chapters based on the comments received in the intervening years since the first edition appeared. These experts have provided information on elements of managing quality as it relates to individual tests or groups of tests extending from nuances of internal quality control to the challenges in many areas where standardization may be absent or inadequate. There is information on all aspects of testing from preanalytic to analytic and results reporting as well as external quality assurance. In addition, chapters are included regarding the development of international guidelines for methods as well as the preparation of international standard plasmas and reagents.

Quality is a changing process, continually striving to improve the product while reducing errors and improving safety. This book represents an event in this continuum, and is intended to capture the elements of quality at all levels of the practice of Laboratory Hemostasis and Thrombosis, bringing these up to date since the construction of the first edition during 2008. We believe that it will continue to provide a useful guide for those involved hemostasis and thrombosis testing, whether very simple, like the point of care, or complex, like the major reference laboratory.

Steve Kitchen
John D. Olson
F. Eric Preston

PART 1

General Quality Program

1 General quality planning in the hemostasis laboratory

John D. Olson[1,2]

[1]Department of Pathology, University of Texas Health Science Center, San Antonio, TX, USA
[2]University Health System, San Antonio, TX, USA

Introduction

Quality:
Invisible when it is good.
Impossible to ignore when it is bad.

"So," you might ask, "What is quality, anyway?" The word quality repeatedly infiltrates our discussions and interactions as we work to produce or choose a product. The *Oxford English Dictionary* devotes more than 3000 words in its effort to define the many variations on the use of this word [1]. We may all have difficulty with a definition, but we do know what we mean. The customer of the product or service defines many aspects of its quality while those who are producing define many others. Stated in its simplest terms, quality is the condition or state of a person, thing, or process.

The principles

As early as the middle of the 1400s, boat makers in Venice, Italy, introduced the principle of "mass production" with the manufacture of boats in the sequential assembly of preproduced parts. This assembly line process was refined in the modern sense by Henry Ford between 1900 and 1910. The scientific elements of quality management systems began in the 1930s with the publication of Shewhart in 1931 [2],

providing a scientific and statistical basis for quality processes. He stated:

> A phenomenon will be said to be controlled when, through the use of past experience, we can predict, at least within limits, how the phenomenon may be expected to vary in the future. Here it is understood that prediction means that we can state, at least approximately, the probability that the observed phenomenon will fall within given limits. [1]

The evolution of quality management systems was influenced by experiences in World War II. During the war, individuals involved in the production of reliable products for the consumer (soldier) to effectively do their job tied the entire system from raw material to the use of the finished product in a unique "team" from start to finish. Few circumstances can link the person in production so directly to the importance of the outcome. The success of the soldier was tied to the long-term well-being of the person making the tools used by that soldier. This ability to build the tight kinship and team performance on the part of people in production to the quality of the product is the goal of quality programs in all sectors of the economy today. It is, of course, very difficult to achieve this attitude in the workplace in the same way that it could be when the outcome could so directly benefit the producers.

Following World War II, the effort of reconstruction of the industry and economy of the affected countries became a major international effort and

Quality in Laboratory Hemostasis and Thrombosis, Second Edition. Edited by Steve Kitchen, John D. Olson and F. Eric Preston.
© 2013 John Wiley & Sons, Ltd. Published 2013 by Blackwell Publishing Ltd.

Table 1.1 Comparison of Deming and traditional management principles

Common company practices	"Deming" company practices
Quality is expensive.	Quality leads to lower costs.
Inspection is the key to quality.	Inspection is too late. If workers can produce defect-free goods, eliminate inspections.
Quality control experts and inspectors can ensure quality.	Quality is made in the boardroom.
Defects are caused by workers.	Most defects are caused by the system.
The manufacturing process can be optimized by outside experts with little or no change in the system afterward.	Process is never optimized; it can always be improved.
Little or no input from workers.	Elimination of all work standards and quotas is necessary. Fear leads to disaster.
Use of work standards, quotas, and goals can help productivity.	People should be made to feel secure in their jobs.
Fear and reward are proper ways to motivate.	Most variation is caused by the system.
Employees can be treated like commodities, buying more when needed and laying off when needing less.	Buy from vendors committed to quality and work with suppliers.
Rewarding the best performers and punishing the worst will lead to greater productivity and creativity.	Invest time and knowledge to help suppliers improve quality and costs. Develop long-term relationships with suppliers.
Buy one supplier off against another and switch suppliers based only on price.	Profits are generated by loyal customers.
Profits are made by keeping revenue high and costs down.	

Source: From Reference 6.

influenced the evolution of quality programs. The work of Deming [3] and Juran [4, 5], both associates of Shewart, extended his work. In 1951, Juran published a seminal book [4] that proposed the key elements for managing quality: quality planning, quality control (QC), and quality improvement. Following World War II, Deming presented a significant departure from the "standard" thinking about quality. He proposed a modification to the real relationships of quality, costs, productivity, and profit. The different approach to quality espoused by Deming is compared to the "standard" thinking in Table 1.1 [6]. Thus, anything that improves the product or service in the eyes of the customer defines the goals of the quality program.

Organizations that follow Deming principles find that good quality is hard to define, but the lack of quality is easily identified. In the "standard" management of a system, the workers ultimately pay for management failure because labor costs are reduced when profits fall. In contrast, moving quality

programs as close to the worker as possible will ultimately lead to lower cost and improved consumer and worker satisfaction.

The clinical laboratory has three "consumers" of their product: (1) the patient who benefits from the best possible quality of care; (2) the ordering clinician who depends upon the right test, at the right time with an accurate result in order to make a clinical decision; (3) the hospital, clinic, or other entity that depends upon the laboratory for a positive margin when comparing cost with revenue. All three consumers benefit when the quality program drives the best possible practice.

Elements of quality in the hemostasis laboratory

When a clinician orders a laboratory test, he/she sets in motion a complex process that involves many individuals. More than two dozen individual actions, involvement of sophisticated instruments, and multiple interfaces of computing devices encompass the

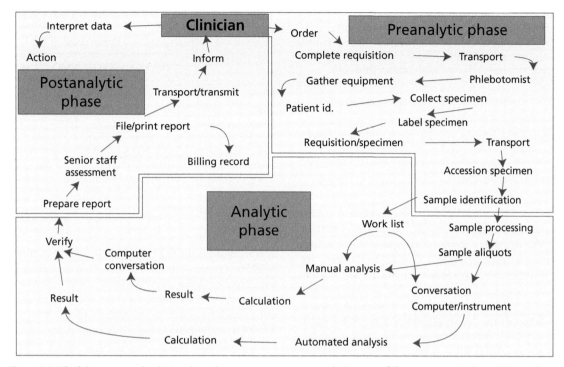

Figure 1.1 The laboratory cycle: depicted are the steps needed to complete a laboratory test, beginning with the ordering clinician and ending with the response of the ordering clinician to the result. Preanalytic, analytic, and postanalytic parts of the process are indicated. More than two dozen steps (arrows) are involved, each of which may be the source of an error. Monitoring all steps by a quality program is required.

three phases: the preanalytic phase (order, collection, and transport); the analytic phase (making the correct measurement); the postanalytic phase (formulating and delivering the data and the action of the clinician in response to the result). Figure 1.1 is a graphic depiction of the laboratory cycle. Examining the figure, one might think that each arrow represents an opportunity for error that could affect the final result. A quality program must encompass all of these events including processes to prevent and detect errors, should they occur.

The tools

Many different quality practices/programs have evolved in the decades since the early work of Shewhart, Juran, and Deming. They all have their acronyms (i.e., TQM, CQI, ISO, IOP, ORYX, SIX SIGMA, Lean, TOC, and others) and a common goal of improving the quality of the performance (and product) of an organization. The discussion of all these individual programs is beyond the scope of this chapter, but many of the principles are addressed below and in other chapters of this book. All programs have great strength, but they also suffer from being proscriptive, an issue that will be discussed later in this chapter.

Currently, *Six Sigma* and *Lean* are programs that are in use in laboratories and merit some description.

Six Sigma

Many industries and some laboratories have adopted control processes that focus on quantifying and reducing errors called *Six Sigma*® [7]. *Six Sigma* was developed by an engineer (Bill Smith) at the Motorola Company and the company began using the program in the mid-1980s. *Six Sigma* is a registered trademark of the Motorola Corporation. Application of the process has become very popular among companies internationally. *Six Sigma* processes can be applied to

Table 1.2 Six Sigma metrics

Measure outcomes	Measure variation
Inspect outcomes and count defects	Measure variation of a process (SD)
Calculate defects per million	Calculate Sigma process capability
Convert DPM to Sigma metric	Determine QC design metric

Source: From Reference 7.

Table 1.3 Sigma metrics for common coagulation tests

Test	Sigma metric			
	TEA (%)	NTQ	NMQ	LMQ
Prothrombin time	15	na	1.77	5.35
INR	20	na	2.39	3.52
Fibrinogen assay	20	1.78	2.01	3.24

TEA, total acceptable error; NTQ, national total quality (all methods); NMQ, national method quality (within method); LMQ, local method quality (single laboratory); na, not available.
Source: From Reference 9.

discrete events (mislabeled specimens, clerical errors, etc.) and to variable events (i.e., variance of a method like the fibrinogen assay). Elements of these activities are depicted in Table 1.2. Discrete elements are expressed in defects per million events (DPM). Achieving the Six Sigma goal means that defects are less than 1:1,000,000, a level achieved in the airline industry. Errors in the healthcare industry are much more frequent with errors causing injury to hospitalized patients at 10,000 DPM (3.8σ), errors in therapeutic drug monitoring 244,000 DPM (2.2σ), or errors of laboratory reporting much better at 447 DPM (4.8σ) [8]. Other aspects of the laboratory activity rely on analysis of the variability of data. This variability can be measured at several levels. The greatest variability is seen in External Quality Assessment (EQA) data regarding the all method variance, referred to as the National Total Quality (NTQ). EQA programs also report data for an analyte comparing many laboratories using the same method, referred to the National Method Quality (NMQ). NMQ is frequently significantly better because variability is only among laboratories using the same methods, but not among methods. The lowest variability is seen with a single method in a single laboratory, referred to as the Local Method Quality (LMQ) [9]. Greater variability occurs with method-specific interlaboratory testing with the greatest variability being observed when all methods are compared. Thus, the degree of variability is best controlled at the local level.

Examples of this degree of variability are shown for prothrombin time, international normalized ratio (INR), and fibrinogen assay in Table 1.3 [9]. The data in Table 1.3 are very specifically based on the data from the 2004 EQA data of the College of American Pathologists, as reported by Westgard [9]. Should a

number of different EQA data sets be analyzed, there would be a range of sigma statistics of a similar magnitude. The low sigma values shown mean that adequate control will demand more rigorous attention to control procedures, often necessitating multiple control rules. Common goals in industry are to strive for 6σ processes and to accept 3σ. At 3σ or below, effective error detection could not be achieved, even with as many as six QC rules. There is much progress yet to be made in the quality of many coagulation procedures.

Lean

Concepts of *Lean* appear to have originated with Henry Ford and his assembly line production. He actually sent engineers to the automobile junkyard to examine automobiles that could no longer function. Two types of information were gathered: first, to determine which parts failed, leading to the failure of the automobile, information used to develop improved parts in order to increase the usable life of the automobile; second, to determine those parts that were not worn out at all (or minimally), information used to examine whether alternative parts of lower cost could suffice. In the latter case, the motive is to provide sufficient performance of the part at the lowest cost to the customer. Representatives of the Toyota Motor Company visited Ford in the early 1930s. They applied and refined the principles, developing the Toyota Production System, later to be known as *Lean* [10]. *Lean* is a business management system designed to improve productivity and quality by elimination of waste. Goals are customer satisfaction; employee satisfaction; increased workplace safety; long-term working relationships with suppliers; improved quality; reduced cost; elimination of waste. Any activity, no matter how trivial, that does not offer benefit to the product (and the customer) is a candidate for elimination. Companies involved with *Lean* are continually examining every process for opportunities to save time and improve quality. Several common activities used in other business models rarely add value. Examples include approval (delegate as much as possible); batching (delay results as little as possible, balance this with cost); searching and walking (keep all supplies immediately at hand, locate tasks as few steps as possible from each other); waiting (work with suppliers for delivery "just in time"). Thus, *Lean* aims to make processes simple enough to understand, do, and manage by the worker.

Organizations using Six Sigma and Lean rely on the common structured problem solving strategy used in business called DMAIC (**D**efine the problem; **M**easure events; **A**nalyze and understand the data; **I**mprove the process; set up **C**ontrols that maintain the improvements). The strategy can be applied to all problem solving; however, more complex issues, such as restructuring a process, require the assembly of a team, the setting of clear goals, and a planned timeline for completion. Further details regarding application of Lean and Six Sigma can be found in George et al. [11].

Error detection and correction

McGregor contrasted two theories of company management that he referred to as X and Y [12]. A company following theory X assumes that the worker prefers to be directed and wants to avoid responsibility. In contrast, a company that is following theory Y assumes the workers enjoy what they do and, in the right conditions, will strive to do their very best. In general, the company that follows theory X manages from the "top down" with dependence of the worker upon management as he/she performs tasks. A hallmark of theory X is toughness, the rules are laid out, and every employee must "obey." The workplace has an element of fear that an error might occur and a reprimand will result. The style of the company that follows theory Y is different. Management works from the "bottom up." The workplace is configured to satisfy the worker and to encourage commitment

to the organization. Workers are encouraged to be self-directed and the management/supervisory style is supportive. Theory Y has been described as operating with a "velvet glove." Stated in another way, management under theory X strives to "drive" the organization and the workers to success, while the management under theory Y strives to "lead" the organization and the workers to success. The goal in both cases is essentially the same, but the means to the goal are very different. This brief description of diverging management styles can impact process improvement within the laboratory.

A later chapter in this book (Chapter 3) addresses the causes of medical errors and reemphasizes the need for a system in the quality program for capturing and categorizing errors. In order for any method, process, or laboratory to improve, it is paramount to correct and understand the cause of the errors that interfere with performance. The laboratory needs a system for capturing and categorizing errors. Such a system becomes the infrastructure for improvement in a quality program. It is obvious that for a system to be successful, there needs to be an aggressive program to identify all errors, optimally at the time of the occurrence. The ideal process is one that looks prospectively at activities seeking to prevent errors. Deming [6] pointed out that inspection is too late. Once again the airline industry provides an example. Considerable effort is applied to understanding what causes the big error, an airplane crash. However, major efforts are now actually directed at the near misses both in the air and on the ground, a proactive effort to understand the "close call" to help prevent the major event. The laboratory needs a similar aggressive approach that must begin with each individual owning their part of an activity and identifying the problems as they occur, or seeing ways to prevent problems by changing procedures. In order for such a process to be most efficient, the worker should not be threatened by the mechanism to report errors. The following examples regarding the differing approaches may be useful.

First, a technologist has just completed a run on an automated instrument using expensive reagents and producing many patient results. He/she notices that two required reagents were placed in the wrong position, causing them to be added in the wrong order. The error caused erroneous patient results, but not to the degree that it would be easily detected. The consequence of repeating the run is twofold: the cost of the reagents and time of the technologist are expensive and the delay in completing the testing results in complaints from clinicians. In this scenario, management under theory X results in a reprimand from the supervisor and a letter being placed in the technologist's personnel file for negative consideration at the next performance evaluation. The consequences may be severe enough for the technologist to consider not reporting the error. In contrast, management under theory Y would result in the supervisor complimenting the technologist for detecting the problem and engaging the technologist in an investigation of the reason that the error occurred. The supervisor and the technologist understand that the goal is to prevent this from happening in the future, whether this person or another performs the procedure. The assumption is that the process contributed to the error.

Second is a case in which the error that occurred above was not detected by the technologist performing the test, but at a later time during the supervisor's inspection of reported results. Managing under theory X, the supervisor will confront the technologist with the data and, just as in the prior example, will issue a reprimand and a letter. Managing under theory Y, the supervisor will present the information to the technologist and ask the technologist to assist in understanding how the problem occurred and how it might be avoided in the future.

Errors like those described that are detected and investigated are most frequently found to be problems in the process, not exclusively with the individual doing the procedure at the time. Improving the process to help workers prevent errors is the goal and can only succeed if errors are detected and investigated. Contrasting the approaches, one can see that punishing the worker and failing to examine process will not improve the quality and the worker will not be enthused about reporting future errors. The second approach engages the workers and rewards activities that improve quality in the laboratory.

Internal quality control

The control of the testing procedure (QC) evolved with the transition of research testing into the clinical arena. In general, internal QC provides a method to verify the imprecision of a test. To be confident that the method returns the correct result requires that steps be taken to ensure all elements are within

the control of the operator. Technologists are taught that instruments/methods are designed to fail and that they can rely upon results only if the entire method performs within defined limits with specimens of known value. The frequency of these control events are method specific and a function of the stability of all of the elements (reagent, specimen, instrument) and must be driven by historical data from the method itself. Internal QC is the grandfather of quality programs in the laboratory and is detailed elsewhere in this book (Chapter 6).

Quality assurance

During the 1980s, laboratories began looking beyond the analytic procedure with quality programs called Quality Assurance. QC remained a part of the Quality Assurance program, but the program expanded to consider such items as laboratory orders, requisitions, collection techniques, and other issues directly impacting the result of the test but not always directly in the control of the laboratory. Preanalytic issues are detailed elsewhere in this book (Chapter 5). Postanalytic issues also became a part of quality initiatives this same era: such issues as reporting formats, verification of calculated results, timely reporting, and even action taken as a result of the data reported. It was during this period that computer applications in both the laboratory and the clinical environments began to grow, requiring the validation and continued verification of computer function and interfaces for electronic result reporting between computers as well as between instruments and computers. Encouraged (or demanded) by accreditation and/or regulatory agencies, laboratory professionals also began asking questions of and listening to clinicians regarding the quality of service and needs to provide new tests shown to have clinical value and to remove antiquated tests that no longer offer added clinical information. These activities started the interaction of the quality programs in the laboratory with similar programs in the rest of the healthcare institutions.

External quality assessment

In the 1930s [13], the need for interlaboratory standardization for public health programs (a method to verify accuracy) led to early efforts at External Quality Assurance. The concept of an unknown specimen being sent from a central EQA agency to the laboratory for testing with the results sent back to the agency for evaluation added an important new level of assurance for the quality of analysis. In addition, results were reported in a way that allowed a laboratory to compare their performance to other laboratories using the same or similar methods. Laboratory participation in EQA programs grew rapidly in the 1950s and 1960s. In large part this growth was due to the development accreditation and regulatory programs requiring EQA; however, the recognition by unregulated laboratories that EQA was vital to the quality of their own programs has also led to widening acceptance.

EQA is generally viewed as a process to examine the analytic phase of testing, offering little or no information regarding the pre- and postanalytic phases. Described below is a method to examine a portion of the preanalytic process and all of the postanalytic process if the laboratory uses a laboratory information system (LIS) with electronic reporting to an electronic medical record (EMR).

Within the LIS and the EMR, one can create an additional floor on the hospital, or clinic in the outpatient department. Doing so allows for development of as many "beds" or clinic visits as necessary to handle all EQA challenges. Next, the Medical Records and/or billing departments assign a block of medical record numbers for laboratory use only. The laboratory then assigns a medical record number and name to each of the EQA challenges to which it subscribes (coagulation limited, coagulation special, etc.). Each challenge may have several analytes.

Having created this for each challenge, when the specimen arrives, the specimen is accessioned into the computer with the same method as a patient, the testing is performed in the same manner as a patient, and the reporting into the LIS and the EMR will occur in the same manner as a patient. The data reported to the EQA provider can be that reported to the EMR.

The advantage of such an approach is that all instrument/computer interfaces are validated and the evaluating, accessioning, and reporting process becomes a part of the EQA program. In addition, with time, the laboratory can query the EMR by the name and medical record number of the EQA challenge to see the longitudinal data reported by analyte.

Detailed discussion of EQA programs is addressed elsewhere in this book (Chapter 7).

The application of the tools in the laboratory

Quality system essentials

Development and maintenance of a quality program in a laboratory requires that there be an infrastructure of support in order for internal and external QC and quality assurance to be successful. The field of hemostasis provides an excellent example of this issue. The hemostasis laboratory has the entire spectrum of testing from the highly automated to the complex manual tests that are time-consuming and demand a different skill set. Thus, in addition to a good QC program, there is need for an effective program for development and continuing education of the staff. The same can be said of a host of essential activities in the laboratory including such things as acquisition and maintenance of capital equipment; supply inventory; safety of staff and patients; and others. In the late 1990s and early 2000s, recommendations began to appear for the comprehensive management of the quality of all aspects of the laboratory operations. International Standards Organization (ISO) developed the ISO 17025 (primarily a laboratory management program) [14] and ISO 15189 (a program specifically for clinical laboratories) [15]. The Clinical Laboratory Standards Institute (CLSI), at the time named NCCLS, published the Quality System Essentials (QSE) [16]. The ISO programs have achieved acceptance in Europe and internationally, while the QSE programs are more commonly in use in North America. Both approach the issues of quality with a very broad perspective, covering all elements of laboratory operations.

The list presented in Table 1.4 is an example of the QSE for a given laboratory. The list is not intended to be the list for use in every laboratory. Each laboratory needs to develop its own essentials, formulated to help manage issues within their own laboratory. The list is ordinarily 9–12 items in length and the types of issues to be addressed are encompassed in Table 1.4. Each of the items on this list will be controlled by a set of three levels of documents:

Policies: Statement of intent with regard to rules and requirements of regulations, accreditation, and standards. Each QSE will have one or a small number of policies that will provide the framework for all activities within the QSE. In the case of test

Table 1.4 Quality system essentials (CLSI—1999)

Purchasing and inventory	Information management
Organization	Deviations, nonconformance
Personnel	Assessments: internal and external
Equipment	Process improvement
Document and records	Customer service
Process control	Facilities and safety

Source: From Reference 14.

development, policies may address such things as validation, QC, EQA, and others.

Process descriptions: This is a description of how the policies are implemented. Process descriptions will often cross more than one department, section of departments, and procedures within a section. Flowcharts and tables are often used to describe processes. An example of a process requiring control is given below.

Procedures and related forms: The standard operating procedure (SOP) is a step-by-step description of how to perform a method or task.

The Policy and the SOP are documents commonly used in all laboratories; however, the process description may not be as familiar. An example is shown in Figure 1.2. The purpose of this process is to provide the surgeon and anesthesiologist with information needed to manage blood transfusion therapy in the rapidly bleeding patient. The data needed are the Prothrombin Time, Fibrinogen, Hemoglobin and Platelet count. The process needs an order, specimen collection, transport, laboratory receipt/accession, testing in two separate sections of the laboratory, reporting, and delivery of the data to the clinician. Ownership of the various steps in this process is in the control of the physician, nurse, and three different sections of the laboratory. In order for this to occur in a meaningful time frame in the clinical setting (less than 15 minutes), there must be well-understood coordination among all of those involved. Each step in the process described has its own SOP for the action taken. In this case, there are at least ten SOPs supporting a single process.

Implementation of a program can be challenging. Most laboratories have a quality program that can provide the beginning for the development of QSE. Most laboratories also have most of the essentials that they will define in their QSE; they are just not under the umbrella of the program and not easily identified. Thus, an initial step in changing the program will be gathering key individuals with knowledge and energy for the process to identify the QSE for the organization. Technologists should also be represented in this process. Once the QSE are identified, teams can be formed to begin drafting of policies. Leadership from the highest levels, supporting the changes that need to be made, and leading the infrastructure of a management structure base upon McGregor's theory Y are crucial elements.

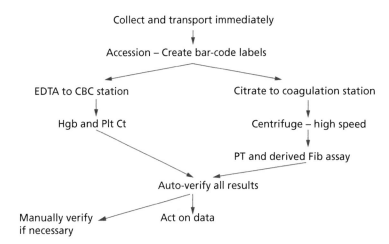

Figure 1.2 Process for the Bleeding Profile: This process for reporting the results of the Prothrombin Time (PT), Fibrinogen Assay (Fib Assay), Platelet Count (Plt Ct), and Hemoglobin (Hgb) involves the activity of at least four different units in the health system and execution of as many as ten SOPs. As a part of the QSE, a process description would be needed to ensure return of results rapidly enough for clinician action when managing an actively bleeding patient.

Possibly the most important issue is putting reality into fault-free reporting of errors, followed by an investigation to improve process to prevent future occurrences.

For many laboratories, instituting the concepts that are described in this chapter would necessitate significant change in the quality program, the perspective of the manager, and the attitude of the employee. Such a change in the culture is difficult. It is tempting to try to "buy, install and run" a program from a quality vendor. Such an approach is likely to meet with resistance from workers who view it as "just another of those quality things that the administration is going to force on us." In the past two decades (or more) most laboratories have instituted more that one new quality program in an effort to find a solution that works well in their setting. One possible difficulty in such an approach is the proscriptive nature of the process. They provide everything that is needed, policies, forms, SOPs, and so on. What they do not provide is the personal ownership that can come from the internal development of the quality process. Managers may find a smoother and more lasting solution in providing policies that allow for each unit to develop their own approach to the gathering of data, the identification of errors, and the many other elements of the quality program.

Summary

Over the course of the past 70 or more years, elements of the quality program have evolved in a somewhat stepwise fashion, beginning with internal QC and progressing to more comprehensive programs that encompass all activities in the workplace. In the remainder of this book you will find information regarding quality in all aspects of the hemostasis laboratory. Experts provide information regarding the highest level of development of standards (both methods and materials) to the finest details of the nuances of selected methods. Integrated into a comprehensive quality program, similar to that described above, the information should help in the development of a "QUALITY HEMOSTASIS LABORATORY."

References

1. Oxford English Dictionary.
2. Shewhart WA. *Economic Control of Quality of Manufactured Product*. New York: D. Van Nostrand; 1931.
3. DeAguayo R. *Deming: The American Who Taught the Japanese about Quality*. New York: Simon & Schuster; 1990:1–66.
4. Juran JM. *Juran's Quality Control Handbook*. 4th ed. New York: McGraw-Hill; 1988.
5. Juran JM. *Juran on Leadership for Quality: An Executive Handbook*. New York: Collier Macmillan; 1989: 1–80.
6. Travers EM, McClatchy KM. Basic laboratory management. In: McClatchy KM, ed. *Clinical Laboratory Medicine*. 2nd ed. Philadelphia, PA: Lippincott Williams & Wilkins; 2002:3–31.
7. Westgard JO. *Six Sigmas Quality Design and Control*. Madison, WI: Westgard QC; 2001:11–22.
8. Nevalainen D, Berte L, Kraft C, Leigh E, Morgan T. Evaluating laboratory performance on quality indicators with the Six Sigma scale. *Arch Pathol Lab Med*. 2000;124:516–519.
9. Westgard JO, Westgard SA. The quality of laboratory testing today: an assessment of σ metrics for analytic quality using performance data from proficiency testing surveys and the clia criteria for acceptable performance. *Am J Clin Pathol*. 2006;125:343–354.
10. Womack JD. The Lean Enterprise Institute. http://www.lean.org; 2009. Accessed 14 Jan 2013.
11. George ML, Rowlands D, Price M, Maxey J. *The Lean Six Sigma Pocket Toolbox*. New York: McGraw-Hill; 2005.
12. McGregor D. *The Human Side of Enterprise*. New York: McGraw-Hill; 1960:1–58.
13. Cumming HS, Hazen HH, Sanford FE, et al. Evaluation of serodiagnostic tests for syphilis in the United States: report of results. *Vener Dis Informat*. 1935;16:189.
14. International Organization for Standardization. ISO/IEC 17025:2005: General requirements for the competence of testing and calibration laboratories. http://www.iso.org/iso/catalogue_detail?csnumber=39883. Accessed 14 Jan 2013.
15. International Organization for Standardization. ISO 15189:2007: Medical laboratories: particular requirements for quality and competence. http://www.iso.org/iso/iso_catalogue/catalogue_tc/catalogue_detail.htm?csnumber=42641. Accessed 14 Jan 2013.
16. National Committee for Clinical Laboratory Standards. *A Quality System Model for Health Care: Approved Guidelines*, Wayne, PA: NCCLS; NCCLS document GP26-A; 1999.

2

Hemostasis test validation, performance, and reference intervals: international recommendations and guidelines

Richard A. Marlar[1,2]

[1]Pathology and Laboratory Medicine, Oklahoma City VA Medical Center, Oklahoma City, OK, USA
[2]Department of Pathology, University of Oklahoma Health Sciences Center, Oklahoma City, OK, USA

The clinical hemostasis or coagulation laboratory is a complex testing arena that does not fit well into the mold of hematology ("counting" of particles—red blood cells or platelets) or chemistry with known concentrations of analytes (sodium charge and albumin mass). The hemostasis or coagulation assay inventory spans multiple test types (from clotting tests to chromogenic and immunologic assays to specialized tests such as electrophoresis, aggregation, and radioactive-based tests) and results are expressed in a wide variety of units: time, percentage, units, mass, optical density units, and even visual interpretation. International standards are available for some analytes (see Chapter 4); however, many still await the development of such standards. As a result, values are based on local or manufacturer's units. These parameters complicate the development, validation, performance of methods in the routine coagulation laboratory, and the more complex methods of the "special" coagulation laboratory.

Modifications of assay methods such as using one manufacturer's kit on another manufacturer's instrument or in-house ("home brew") tests or components lead to many challenges of method standardization and validation to produce accurate diagnostic, monitoring, or therapeutic information. Before a new method can be introduced into clinical use, both analytical and clinical performances must be verified under standard operating parameters of the laboratory. This chapter is intended to review the validation procedure and outline a systematic approach for hemostatic assay validation, helping laboratories meet the daily needs of internal quality standards and external certification requirements.

The general and continuing assessment of clinical coagulation testing falls to accrediting agencies sanctioned by each country. The accreditation requirements of "good laboratory practices" vary for each oversight agency. For many hemostasis tests, significant problems are encountered: differences in reagents generating results in different arbitrary units (prothrombin time (PT) and activated partial thromboplastin time (aPTT)); tests with multiple protocols (Bethesda vs. Nijmegen inhibitor assays); and test results based on experience or visual interpretation (platelet aggregation or von Willebrand factor (vWF) multimers).

The processes of validation and performance evaluation are presented followed by a discussion of the reference interval, a difficult concept in hemostasis and coagulation. The use of a standardized validation protocol will help to objectively evaluate method performance. The parameters of this validation protocol must be established prior to any studies better defining the limits of the method, reference interval, and certainly its use in the clinical laboratory (Table 2.1). Validation is the process of proving that a procedure, process, system, equipment, reagents, and methods work singly and together as expected to achieve the intended result. Method validation assesses not only

Quality in Laboratory Hemostasis and Thrombosis, Second Edition. Edited by Steve Kitchen, John D. Olson and F. Eric Preston.
© 2013 John Wiley & Sons, Ltd. Published 2013 by Blackwell Publishing Ltd.

Table 2.1 The basic components and responsibilities of a validation study for new or modified coagulation assay

---

Supervisor responsibilities

Confirmation of no existing patents (if applicable)

Written laboratory procedure (CLSI GP2-A5 format)

Validation study: accuracy, precision, analytical sensitivity and specificity

Interferences, LOD, limit of quantification

RR

Quality control procedure

MSDS update

Training plan: training method, list of staff requiring training, competency

Assessment, new-employee training

Prepare memo to announce availability of test

Cost analysis of test and recommended test charge

Laboratory information manager
Establish "test definition"

Add test to LIS and HIS files

Verify report format is acceptable in all systems

QA supervisor

Add document-to-document inventory log and assign number

Add test to specimen collection manual

Add test to activity menu

Order proficiency testing materials

Laboratory director
Written approval of test establishment

Summary statement with director signature and date of implementation

---

Not all the listed components may be needed for every assay. The laboratory director must decide which aspects are relevant.

the major characteristics of the method but also continues assay performance over time assuring the same characteristics as initially assigned. After the assay has been deemed valid and the performance characteristics established, the final aspect of method characterization is to determine the value range(s) present in the populations in which the assay will be used. This concept of reference range evaluation and population

sampling in conjunction with the reference interval establishment methods will be discussed.

Hemostatic test validation concepts

The purpose of test method validation is to ensure high-quality data for the accurate diagnosis of disease. The time invested in the initial validation of an analytical method will ultimately provide the necessary diagnostic advantages in the long run. Procedural, methodological, or instrumentation validation will demonstrate that the procedure, method, or instrument, respectively, is acceptable for the overall intended use. The validation steps must be thorough for each aspect of the process. The validation components should include (but not limited to) specificity, accuracy, precision, limits, linearity, and robustness (Table 2.1). Validation of coagulation methods, whether assays, instruments, or reagents, is the cornerstone of coagulation laboratory diagnostics and is the process to determine acceptability of the analytical method.

The validation protocol is necessary for the determination of the performance characteristics. A written procedure (protocol) detailing the validation process should include (1) procedural steps necessary to perform the test; (2) necessary instrumentation, reagents, and samples; (3) method for calibration; (4) formulae for generating results; and (5) source of reference standards and controls (Table 2.1). In addition, the common statistics (see Appendix) used in assay validation must also be incorporated. The typical validation parameters are discussed below using descriptions from formal definitions but slanted toward hemostatic testing [1, 2]. These include specificity, accuracy, precision, linearity, limit of detection (LOD), limit of quantitation (LOQ), and robustness.

A validation process for hemostasis/coagulation methods must be designed to ensure that the result of the method will accurately support the diagnosis of patients with coagulation defects. The samples, reagents, controls, calibrators, and instruments to be used for validation purposes should be carefully selected. Samples and specimens for validation must be collected, processed, and stored by established guidelines and identical to routine collection and storage methods used in the laboratory [3]. In the validation process for diagnostic and/or therapeutic control methods, the reagent lots and instruments must be those that will be used in the laboratory when the methods are put in place [2, 3].

Specificity is the ability to unequivocally assess the analyte in a standard specimen in the presence of components that may be expected to be present [2, 4]. Typically this includes such components like the plasma (matrix) and degraded or inactive components. The method should be capable of the differentiation of similar analytes or interfering substances that could have a significant effect on the value. In commercially available methods (in the United States, especially FDA-approved methods), these evaluations should have been performed by the manufacturer. In "home-brew" assays, the user must demonstrate specificity, a task that may be a very difficult.

Accuracy is the closeness of agreement between the test value and the true value [5]. In hemostasis testing, this can be one of the most difficult or even impossible parameters to determine; in fact the concept of "true value" may not even apply to many coagulation tests especially those that report results as time values (PT, aPTT, and thrombin time) [2, 6]. In addition, the majority of hemostasis/coagulation tests has no "gold" standards or even established true values. This concept is changing as international standards are being developed and accepted (fibrinogen, factor VIII, protein C, antithrombin, and vWF) [7, 8]. For some standards (fibrinogen, protein C, protein S, antithrombin, and factor VIII), accuracy issues still arise due to differences in the methods used (clotting vs. chromogenic assays). The laboratory must make certain that their standards are linked, if available, to the international standard through a secondary standard of the manufacturer [2, 6]. Preparation of international standards is addressed elsewhere in this book (Chapter 4).

Precision is defined as the closeness of agreement (degree of variability) among a series of measurements obtained from multiple sampling from a single sample or reference material [2, 9]. Imprecision is measured using within-assay variability (intra-assay) and day-to-day variability (inter-assay). Intra-assay variability is the imprecision determined under the same operating conditions. Inter-assay reproducibility is the imprecision of the method when the assay components may be slightly different (different days, different operators, and different reagent vials). Precision is established irrespective of accuracy since it is the closeness of the reproducibility of the result data that

is important. The imprecision is usually expressed as coefficient of variation (CV).

Imprecision evaluation consists of a two-prong assessment: within-run variation and between-run or day-to-day variation. Variation for the within-run assessment is determined by performing the assay on the same specimen or control sample within a single run using the same reagent batch for a minimum of 20 measurements. The CV should usually be 3–6% for clotting, chromogenic, and most immunologic analytes but never more than 10%. However, for the more complex assays (platelet aggregation, vWF, and lupus anticoagulant), the imprecision in terms of CV may be 10–20%.

Between-run precision is evaluated by repeating the same specimen (usually controls) on the same instrument but with other variables (such as new reagent vials, different operators, and different environmental conditions) for a minimum of 10 runs. In general, the precision for between-run studies is greater than that observed for within-run precision studies. Usually, the CV for between-run studies is 4–8% but never more than 12%. Again for the more complex assays, the precision can increase to a significant 20–40%. The acceptable limits of precision during the validation phase is difficult to define and will vary among laboratories. No hard and fast rules apply for acceptability of coagulation testing precision; however, the laboratory must decide on the acceptable limits of precision based on publications, manufacturer's data, or published guidelines. At least three samples that span the reportable range ((RR) including normal and abnormal values) must be used as part of the precision study. The acceptable levels of precision may be different between normal and abnormal samples, the type of assay, and the reagent–instrument combinations. The precision results should mirror the values reported by the reagent and/or instrument manufacturer. Precision within the manufacturer's reported limits are acceptable. If the precision value obtained is greater than the manufacturer's reported values, then the laboratory may still accept the results if their method parameters justify the increased imprecision.

Limits

In the validation of an assay's performance, two types of "limits" must be evaluated: LOD and LOQ [2, 6, 10]. The LOD of a method is the level at which the assay can distinguish a sample without analyte present (blank) from the sample with analyte present; however, the assay may not accurately quantify the amount [10]. The LOD is usually defined as 3 standard deviation (SD) above the mean of the blank, making the limit above the "noise" of the method, thus the probability of a false positive is minimal (<1%). The accuracy and precision of the method (including all components and reagents) and pre-analytical variables play an important role in determining the LOD. Although these components are important for a coagulation assay, an added layer of assay complexity occurs with the time-based result assays (PT and aPTT) as these methods have no specific analyte to determine. Some coagulation methods have poor LOD due to imprecision including poor differentiation at levels that are clinically relevant. The standard protocol for determining the lower LOD is to measure a zero standard (no analyte present) multiple times (20 replicates) and calculate the standard deviation. The 3 SD range is considered "noise" and the value at the upper end of the 3 SD is the lower LOD. In coagulation, this lower limit is sometimes difficult to ascertain since finding a true "zero" standard that is plasma-based is not available. Usually, the "zero" standard plasma is an artificially created sample since clinically relevant "zero" samples are not available. It is important to understand the lower LOD of the assay in relation to the clinical use of the assay. A good example of this relationship is found in hemophilia testing in which it is important to clinically distinguish between a level of <1% and 3%. If the lower LOD is only 3%, then patients with severe hemophilia (major bleeding symptoms) cannot be differentiated from moderate hemophilia (milder bleeding symptoms). The laboratory must decide what analyte level is necessary for clinical utility for each method and then make sure the assay meets those criteria.

There are a number of different "detection limits" that must be taken into account in the overall evaluation of the coagulation assay method (instrument LOD, method LOD, reagent LOD, and plasma substrate LOD). Both the instrument detection limit and the method detection limit are the main parameters for the evaluation of a new method or new reagent–instrument system. This information is usually supplied by the manufacturer but should be verified by the laboratory before using the assay. Confirmation studies must be performed.

LOQs define the lowest amount of analyte that is quantifiable in the assay, and in addition, the LOQ defines the level at which two values can be distinguished with acceptable precision and accuracy [10]. In standard practice, the lower LOQ is statistically defined as 5–10 SD from the "zero" standard control value; however, each method must be evaluated independently to determine the lowest level of the LOQ.

The laboratory in consultation with the clinical staff must determine the clinically relevant lower LOQ for each assay. For clinical purposes, the assay must be able to accurately differentiate the medical decision points. However, the LOQ can be drastically different among methods, types of methods, types of results reported, and among laboratories. Coagulation assays such as the PT, aPTT, and some lupus anticoagulant tests have a large difference in LOQ since they are global assays measuring multiple factors.

The analytical measurement range (AMR) of an analytical method is the interval between the upper and lower analyte concentrations for which the analytical method has demonstrated a suitable level of precision, accuracy, and linearity without pretreatment (dilutions) [2, 10]. Whereas the RR is the range of analyte concentration in which the analytical method demonstrates suitable precision, accuracy, and linearity with pretreatment (dilutions or concentration). For RR, recovery studies are required to verify that pretreatment (dilution or concentration) does not affect the reported value. The precision and accuracy of a method at the lower and upper limits of the RR and AMR are important, but even more important are the clinical needs (medical decision points) for the specific analyte. The lower end of the linear range is usually the most important in coagulation, but may be the most difficult to establish at a clinically relevant level. The laboratory cannot report values lower than the lowest standard of the calibration curve. If the test method cannot be reported to the level necessary for clinical utility, then modifications of the method or alternative methods must be used to achieve the desired level including curves established for lower ranges, different dilutions of the standards or other methods [2, 11].

The linearity is the ability to obtain results that are directly proportional between the instrument response and the concentration of analyte within a given range [2, 12]. Linearity acceptance criteria are usually based on the statistical correlation coefficient of linear regression. Mathematical transformations of data can help to promote linearity if there is scientific evidence that transformation is appropriate for the method. A good example is the factor assay that may use semi-log or log–log transformations. It is important not to force the origin to zero in the calculation as this may skew the actual best-fit slope through the clinically relevant range of use. For quantitative coagulation methods used for diagnosis and monitoring, the analytical method must have a good proportional relationship between analyte concentration and instrument response. The limit for the upper range must not exceed the level of the highest linear standard.

Methods for linearity determination of a coagulation quantitative method have changed over the last decade [2]. Linearity computations have evolved from visual assessment of the line to statistical analysis via linear regression [2]. However, linear regression will not readily define acceptable limits because many of the quantitative coagulation assays may be imprecise and have a poor linear fit. In the future, refined statistical methods including polynomial analysis will be a standard linearity assessment tool.

The robustness of an analytical procedure is a measure of its capacity to remain unaffected by small to moderate variations in method parameters and preanalytical variables [13, 14]. It provides an indication of the assay's reliability during normal usage [13, 14]. The important analytical parameters include different machines, operators, reagent lots, and sample preparation, among a host of others.

Robustness is difficult to truly assess and is generally associated with more problems with increasing complexity of the analytical system. The majority of the analysis for robustness is determined by the manufacturer and usually approved by a regulatory agency such as the FDA. However, if the reagents are not designed and evaluated by the manufacturer or used differently than intended, then stated claims of the method are not validated. In this case, the coagulation laboratory must assume responsibility for determining robustness. The pre-analytical variables that the laboratory must evaluate are those encountered in the clinical setting, whereas the analytical parameters are evaluated based on the assay's method, equipment, and reagents.

Ideally, robustness should be explored during the development of the assay method through the use of a

protocol. For such a protocol, one must first identify variables in the method that may influence the results. One might expect storage conditions and processing of the sample, minimal and maximal dilution, and the type of dilutant; level of interference (hemolysis, lipemia, etc.) to have an effect on the assay. The pre-analytic issues are addressed elsewhere in this book (Chapter 4). This type of method manipulation will ensure that the system components are robust.

Protocol

Before initiating any validation study, whether establishing a new test, changing reagents or instruments, or changing methodology, a well-planned validation protocol must be developed using sound scientific and clinical criteria [2, 15]. Commercial companies that supply the reagents and/or instruments typically provide protocol outlines. The major components of a validation protocol are presented in Table 2.1. The protocol must describe in detail the planned studies including the statistics and defined acceptance criteria [15]. The protocol must be performed in a timely manner with adequate samples, standards, and calibrators. Much of the general information on validation protocols is described in documents provided by accrediting and standards organizations [1, 2, 6, 15].

After performing the validation protocol, the data must be analyzed with predetermined statistical methods such that the results and conclusions are presented in a validation summary report. If the defined criteria established in the protocol are met or any variations that might affect the overall conclusions are justified, then the method can be considered valid. The final validation report, along with all the data, statistical analyses, and the signatures and titles of all participants, including supervisors, laboratory director, section director, administrators, consultants, and reviewers are placed in the official standard operating procedure manual or kept readily available for inspection.

Continued performance of coagulation/hemostasis assays

To ensure the continued accurate diagnosis and treatment of hemostatic disorders, long-term consistent assay precision and accuracy is necessary. For each assay, consistency and reproducibility over time in conjunction with accurate results are required for every coagulation/hemostasis assay. This requires ongoing evaluation of the assay methodology not only during each performance run (internal quality control) but also periodic comparison with other laboratories for continual accuracy (external quality assurance).

Internal quality control

A good quality control program maintains an ongoing statistical analysis of control material for each assay method. This is usually mandated by regulatory agencies, government regulations, and/or published standards or guidelines. The main aim of an internal quality assessment program is to confirm that generated results remain consistent over time (a measure of imprecision). Internal quality control is discussed in detail elsewhere in this book (Chapter 6).

External quality assessment

External quality assessment (a measure of accuracy) is a critical element in any laboratory quality program [16, 17]. Currently, in many countries, laboratories are required to participate in external quality programs to promote accurate and consistent test results. External quality assessment is discussed in detail elsewhere in this book (Chapter 7).

Reference interval

The interpretation of coagulation test data from a patient is a comparative decision-making process, that is, a patient's result is compared to a "reference interval" for making diagnostic and/or therapeutic decisions. Therefore, the determination of the correct reference interval is of the utmost importance. In the past, ranges have been poorly defined without a consistent process for determination. With the broad spectrum of coagulation testing methods, a systematic and consistent process must be used to establish the proper reference interval for the population in question. The reference interval criteria and methodology can be found in a variety of publications and guidelines from various organizations [18]. The criteria and protocols

Table 2.2 Types and requirements for reference intervals in coagulation

Reference interval	Criteria definition
New analyte	Measurement of reference interval is difficult, lack of established data on physiology and medical aspects
New analyte method	Measurement of reference interval is easier as physiological and medical information is established
Transference of reference values	Same analyte with same method utilizing new lot or instrument; however, difficult to establish evaluation of standards

for reference interval determination fall into three categories (Table 2.2), each requiring different method requirements. A therapeutic reference interval such as for heparin therapy must be determined in a similar manner as the reference interval.

For reference intervals, specific definition of terms is required. A reference population is the population consisting of all the reference individuals [16, 17]. This is usually a very large and hypothetical group. The reference sample group is a selected group of individuals representing the reference population. The size of the sample is determined based on statistical probability. The reference distribution is the range of reference values with the reference limits determined by a statistical evaluation of the reference sample group, and the reference interval is the set of values between the upper and lower reference limits [18, 19]. Reference intervals can be associated with "normal" or good health, gender, various age groups, pathological conditions, and therapeutic interventions.

To establish a reference interval, a well-defined protocol must be followed. An outline of a reference interval protocol for new analytes and/or new methods is presented in Table 2.3; however, more detailed protocols for reference intervals for the general laboratory have been published elsewhere [17]. These can be tailored to coagulation testing using published protocols [2, 6].

One of the most difficult aspects of reference interval determination for coagulation testing is the

Table 2.3 Basic protocol for establishing reference interval for a new analyte or new analyte method

1 Establish biological variations and analytical interferences from the literature.
2 Establish selection (or exclusion) criteria and develop questionnaires and consent forms.
3 Determine potential reference individuals (exclude as necessary).
4 Determine the appropriate number of reference individuals.
5 Collect appropriate samples under appropriate pre-analytical conditions.
6 Determine the reference values and review for data distribution, errors, or outliers.
7 Analyze reference values into appropriate categories and determine reference interval(s) as predefined in protocol.
8 Document all the steps and procedures.

inclusion and exclusion of potential individuals. Many factors influence the levels of hemostatic parameters and factors. In addition, changes in these individual factors will influence not only the results of specific factor levels but also global-type assays. As an example, exercise, hormonal therapy, and pregnancy can increase factor VIII levels to an extent that the aPTT value can be shortened. It is important to develop a questionnaire to exclude inappropriate individuals from the reference interval determination. The individuals used to establish the reference interval should reflect the population that will be the primary group being evaluated. Also important is the consideration of pre-analytical and analytical variables. The results from the reference population values must reflect the variables encountered in the patient samples [2, 3]. The same considerations for sample collection, processing, and storage must be employed [3]. It is unacceptable to determine the reference interval using a different method, protocol, manufacturer, and even reagent lots than what will be used for patient testing [2, 3, 6].

The reference interval is defined as the interval between the upper and lower reference limits. The assignment of those limits is established as an a priori statistical value. For most coagulation testing, those limits are 2 SD from the mean for a normally distributed (Gaussian) population. Limits for a non-Gaussian distribution are established by more complex methods. The reference limits become more accurate and closer to the true reference population values with a larger sample group. In practice, it is usually difficult to procure a large set of qualifying reference individuals [2, 6]. A minimum of 40 individuals should be used to establish the reference interval. If that is too difficult or impossible to obtain, then a group as few as 20 individuals may be tested but greater care must be taken when computing the values and determining the limits [2, 6]. The calculated reference limits should be compared with other laboratories using the same method, reagents, and instruments. For some coagulation reference intervals, subdivisions of specific groups may be necessary, such as newborn reference interval or vWF and blood type. It is the responsibility of the laboratory to set the appropriate number of samples for each subgroup to establish group-specific ranges.

Establishing a new reference interval for a new test or change in methodology can be difficult and costly; therefore, some laboratories consider "transferring" the reference interval from their previous method, using the range of another laboratory, the manufacturer-suggested range, or a range obtained from the literature. The methods to transfer reference values are not soundly established [2, 18, 19]. Much effort has been attempted in the establishment of protocols for transference; however, a variety of scenarios make the effort complex: different reference populations from another laboratory, literature or manufacturer, slightly different analytical methods, and different pre-analytical problems [18, 19]. Although not recommended, transference has been used quite frequently but two major issues must be taken into account: comparability of analytical methods and comparability of reference population [18, 19]. Even using the same population (age, gender, regional location, demographics, and pre-analytical variables), it may be very difficult or even impossible to arrive at the same reference interval. If the method has the same characteristics and values (imprecision, interferences, standards, secondary reference standards, calibrators, and units), then the assay method can be considered similar and possibly the same range could be used. Several approaches can be utilized to judge the acceptability of reference interval transference [18]:

1 Use inspection and subjectivity of the original method reference range (demographics and pre-analytical variables) and the new method. Based on the judgment of consistent method similarities, the reference interval can be transferred without validation studies. Unfortunately, many coagulation laboratories that do not have the ability to acquire appropriate samples from the population use this method. This method is used especially for unique populations such as newborn infants and pediatrics. However, it is not recommended.

2 Validation of the reference range provided by the manufacturer or another laboratory using a small number of reference individuals (usually a minimum of 20 from the same population) to compare to a larger study performed by the original laboratory or manufacturer. Again problems can occur because of the differences in pre-analytical variables, population, and regional demographics. After testing the 20 specimens, the results are statistically evaluated (based on predefined criteria with no outliers present), and then the reference interval can be accepted. If the values are outside of the reference range, then the outlier(s) should be evaluated for cause, but in all likelihood, the reference interval should not be accepted and a full determination of a reference interval must be undertaken.

The majority of information and theories dealing with transference of reference intervals has been established for analytes with known quantities such as cell number and mass per volume [18, 19]. For analytes such as clotting factors and coagulation tests reported in time intervals, transference methods have not been validated [6]. More detailed methodology for transference of reference intervals can be found in general guidelines [18, 19]. As with any established reference interval, they must be periodically re-evaluated and confirmed [2, 18].

The majority of reference intervals are established to compare a patient's value with the appropriate population. The patient result is usually reported as "within normal limits," "high" (above the reference interval), or "low" (below the reference interval). Clinical interpretation of the value as either above or below the reference interval is the responsibility of the health care provider; however, it may be the responsibility of the laboratory director to assign the importance of a value that does not fall within the reference interval.

In consultation with clinical staff, the levels that are critical for disease diagnosis or therapeutic use must be established and designated in the computer system and/or on a written report.

Appendix: Standards and guideline developing organizations

A number of international organizations (usually non-profit) develop consensus guidelines and standards as a concise and cost-effective laboratory medicine process to improve and standardize patient testing. Most of these organizations derive their guidelines and standards from consensus written documents from experts followed by open and unbiased input from the laboratory and manufacturing communities. "Standards" documents developed through this consensus process help to clearly identify the specific and essential requirements for the material, method, or practice of laboratory testing. Whereas "guideline" documents are developed through a similar consensus process for general criteria of a material, method, or practice of laboratory testing that may be used as written or modified to fit the user's needs upon their own validation program. The most well-known organization is Clinical and Laboratory Standards Institute (CLSI). It is an international nonprofit organization that uses voluntary experts from the laboratory community, manufacturers, and regulators input to develop these standards and guidelines in all areas of patient testing and other health care issues.

Statistics

The evaluation and subsequent interpretation of the coagulation data (reference intervals, standard curves, and comparison of patient results) uses the field of statistics. In general, statistical evaluations are divided into two groups: descriptive statistics that define a population based on data from a sample set and comparative statistics that evaluates the difference or similarity of two groups of data. Different types of data call for different statistical evaluations. This appendix summarizes the basic statistical methods used in the coagulation laboratory. More in-depth information on statistical methods and performing statistical tests are available in many books and computer programs [19–21].

Descriptive statistics are used to "describe" the data, that is, evaluate the sample to assess the representation of a specific population. The mean, median, SD, range for minimum and maximum values, the 95% confidence interval and CV are the most important descriptive statistics. This summary information provides an initial assessment of the test data compared to the population. In addition, these statistics may indicate poor population sampling, outliers, or data entry errors.

The concept of comparative statistics is to compare and contrast differences between two sets of data. In the statistical comparison of two groups of data, the data are considered the same (termed the null hypothesis) and then tested to determine whether they are statistically different. Usually the 95% confidence limit is used as the differentiating point, that is, if greater than 95%, then the two means are considered different between the two groups or populations. In a cautionary note, it is very easy to read too much into the term significant, as an example two groups of data may be statistically significantly different but are not clinically different. Statistical significance and clinical significance are two unrelated interpretations of the data. Asking how the data will be used from a clinical perspective (will these data change the treatment plan?) may be as important as statistical significance.

Statistics are important in the evaluation and performance of methods and instruments as it is for determining reference intervals. The laboratory personnel must be able to analyze the results using the proper statistical methods. The p value, which stands for probability value, has a value ranging from 0 to 1.0. It is useful in the interpretation of many statistical tests like the Student's t-test. If the p value is small (usually <0.05), then the difference between sample means is not likely the same population. Again the p value is a statistical result and does not necessarily reflect the "clinical difference."

The Student's t-test compares the means of two groups of data. As an example, comparison of the PT/INR results from normal individuals obtained with two reagent–instrument combinations. To use the Student's t-test, the same variables must be compared. The result is a p value that determines whether the comparison is statistically the same or different.

Linear regression is the statistical method used to describe the "best fit" of two sets of continuous data. For example, linear regression is used to find the relationship between two instruments when comparing a large number of quantitative values over a wide range. For these types of method comparisons, theoretically, the slope should be 1.0 with the "best fit" line crossing the x and y axes at 0. When the slope is outside the range of 0.95–1.05, a true difference or bias between the methods being compared is a possibility. It is the responsibility of the laboratory to determine whether this difference is clinically important.

Linear regression is used to create a standard curve for clotting factor, ELISA, or chromogenic assays. Standards with known values are analyzed and the instrument data are recorded. These two data sets (concentration and instrument output data) are compared to generate the "best fit" line. The instrument output data for an unknown sample is then used to find the unknown sample's concentration or activity from this curve. Linear correlation quantifies how well two sets of data vary together. The statistical correlation coefficient (r value between 0.0 and 1.0) indicates the amount of random error (variation) between the two sets of data. The correlation coefficient is a semiquantitative indication of imprecision. These r values are helpful with standard curves, such as clotting factor or ELISA assays. For most coagulation studies, an r value of less than 0.9 is not optimum.

From the laboratory perspective, one of the best statistical methods for comparing two measurements between two techniques, instruments, or methods is the Bland–Altman plot, a graphical representation of the absolute differences, differences as percentage of the mean, or ratios of different comparisons of methods and/or components. The results are a scatter diagram of the differences plotted against the average. This evaluation method will elucidate the differences in means and determine systematic bias and identify outliers. If there is no detectable statistical bias and no clinical differences, then the two methods can be considered the same.

From a clinical or disease-related perspective, sensitivity and specificity are two of the most widely used statistics describing a diagnostic test, but must be interpreted with caution. Clinical sensitivity is defined as the probability of a positive test among patients with disease; whereas clinical specificity is the probability of a negative test present in patients without disease [19–21]. Measurements of test performance may not take into account the level at which a test is clinically positive. Receiver–operator characteristics curves (ROC curves), a complex statistical analytical method that is underutilized in coagulation work, assess the performance of a test throughout the assay's range of values observed in disease states. As the ROC curve approaches 1.0, the better the clinical diagnostic ability of the assay, while a truly random test parameter for predicting disease has the ROC curve of ∼0.5.

Acknowledgments

This work was supported in part by a MERIT Review grant from the Department of Veteran's Affairs.

References

1. Clinical and Laboratory Standards Institute (CLSI) Evaluation Protocols (EP05 through EP21). The Clinical and Laboratory Standards Institute Web Site (Wayne, PA: 2004); www.nccls.org.
2. Clinical and Laboratory Standards Institute (CLSI). Protocol for the Evaluation, Validation, and Implementation of Coagulometers. CLSI document H57-P, 2008.
3. Clinical and Laboratory Standards Institute (CLSI). Collection, Transport, and Processing of Blood Specimens for Testing Plasma-Based Coagulation Assays and Molecular Hemostasis Assays. H21-A5. 2008.
4. McPherson RA. Laboratory statistics. In: McPherson RA, Pincus MR, eds. Henry's Clinical Diagnosis and Management by Laboratory Methods. 22nd ed. Philadelphia, PA: Saunders; 2011:109–118.
5. Clinical and Laboratory Standards Institute (CLSI). User Demonstration of Performance for Precision and Accuracy. EP15-A. 2001.
6. Clinical and Laboratory Standards Institute (CLSI). One-Stage Prothrombin Time (PT) Test and Activated Partial Thromboplastin Time (aPTT) Test. H47-A2. 2008.
7. Hubbard AR. International biological standards for coagulation factors and inhibitors. Sem Thromb Hemost. 2007;33:283–289.
8. Hubbard AR. Heath AB. Standardization of factor VIII and von Willebrand factor in plasma: calibration of the WHO 5th International Standard. J Thromb Haemost. 2004;2:1380–1384.
9. Clinical and Laboratory Standards Institute (CLSI). Evaluation of Precision Performance of Quantitative Measurement Methods. EP5-A2. 2004.
10. Clinical and Laboratory Standards Institute (CLSI). Protocols for Determination of Detection and Limits of Quantitation. EP17-A. 2004.
11. Clinical and Laboratory Standards Institute (CLSI). Statistical Quality Control for Quantitative Measurement Procedures: Principles and Definitions; Approved Guideline-Third Edition C24-A3, 2004.
12. Clinical and Laboratory Standards Institute (CLSI): Evaluation of the Linearity of Quantitative Measurement Procedures. EP6-A. 2003.
13. Kroll M, Gilstad C, Gochman G, et al., eds. Laboratory Instrument Evaluation, Verification and Maintenance Manual. 5th ed. Northfield, IL: College of American Pathologists; 1999.
14. Clinical and Laboratory Standards Institute (CLSI). Method Comparison and Bias Estimation Using Patient Samples. EP9-A2. 2002.
15. Lott JA. Process control and method evaluation. In: Snyder JR, Wilkinson DS eds. Management in Laboratory Medicine. 3rd ed. Philadelphia, PA: Lippincott; 1998:293–325.
16. World Health Organization. Requirements and Guidance for External Quality Assessment Schemes for Health Laboratories. 1999.
17. Clinical and Laboratory Standards Institute (CLSI). Validation of Laboratory Tests When Proficiency Testing is Not Available. GP29-P. 2001.
18. Clinical and Laboratory Standards Institute (CLSI). How to Define and Determine Reference Intervals in the Clinical Laboratory. C28-A2. 2000.
19. Daniel WW. Biostatistics: A Foundation for Analysis in the Health Sciences. 7th ed. New York: John Wiley & Sons; 1999.
20. Dawson B, Trapp RG. Basic & Clinical Biostatistics. 3rd ed. London: Lange Medical/McGraw-Hill; 2001.
21. Jhang J, Sireci AN, Kratz A. Post-analysis: medical decision making. In: McPherson RA, Pincus MR, eds. Henry's Clinical Diagnosis and Management by Laboratory Methods. 22nd ed. Philadelphia, PA: Saunders; 2011:80–90.

3

Causes of errors in medical laboratories

Giuseppe Lippi[1] *& Emmanuel J. Favaloro*[2]

[1]Clinical Chemistry and Haematology Laboratory, Department of Pathology and Laboratory Medicine, Academic Hospital of Parma, Parma, Italy

[2]Department of Hematology, ICPMR, Westmead Hospital, Westmead, NSW, Australia

Overview on medical errors

In the United States in 2006 12,791 firearm homicides were reported, while the overall number of firearms available in the country has been estimated at 223 million. In the same year, the number of physicians working in the United States was 794,893, whereas preventable medical harm accounts for ~100,000 deaths yearly according to the Institute of Medicine (IOM) report "To Err Is Human" [1]. Accordingly, the chance of dying needlessly because of preventable medical errors in the United States each year is more than 2000 times as likely as the probability of being killed by gunshot (1:8 vs. 1:17,434). Although this premise can be challenged, the burden of medical errors, and the potential harm that these might cause to patients, is indeed alarming. According to the HealthGrades study, which assessed the mortality and economic impact of medical errors and injuries that occurred during Medicare hospital admissions nationwide from 2000 to 2002, double the number of people than that reported by the IOM (i.e., 195,000 people; the equivalent of 390 full jumbo jets) would die each year due to likely preventable, in-hospital medical errors, making this one of the leading killers in the United States, and with an associated cost of more than $6 billion per year [2]. In another article, Dr. Barbara Starfield reported that medical errors may cause up to 225,000 deaths per year, thus representing the third leading cause of death in the United States. The figures included 2000 deaths/year from unnecessary surgery; 7000 deaths/year from medication errors in hospitals; 20,000 deaths/year from other errors in hospitals; 80,000 deaths/year from infections in hospitals; 106,000 deaths/year from non-error, adverse effects of medications [3].

At variance with aircraft crashes—which have high public visibility, often involving loss of many lives at once, and thus given worldwide publicity, resulting in exhaustive investigations into causal factors, public reports, and remedial action—medical errors occur to individual patients, rarely receive broad media coverage, and quite likely represent just the tip of the iceberg, since there is little standardized method of investigation and reporting. Although several definitions of medical errors have been provided to date, a reliable one is that of " . . . a preventable adverse effect of care, whether or not it is evident or harmful to the patient, which might include an inaccurate or incomplete diagnosis or treatment of a disease, injury, syndrome behaviour, infection, or other ailment" [4]. According to this definition, a medical error might arise from any single part of the clinical reasoning and decision making (i.e., from the diagnosis to the therapy of diseases). While major attention has been historically focused on therapeutic errors (i.e., inappropriate medical therapy or mishandled surgery), the undeniable evidence that laboratory data substantially contribute to the clinical decision making (in up to 70% of the cases) provides mounting evidence that diagnostics (laboratory) errors might have a substantial, negative impact on the effectiveness of care, economically wasting a huge amount of resources and, especially, contributing to produce adverse clinical outcomes [4].

Diagnostic errors: the laboratory scenario

Laboratory medicine has undergone a dramatic revolution over past decades, moving forward from a traditional clinical science focused on providing diagnostic information, to a broadened scientific enterprise aimed at investigating biochemical pathways, unveiling the pathogenesis of disease, discovering innovative biomarkers, and developing and introducing innovative analytical technologies into practice. Propelled by the ongoing economic crisis and the consequent shortage of public funding, the organization of clinical laboratories has also undergone a substantial revolution worldwide, with two apparently opposite trends—i.e., the coexistence of centralization of testing in automated mega-structures that perform enormous test volumes plus widespread introduction of decentralized and point-of-care testing (POCT) options [5]. While this evolutionary process has been the catalyst for several changes in the network of laboratory services, several new challenges have also been raised that might disrupt both the effectiveness and efficacy of laboratory testing, as well as introducing additional possibilities of diagnostics (i.e., laboratory) errors.

The definition of laboratory error

In order to arrive at the most suitable definition of laboratory error, it must be first kept in mind that diagnostics always develops through a complex pathway of actions, some of them occurring outside the traditional laboratory environment and thereby beyond the direct control and jurisdiction of laboratory professionals. This path has originally been described by Prof. George Lundberg, as the well-known "brain-to-brain turnaround time loop" [6], where laboratory tests consist of nine steps including ordering, collection, identification, transportation, preparation, analysis, reporting, interpretation, and action. In particular, all these activities have been classically "clustered" within five leading sections of the total testing process,

namely "pre-preanalytical," "preanalytical," "analytical," "postanalytical," and "post-postanalytical." It is thereby readily understandable that the most suitable definition of laboratory error must be based on the clear concept that laboratory mistakes might arise from any step of the "loop," that is, from test ordering to the final (medical) action(s) undertaken on the basis of test results. As such, the first trustworthy definition of laboratory errors was originally provided by Bonini et al. in 2002, as "a diagnosis that is missed, wrong, or delayed, as detected by some subsequent definitive test or finding" [7], which has been formally recognized and slightly modified in the International Organization for Standardization (ISO) Technical Report 22367, as "a defect occurring at any part of the laboratory cycle, from ordering tests to reporting, interpreting, and reacting to results" [8].

Exploring the iceberg of laboratory errors

A primary, pivotal concept is that diagnostic errors, likewise medical errors in general, typically represent the "tip of the iceberg," whereby most problems go undetected for several reasons, including lack of automatic translation into a real harm for the patient (except in some circumstances) and underidentification as well as underreporting (Figure 3.1). Although laboratory errors are typically recognized as "analytical," a comprehensive review of early and recent literature data confirms that the vast majority of such errors occur in the extra-analytical phases of the total testing process and—even more notably—they principally occur in the manually intensive activities of the preanalytical phase, from test request to the analysis of the sample(s) [9, 10]. As such, the current concept of "total error" (or "total allowable error" as currently portrayed by James Westgard) might be misleading since it only considers the analytical performances of laboratory testing, ignoring the remaining steps of the brain-to-brain loop and finally missing the real "quality goal" of laboratory diagnostics, that is the improvement of patient safety and outcome.

As regards coagulation testing, the consequences of errors in routine (e.g., screening) tests might potentially generate several negative outcomes, since they may affect the clinical decision making in terms of (i) misdiagnosis (e.g., a falsely normal coagulation screening might expose patients carrying inherited disorders such as hemophilia or von Willebrand disease

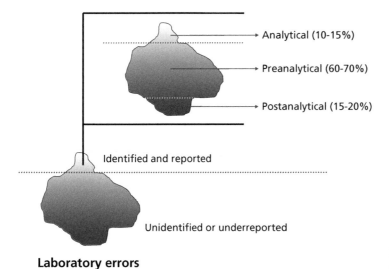

Analytical (10-15%)

Preanalytical (60-70%)

Postanalytical (15-20%)

Identified and reported

Unidentified or underreported

Laboratory errors

Figure 3.1 Types and potential outcomes of laboratory errors.

to invasive procedures without appropriate prophylaxis); (ii) delayed care (e.g., a falsely abnormal coagulation screening would unnecessarily delay invasive procedures or anticoagulant/antiplatelet therapy); (iii) prevention (i.e., falsely normal screening) or triggering (i.e., falsely abnormal screening) of further specific (second- and third-line), occasionally invasive but always expensive and time-consuming, testing; (iv) inappropriate variation of the therapeutic regimen in patients undergoing anticoagulant/antiplatelet therapy and thereby exposing patients to the risk of bleeding or thrombosis according to the direction of change [11, 12].

Preanalytical errors

As previously mentioned, the preanalytical phase is the most vulnerable part of the total testing process, since it is still based on a variety of manually intensive activities and it mostly develops outside the traditional laboratory environment, so that laboratory personnel cannot always exert a direct control on all these activities. The vast majority of preanalytical errors arise from unsuitable, inappropriate, or mishandled procedures during collection and handling of the specimen. Thus, problems during collection of biological samples—especially blood specimens—include identification errors; use of incorrect devices (i.e., butterfly needles or IV catheters) or needles (e.g.,

small gauge needles); prolonged tourniquet placing; unsuccessful attempts to locate the vein; collection of unsuitable samples for quality (e.g., hemolyzed, contaminated) or quantity (e.g., insufficient amount of blood or inappropriate blood-to-anticoagulant ratio); inappropriate mixing of the sample; and inappropriate procedures for transportation, preparation (e.g., centrifugation), and storage (Figure 3.2). As regards coagulation testing, preanalytical variability is considered a leading issue affecting the overall quality of the specimens. Recent data have determined that preanalytical problems can be identified in up to 5.5% of coagulation specimens, the more frequent being samples not received in the laboratory after physician's order (49%), hemolysis (20%), sample clotting (14%), and inappropriate blood-to-anticoagulant ratio (14%) [13]. While misidentification rarely occurs or—at least—is underidentified and underreported for reasons discussed elsewhere [14, 15], errors of identification are, however, an important issue for patient safety in both transfusion as well as in laboratory medicine, since they might expose the patients to serious diagnostic and therapeutic errors [14, 15].

Although it is always difficult to establish a direct relationship between spurious results and patients' outcome, the adverse consequences of laboratory errors might often be serious, especially for those related to specialized tests, as these are often considered as "diagnostic." Thus, patients might be diagnosed with a particular disorder, when in fact they do

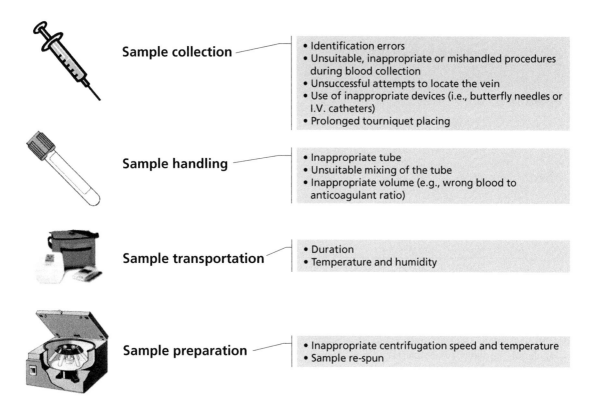

Sample collection
- Identification errors
- Unsuitable, inappropriate or mishandled procedures during blood collection
- Unsuccessful attempts to locate the vein
- Use of inappropriate devices (i.e., butterfly needles or I.V. catheters)
- Prolonged tourniquet placing

Sample handling
- Inappropriate tube
- Unsuitable mixing of the tube
- Inappropriate volume (e.g., wrong blood to anticoagulant ratio)

Sample transportation
- Duration
- Temperature and humidity

Sample preparation
- Inappropriate centrifugation speed and temperature
- Sample re-spun

Figure 3.2 Leading causes of preanalytical errors.

not have it (i.e., "false positive" test result is obtained), or else a patient with a true disorder might be missed (i.e., "false negative" test result is obtained), both circumstances jeopardizing the patient's health, identifying serious organizational problems, and producing unnecessary costs to the healthcare system. As regards the first aspect (i.e., the clinical consequences of laboratory errors), a significant impact on patient care of a laboratory error has been reported to range between 9% and 15%, whereas the risk of inappropriate care ranges between 2% and 7% [16]. In two seminal articles by Plebani and Carraro on types and frequencies of mistakes in a clinical laboratory, the percentage of errors translating into a real patient harm has been reported to be ∼25%. In the former article, published in 1997, the most frequent inappropriate care was identified as further inappropriate investigations (19.6%), inappropriate transfusion or inappropriate modification of anticoagulant therapy (2.2%), inappropriate infusion of electrolyte solutions, or unjustified modification of digoxin therapy (1%) [17]. In

the latter paper, published 10 years later, laboratory test repetition accounted for 16.9% of the unwelcome outcome, followed by further inappropriate investigations (5.6%), inappropriate transfusions (1.3%), and unjustified admission to the intensive care unit (0.6%) [18]. The negative economical impact of laboratory errors based on current costs in western Europe is also remarkable and can be roughly estimated considering that a repeated collection of a blood tube would cost approximately US $0.10 and require nearly 0.25 minutes plus repeat or additional testing (Figure 3.3).

Specific preanalytical issues related to coagulation testing

The kaleidoscope of first- and second-line coagulation tests, often requiring different techniques, methodologies, and instrumentation, is plagued by significant problems when samples are provided in an unsuitable presentation. Although there are guidelines available for how to manage unsuitable specimens, and

25

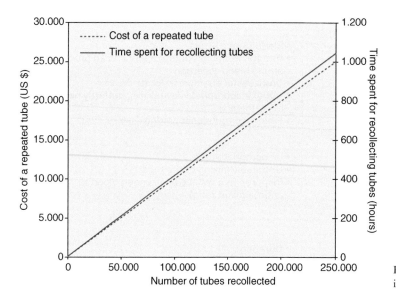

Figure 3.3 The negative economical impact of laboratory errors.

for deciding when to reject poor quality specimens [19, 20], it is often challenging to establish whether a coagulation specimen is suitable for testing. Moreover, preanalytical problems and errors can arise throughout the preanalytical phase, and thereby during sample collection, handling, transportation, processing, and storage.

Analogous to other area of laboratory diagnostics, all coagulation tests have detailed collection requirements, the vast majority of these samples should be collected into citrate-based anticoagulant tubes. The Clinical and Laboratory Standards Institute (CLSI) guidelines advise the use of 105–109 mmol/L (or 3.2%) tubes [20]. A higher citrate concentration (i.e., 129 mmol/L or 3.8%) is however also available, so the consensus recommendation suggests that laboratories should standardize to one citrate concentration and develop normal ranges appropriate for that concentration. Regardless of the citrate concentration used by laboratories, sometimes samples might be collected in the wrong tube (e.g., serum or EDTA-plasma) or inappropriately mixed (e.g., left for a long time unmixed, thereby avoiding the full contact of the blood with the anticoagulant which determines partial clotting; or too vigorously shacked, thereby causing breakdown of blood cells). Owing to the developments of large laboratory networks where collection of the specimens is outside the control of the core lab, the prevalence of blood collected off-site, and thus into

inappropriate containers, separated, aliquoted, and then shipped to the actual test facility, is expected to increase further in the near future—making the identification of the unsuitable matrix even more challenging [5]. To overcome this problem, two algorithms were recently developed—one based on the sequential measurement of potassium, calcium, and sodium, the second on potassium and sodium—for differential identification of citrated plasma versus other samples, and displaying almost 100% sensitivity and specificity [21]. While it has once been suggested that a first collection tube be discarded before drawing that for coagulation testing, this may not be required [20]. A discard tube is instead required when drawing blood from butterfly devices or IV catheters, since air contained in the tubing might be introduced into the vacuum tube, leading to under-filling—another important source of error since it provides an insufficient volume for testing and, more importantly, modifies the fixed blood-to-anticoagulant ratio, essential to enable reliable results on citrated plasma (e.g., tubes should be filled up to 90% of the nominal volume) [11]. Transportation might also strongly affect sample quality, so that specimens should be shipped from peripheral collection facilities to the core laboratory utilizing current CLSI guidelines [20]. The samples should hence be preferably delivered non-refrigerated, at ambient temperature (15–22°C) and in the shortest possible time. There is, however, evidence that some transport boxes typically used for shipping the specimens might not be suitable for all conditions, especially during long transports, under extreme external conditions of temperature and humidity [22]. Whenever a delay in transport is expected, it might be advisable to perform local centrifugation, separation, and production of secondary aliquots of plasma followed by freezing and frozen delivery. A final issue in coagulation testing is the effect of freeze-thawing of plasma, which is actually not recommended since it might determine the loss of some labile factors, especially factors V and VIII. However, frozen aliquots of citrate plasma should also be warmed to 37°C for at least 5–10 minutes before testing, to enable reversal of cryoprecipitates potentially generated during freezing and which might influence factor VIII and von Willebrand factor (VWF) testing.

The most widely used definition of "interference" is the presence of one or more substances which alter the measurable concentration of an analyte [23]. The interferences are typically classified according to their origin, and the more common endogenous interferents include hemolysis, hyperbilirubinemia, lipemia, and paraproteinemia, while exogenous substances that can act as interferents include drugs as well as chemical additives [24]. An important problem, which has plagued clinical laboratories for long, is the receipt of hemolyzed specimens. The CLSI-approved guideline for "Collection, Transport, and Processing of Blood Specimens for Testing Plasma-Based Coagulation Assays and Molecular Hemostasis Assays" currently recommends that samples with visible hemolysis should not be used because of possible clotting factor activation and interference with end point measurement interference [20]. Basically, the presence of hemolysis in the specimen might strongly influence several coagulation tests, since the lysis of erythrocytes produces stroma and triggers the release of ADP and other pro-coagulant factors which thereby activate the platelets and, subsequently, the coagulation cascade [25]. As such, the potential interference due to *in vitro* hemolysis is thereby not completely due to the presence of cell-free hemoglobin in plasma, because many other substances involved in the activation of blood coagulation can be released from blood cells so that it is more likely that the source of bias in hemostasis assay would arise mainly from the release of intracellular and thromboplastic substances from erythrocytes, leukocytes, and platelets. Lippi et al.

observed prolongations in prothrombin time (PT) and increased levels of D-dimer in samples containing final lysate concentrations (obtained by freezing and thawing whole blood samples) of 0.5% and 2.7%, respectively, whereas significant shortenings of activated partial thromboplastin time (APTT) and decreased values of fibrinogen have instead been found in samples containing a final lysate concentration of 0.9% [26]. Laga et al. also performed a prospective study to establish whether a difference in PT, APTT, and selected factor assays can arise between hemolyzed and subsequently re-collected nonhemolyzed specimens from the same patient [27]. In the latter phase, the samples were obtained from healthy volunteers and *in vitro* hemolysis was experimentally generated by means of a tissue homogenizer. A nonsignificant trend toward shortening of PT was observed, whereas the values of APTT were instead significantly prolonged in hemolyzed specimens, by 3% of the value in nonhemolyzed samples. This bias was, however, judged to be not clinically meaningful. Significant differences were also recoded for clotting factors of the extrinsic pathway (factor VIIa, V, X), but not for those of intrinsic pathway (factor XIIa, VIII). At variance with the study of Lippi et al., who used freezing-thawing to generate the lysis of blood cells, a modest and nonsignificant trend for change was apparent in the PT despite a progressive increase of cell-free hemoglobin in the supernatant, whereas a progressive, statistically but not clinically significant lengthening of the APTT was recorded. Finally, a significant decrease of antithrombin measured with a chromogenic assay was also observed in hemolyzed specimens. A preliminary study also reported that platelet function testing (i.e., by PFA-100) might be substantially biased by the presence of hemolysis in the sample, since results of both collagen/ADP and collagen/epinephrine cartridges were flagged as "flow obstruction" or yielded dramatic prolongations of the closure times in even modestly hemolyzed specimens (Lippi et al., personal data, in press).

Dealing with preanalytical errors

The most reliable strategy to limit the burden as well as the potential adverse consequences of preanalytical errors on patient's safety is that based on a multifaceted approach to intercept all potential incidents throughout the preanalytical phase, and thereby encompassing analysis, standardization, and monitoring of all preanalytical activities [28]. As such, it is essential to adopt a comprehensive risk management policy, which would include systematic analysis of workflows, weakness, and bottlenecks; eradication or remodeling of the most vulnerable procedures; identification of local organizational changes in the pathway of collecting, handling, transporting, and processing samples; implementation of customized "error identification and recording systems"; continuous education of operators (both inside and outside the laboratory) by dissemination of best practice recommendations; and definition and implementation of representative quality indicators and outcome measures that would enable continuous monitoring and benchmark of all changes. There are several technological advances in technology and computer sciences that might help this process, including Computerized Physician Order Entry (CPOE), positive patient identification by barcode technology, smart cards, radio-frequency identification, the use of lab-on-a-chip integrated tubes, pneumatic tube conveyers or robots for transporting specimens, transportation monitoring systems (e.g., time of transportation, temperature, humidity, etc.), query-host communication, primary tube processing, volume/clotting/bubbles sensors, and serum indices. This last opportunity has become already available on a variety of clinical chemistry instruments, but it is still unavailable on most coagulometers due to inherent technical limitations. It is thereby advisable that all manufacturers of coagulation testing instrumentation rapidly fill this gap, since the assessment of the indices of plasma is so far the gold standard to establish the quality of the specimens and their suitability to be tested.

As regards the continuous monitoring of the implemented changes, which is necessary to establish whether the various adjustments in the pathways have been associated with a real improvement throughout the preanalytical phase (i.e., error reduction), the identification and implementation of a reliable set of preanalytical quality indicators represent a pivotal aspect. Several international and nationwide experiences are ongoing and consistent data on this issue have already been collected. Along with the worldwide projects, such as those of the International Federation of Clinical Chemistry and Laboratory Medicine (IFCC) Working Group on "Laboratory errors and patient safety" [29] and of the Global Preanalytical Scientific Committee (GPSC) [30], other valuable experiences in several countries include those supported by the Association for Clinical Biochemistry in UK and Eire [31], the Sociedad Española de Bioquímica Clínica y Patología Molecular (SEQC) [32], the External Quality Assessment (EQA) scheme developed in Croatia for monitoring the extra-analytical areas of testing [33], as well as the over 12-year series of pilot pre- and postanalytical programs that have been developed and trialed in volunteer pathology laboratories throughout Australia and New Zealand [34]. The Institute for Quality in Laboratory Medicine (IQLM) is also preparing a set of quality indicators, as well as a list of aspects that physicians do not like about laboratorians and a list of things that laboratorians do not like about physicians [35]. Although most of these worldwide efforts recognize similar patterns and are based on nearly identical quality indicators, a major standardization is, however, needed, most advisably under the auspices of the IFCC, to develop measures of quality than can be applied internationally for benchmarking and defining best practices [36].

Analytical errors

Although the prevalence of analytical errors has substantially decreased over the past decades due to the major focus placed on this problem as well as to remarkable technological advances (e.g., automation, query-host communication, processing of primary tube, volume/clotting/bubbles sensors, and serum indices), the laboratory testing process cannot as yet be considered completely safe. Most of the problems are attributable to equipment malfunction, release of results despite poor quality controls, inappropriate reagent/instrument calibrations, reagent problems (e.g., not properly reconstituted or used beyond stability), methodological issues (poor methodologies), analytical interferences, and poor standardization of the tests [12].

As such, since several steps during analysis might go awry, they must be strictly monitored. Systematic quality monitoring should therefore be established, with internal quality control (IQC), external quality assurance (EQA), and/or proficiency testing [PC]. IQC is useful to assess ongoing assay performance, ensures that the test is performing according to the required specifications, and finally certifies that test results are accurate and reliable. Typically, IQC includes both normal (i.e., analyte concentration within the reference range of the test) and abnormal (i.e., analyte concentration above or below the reference range of the test) materials. Results of IQC are typically plotted and statistically analyzed (e.g., by using Levey-Jennings charts). The process should encompass all the analytes tested by using a specific time frame according to number and type of tests. At variance with IQC, the EQA and PT processes represent a different and supplementary approach to validate the quality of testing. Basically, EQA is a peer group assessment process that enables the laboratory to assess test results against those of other laboratories that use the same or different reagents or instrumentation. Interestingly, along with IQC, EQA is also a reliable mean to assess local accuracy and precision as well as long-term performance and thereby timely identify potential instrument drifts. Although there are already several internationally recognized EQA ongoing programs such as the RCPA Haematology QAP, the UK-based NEQAS (National External Quality Assurance Scheme), the European-based ECAT, and the US-based CAP (College of American Pathologists) and NASCOLA (North American Specialized Coagulation Laboratory Association), national programs within more localized regions such as individual countries are also available.

Analytically, it has also been recently reported that a citrated plasma layer stratification might occur after conventional centrifugation in primary tubes for coagulation testing, thereby introducing a bias in the measurement (i.e., shortened PT values and higher fibrinogen levels) when the instrument needle collects an aliquot in the lower rather than in the upper part of the tube. This aspect might be analytically noteworthy and can even be magnified when preparing multiple aliquots from an original primary collection tube (e.g., for storage and delayed analysis of samples) [37]. As such, it is advisable that laboratories separate the citrated plasma from the pellet immediately after centrifugation and this be appropriately mixed before delayed/repeated analysis or aliquoting is undertaken.

Postanalytical errors

Postanalytical (e.g., inappropriate reporting or analysis, improper data entry, high turnaround times,

failure to notify critical values) and interpretative issues related to the interpretation of the test result by the laboratory (including the issued report) and/or the clinician (who interprets the reported test results) represent other important issues. Here, both the laboratory and the clinician may be at fault. Thus, how the laboratory reports its test results can have significant adverse consequences if clinicians base treatment on the test report and this report fails to appropriately identify the significance or nonsignificance of test results, or indeed the possibility of false values arising from preanalytical events and analytical peculiarities [38]. Similarly, the clinician may inappropriately base treatment on this test result without understanding that this test result may not be "true." This point in the brain-to-brain loop process therefore represents the final opportunity for laboratories to advise clinicians regarding the interpretation of results or the possibility of factors that may have inappropriately influenced results (e.g., preanalytical issues).

Several examples can be highlighted for hemostasis here. Laboratories may issue results for rare congenital thrombophilia markers such as protein C, protein S, and antithrombin without appropriate comments to indicate that such deficiencies are rare and that low reported values may (more likely) arise from "acquired deficiencies" post-thrombotic event "consumption" or due to concomitant anticoagulant therapy (e.g., coumarins such as warfarin decrease the vitamin K-dependent factors II, VII, IX, and X, as well as protein C and S, whereas high-dose heparin reduces the concentration of antithrombin), with the consequence that patients may be inappropriately labeled as having a congenital disorder and possibly placed on extended anticoagulant therapy with increased risk of bleeding. As a second example, inappropriate processing of normal blood can easily give rise to result patterns suggestive of von Willebrand disease. Therefore, should laboratories report abnormal test results for these investigations, without advising of the need to repeat test for confirmation, then patients may be inappropriately labeled as having a congenital bleeding disorder. A third example relates to the standardization/harmonization of reported test results. D-dimer resulting is paradigmatic, with multiple measure units being available (e.g., D-dimer units or fibrinogen equivalent units [FEU] in ng/mL, mg/dL, or g/L [39, 40]. Thus, specific guidance is required to clearly identify normal or raised levels, particularly if clinicians access results from several distinct providers.

Therefore, the inclusion of interpretative comments on laboratory reports provides added diagnostic value and greatly enhances visibility and competency of laboratory activities [11, 38]. Such interpretative comments might be particularly advisable when reporting results of hemostasis testing, given the large number of potential issues that impact on test results, as highlighted here and elsewhere. Extensive examples of appropriate interpretative comments are also available in previous publications [11, 38].

Conclusion

Quality in laboratory as well as in coagulation testing is often taken for granted rather than thoughtfully pursued. The rather impressive advances of analytical quality achieved by the implementation of reliable internal and external programs for assessing analytical quality have allowed to dramatically decrease the bias and uncertainty in this phase of the testing process. Nevertheless, several pre- and postanalytical issues still plague coagulation testing, and they should be the leading targets of further improvement actions. In this respect, the adoption of quality requirements and indicators, which strictly monitor each phase of the testing process (from test prescription to result reporting) and that can be universally adopted, is the cornerstone for ensuring high-quality, reliable, and safe diagnostics [36].

References

1. Kohn KT, Corrigan JM, Donaldson MS. *To Err Is Human: Building a Safer Health System*. Washington, DC: National Academy Press; 1999.
2. Krumholz HM, Rathore SS, Chen J, Wang Y, Radford MJ. Evaluation of a consumer-oriented internet health care report card: the risk of quality ratings based on mortality data. *JAMA*. 2002;287:1277–1287.
3. Starfield B. Is US health really the best in the world? *JAMA*. 2000;284:483–485.
4. Lippi G, Simundic AM, Mattiuzzi C. Overview on patient safety in healthcare and laboratory diagnostics. *Biochem Med*. 2010;20:131–143.
5. Plebani M, Lippi G. Is laboratory medicine a dying profession? Blessed are those who have not seen and yet have believed. *Clin Biochem*. 2010;43:939–941.
6. Lundberg GD. Acting on significant laboratory results. *JAMA*. 1981;245:1762–1763.
7. Bonini P, Plebani M, Ceriotti F, Rubboli F. Errors in laboratory medicine. *Clin Chem*. 2002;48:691–698.
8. International Organization for Standardization. ISO/PDTS 22367. *Medical Laboratories: Reducing Error Through Risk Management and Continual Improvement: Complementary Element*. Geneva, Switzerland: ISO; 2005:9.
9. Lippi G, Guidi GC, Mattiuzzi C, Plebani M. Preanalytical variability: the dark side of the moon in laboratory testing. *Clin Chem Lab Med*. 2006;44:358–365.
10. Plebani M. Exploring the iceberg of errors in laboratory medicine. *Clin Chim Acta*. 2009;404:16–23.
11. Favaloro EJ, Lippi G, Adcock DM. Preanalytical and postanalytical variables: the leading causes of diagnostic error in haemostasis? *Semin Thromb Hemost*. 2008;34:612–634.
12. Preston FE, Lippi G, Favaloro EJ, Jayandharan GR, Edison ES, Srivastava A. Quality issues in laboratory haemostasis. *Haemophilia*. 2010;16(suppl 5):93–99.
13. Salvagno GL, Lippi G, Bassi A, Poli G, Guidi GC. Prevalence and type of pre-analytical problems for inpatients samples in coagulation laboratory. *J Eval Clin Pract*. 2008;14:351–353.
14. Lippi G, Blanckaert N, Bonini P, et al. Causes, consequences, detection, and prevention of identification errors in laboratory diagnostics. *Clin Chem Lab Med*. 2009;47:143–153.
15. Lippi G, Plebani M. Identification errors in the blood transfusion laboratory: a still relevant issue for patient safety. *Transfus Apher Sci*. 2011;44:231–233.
16. Plebani M. Errors in clinical laboratories or errors in laboratory medicine? *Clin Chem Lab Med*. 2006;44:750–759.
17. Plebani M, Carraro P. Mistakes in a stat laboratory: types and frequency. *Clin Chem*. 1997;43:1348–1351.
18. Carraro P, Plebani M. Errors in a stat laboratory: types and frequencies 10 years later. *Clin Chem*. 2007;53:1338–1342.
19. Lippi G, Banfi G, Buttarello M, et al. For the Italian Intersociety SIBioC-SIMeL-CISMEL Study Group on Extraanalytical Variability. Recommendations for detection and management of unsuitable samples in clinical laboratories. *Clin Chem Lab Med*. 2007;45:728–736.
20. Adcock DM, Hoefner DM, Kottke-Marchant K, Marlar RA, Szamosi DI, Warunek DJ. *Collection, Transport, and Processing of Blood Specimens for Testing Plasma-Based Coagulation Assays and Molecular Hemostasis*

Assays: Approved Guideline. 5th ed. Wayne, PA: Clinical Laboratory Standards Institute; CLSI document H21-A5; 2008.

21. Lippi G, Salvagno GL, Adcock DM, Gelati M, Guidi GC, Favaloro EJ. Right or wrong sample received for coagulation testing? Tentative algorithms for detection of an incorrect type of sample. *Int J Lab Hematol.* 2010;32:132–138.

22. Lippi G, Lima-Oliveira G, Nazer SC, et al. Suitability of a transport box for blood sample shipment over a long period. *Clin Biochem.* 2011;44:1028–1029.

23. Tate J, Ward G. Interferences in immunoassay. *Clin Biochem Rev.* 2004;25:105–120.

24. Kazmierczak SC, Catrou PG. Analytical interference. More than just a laboratory problem. *Am J Clin Pathol.* 2000;113:9–11.

25. Lippi G, Blanckaert N, Bonini P, et al. Haemolysis: an overview of the leading cause of unsuitable specimens in clinical laboratories. *Clin Chem Lab Med.* 2008;46:764–772.

26. Lippi G, Salvagno GL, Montagnana M, Poli G, Guidi GC. Influence of the needle bore size on platelet count and routine coagulation testing. *Blood Coagul Fibrinolysis.* 2006;17:557–561.

27. Laga AC, Cheves TA, Sweeney JD. The effect of specimen hemolysis on coagulation test results. *Am J Clin Pathol.* 2006;126748–126755.

28. Lippi G, Guidi GC. Risk management in the preanalytical phase of laboratory testing. *Clin Chem Lab Med.* 2007;45:720–727.

29. Sciacovelli L, Plebani M. The IFCC Working Group on laboratory errors and patient safety. *Clin Chim Acta.* 2009;404:79–85.

30. Global Preanalytical Scientific Committee (GPSC). Available at: http://www.specimencare.com/index.asp. Accessed 15 November 2012.

31. Barth JH. Clinical quality indicators in laboratory medicine: a survey of current practice in the UK. *Ann Clin Biochem.* 2011;48:238–240.

32. Alsina MJ, Alvarez V, Barba N, et al. Preanalytical quality control program—an overview of results (2001-2005 summary). *Clin Chem Lab Med.* 2008;46:849–854.

33. Bilic-Zulle L, Simundic AM, Supak Smolcic V, Nikolac N, Honovic L. Self reported routines and procedures for the extra-analytical phase of laboratory practice in Croatia—cross-sectional survey study. *Biochem Med.* 2010;20:64–74.

34. Khoury M, Burnett L, Mackay M. Error rates in Australian chemical pathology laboratories. *Med J Aust.* 1996;165:128–130.

35. Hilbourne L, Meier F. Quality Indicators Workgroup Report. Personal communication at the IQLM Conference, April 29, 2005, Atlanta, GA.

36. Plebani M, Sciacovelli L, Lippi G. Quality indicators for laboratory diagnostics: consensus is needed. *Ann Clin Biochem.* 2011;48:479.

37. Lippi G, Salvagno GL, Bassi A, Montagnana M, Poli G, Guidi GC. Dishomogeneous separation of citrated plasma in primary collection tubes for routine coagulation testing. *Blood Coagul Fibrinolysis.* 2008;19:330–332.

38. Favaloro EJ, Lippi G. Laboratory reporting of haemostasis assays: the final post-analytical opportunity to reduce errors of clinical diagnosis in hemostasis? *Clin Chem Lab Med.* 2010;48:309–321.

39. Jennings I, Woods TA, Kitchen DP, Kitchen S, Walker ID. Laboratory D-dimer measurement: improved agreement between methods through calibration. *Thromb Haemost.* 2007;98:1127–1135.

40. Lippi G, Franchini M, Targher G, Favaloro EJ. Help me, Doctor! My D-dimer is raised. *Ann Med.* 2008;40:594–605.

4

International standards in hemostasis

Trevor W. Barrowcliffe[1] & Anthony R. Hubbard[2]
[1]Formerly National Institute for Biological Standards and Control (NIBSC), Potters Bar, Hertfordshire, UK
[2]National Institute for Biological Standards and Control, Hertfordshire, UK

Introduction

Assays of most components of the hemostatic system, and of many therapeutic materials used to treat disorders of hemostasis, are carried out on a comparative basis, relative to a standard of known potency. This is true of many other biological materials such as hormones and cytokines, and such comparative assays have many advantages over direct determinations without reference to a standard, which in any case are either difficult or impossible in complex biological matrices such as plasma.

In order to relate results in one laboratory to those in other laboratories there must be some means of linking the standards used in local laboratory assays. The concept of a single biological standard that could provide such a link was first established for insulin in the early twentieth century by Sir Henry Dale [1], and this has been developed into a well-established international system for many biological components under the auspices of the World Health Organization (WHO).

The first international standard in the area of hemostasis was for heparin, established in 1942 by the League of Nations, which subsequently became WHO [2]. In the 1960s work commenced on establishing WHO Reference Preparations for thromboplastin reagents, because of their widespread use in control of oral anticoagulation [3], and this was soon followed by the establishment of the first international standard

for one of the clotting factors, factor VIII (FVIII) [4]. Since then international standards have been established for most of the components of the hemostatic system; Tables 4.1–4.3 and 4.5 give an up-to-date summary of the international standards that are currently available. Further information about these and other standards can be found on the WHO website (www.who.int/biologicals).

This chapter describes the establishment and use of international standards in the field of hemostasis and thrombosis, with particular emphasis on their role in quality control (QC) of clinical samples.

International standards and international units

Units of activity

For most biological materials, including those involved in hemostasis, units of biological activity are defined soon after their discovery, and well before the establishment of international standards. The definition of the unit is usually related to the type of activity, for example, anticoagulant or procoagulant, and the method of measurement. Thus the unit of activity for heparin was first defined in terms of its ability to delay clotting of cats' blood [5], and that for thrombin in terms of the clotting time of a preparation of fibrinogen [6]. For most clotting factors in plasma, the unit

Quality in Laboratory Hemostasis and Thrombosis, Second Edition. Edited by Steve Kitchen, John D. Olson and F. Eric Preston.
© 2013 John Wiley & Sons, Ltd. Published 2013 by Blackwell Publishing Ltd.

Table 4.1 WHO standards for therapeutic concentrates of coagulation factors and inhibitors

Clotting factor	2011 standard
Factors II & X	3rd
Factor VII	1st
Factor VIIa	2nd
Factor VIII	8th
Fibrinogen	1st
von Willebrand factor	2nd
Factor IX	4th
Antithrombin	3rd
Protein C	1st

of activity was first defined as the amount in "average normal plasma." Such units may have practicability initially, but are not a very good basis for standardization of results among different laboratories.

International units

When international standards have been established for the first time, they are usually calibrated using the preexisting units, in order to provide continuity of measurement. Once the first international standard has been calibrated it is assigned a value in international units (IUs), and from then on the unit of activity for that particular analyte is defined only in terms of the amount of activity in the international standard. Subsequent batches of international standards are calibrated in IUs against the previous standard, although there may be ongoing studies of the relationship between the IU and the preexisting unit, as has

Table 4.2 WHO standards for coagulation factors and inhibitors in plasma

Clotting factor	2011 standard
Factors II, VII, IX, X	4th
Factor V	1st
Factor VIII/VWF	6th
Factor XI	1st
Factor XIII	1st
Fibrinogen	2nd
Antithrombin	3rd
Protein C	2nd
Protein S	2nd

Table 4.3 Other WHO standards and reference reagents used in hemostasis

Material	2011 standard or reference reagent
Ancrod	1st
β-Thromboglobulin	1st
Factor IXa	1st
Thrombin	2nd
Factor V Leiden (DNA reference panel)	1st
Prothrombin mutation G20210A (DNA reference panel)	1st
Heparin	6th
LMW heparin	2nd
Platelet factor 4	1st
Thromboplastin, human	4th
Thromboplastin, rabbit	4th

been the case for several of the clotting factor plasma standards (see subsequent section).

Establishment of international standards

The procedure for establishment of international standards has evolved over the last 60 years, and although it has tended to become more complex and sophisticated in recent years, many of the basic principles remain unchanged. The process is described in detail by WHO [7], but a brief outline will be given here, because it is common to many of the standards in hemostasis.

Choice of materials

For establishment of the first international standard for any analyte, it may be necessary to investigate a number of potential candidate materials in preliminary studies, and to include more than one candidate in the collaborative study. The type of material is chosen on the basis of its intended use, with application of the "like versus like" principle (see next section), and consideration of its stability. For replacement standards it is usually possible to select only one candidate on the basis of previous experience, though there are exceptions, notably low molecular weight (LMW) heparin (see subsequent section).

"Like versus like"

A basic tenet of biological standardization is the principle of "like versus like," that is, the test sample should be of similar composition to that of the standard against which it is assayed. This follows from one of the assumptions of comparative bioassays, namely, that the test sample should behave like a dilution of the standard. This is most likely if the standard and test are very similar to one another. Differences in composition would have little impact if coagulation assays were completely specific and unaffected by the type of matrix, but in practice this is not the case, and comparison of unlike materials, such as plasma and concentrates, tends to give high variability and differences among methods. Therefore for most coagulation factors international standards have been established for both plasma and concentrates (see subsequent section).

Physical attributes

Certain physical requirements must be fulfilled for preparations to serve as international standards. These include homogeneity (interampoule variability) of the preparation and characteristics consistent with long-term stability, such as low residual moisture and oxygen content [8, 9]. International standards exist as multiple sealed glass ampoules containing the freeze-dried physical material (the standard), and it is essential that all ampoule contents be as near identical as possible. This is achieved by extremely precise liquid filling, which is monitored through numerous check-weights evenly spaced throughout the total fill. Although the WHO guidelines quote interampoule variability (coefficient of variation [CV]) of <0.25% for liquid fills and <1% for viscous fills (e.g., plasma), CVs below 0.2% are routinely achieved for both plasma and concentrates. In practice, this corresponds to an extreme range of liquid filling weights less than $\pm 1\%$ of the mean filling weight.

Low residual moisture and low oxygen content, which improve long-term stability, are controlled during the manufacturing process by the use of efficient freeze-drying cycles, which routinely achieve residual moisture levels below 0.2% w/w (considerably below the WHO recommendation of <1% w/w) and by the backfilling of ampoules with nitrogen gas before sealing. Sealed glass ampoules are preferred for most international standards to ensure no ingress of atmospheric gases during long-term use, which may be over ten

years, but for materials that are very stable and are replaced over a shorter time frame, stoppered vials may be acceptable (e.g., FIX concentrate).

Collaborative study

International standards undergo calibration in extensive multicenter international collaborative studies, often involving more than 20 different laboratories. Collaborative studies are planned carefully to include relevant expert laboratories (clinical, academic, and commercial) and to represent the current methodologies.

Organization and analysis of such studies is quite complex and time-consuming, and it is essential to have an experienced central organization to undertake this. For virtually all WHO standards in the hemostasis area this task has been undertaken by the National Institute for Biological Standards and Control (NIBSC), which also acts as the custodian for the great majority of WHO standards (for further details and information on ordering standards see the website www.nibsc.ac.uk).

Proposed assigned potencies are usually based on the consensus overall mean estimates, and these require endorsement by study participants and by the Scientific and Standardisation Committee (SSC) of the International Society on Thrombosis and Haemostasis (ISTH) before they are submitted to the WHO Expert Committee on Biological Standardization for formal establishment of the standard.

In some cases excessive variability in the estimates from different laboratories that contribute to the consensus mean, or significant differences between methods, can preclude the assignment of a mean value. This was found to be the case for the calibration of the first international standard for LMW heparin against the unfractionated heparin (UFH) standard. Fortunately, such occurrences are rare and it is usually possible to assign a single value acceptable for all methods relating to a given analyte (e.g., FVIII:coagulant activity, protein S function).

Stability studies

International standards may be used for many years, and it is therefore essential that the preparations remain stable and the assigned values valid for the period of use. This property is also critical for maintaining the continuity of the IU, given that replacements are calibrated relative to previous standards.

Assessment of stability relies on two approaches: the accelerated degradation study and real-time stability.

Accelerated degradation studies have been used to predict the degradation rates of lyophilized coagulation factors for more than 30 years [10, 11]. These studies are based on the measurement of residual potency of ampoules stored at elevated temperatures (e.g., $4°C, 20°C, 37°C,$ and $45°C$) relative to ampoules stored at the bulk storage temperature (e.g., $-20°C$). The predictive model is based on the assumption that degradation is caused by unimolecular decay, with the probability of any intact molecule changing state in any unit of time remaining constant. In addition, the degradation rate must also follow a fixed law of temperature dependency, as described in the Arrhenius equation; hence, the degradation occurring at higher temperatures only differs from the degradation at lower temperatures in terms of rate. This allows the measured relative loss of activity observed for samples stored at elevated temperatures to be used to predict the degradation rate for samples stored at the bulk storage temperature of $-20°C$.

Results from accelerated degradation studies have indicated that the international standards for coagulation factors should be remarkably stable when stored at $-20°C$. For example, studies on even the more labile factors, FV:C and FVIII:C, have returned extremely low predicted losses of <0.1% per year [12].

Real-time studies provide a more objective assessment of the stability of ampoules in bulk storage by direct comparison with ampoules stored at lower temperatures (e.g., $-70°C$ or $-150°C$) and are most useful when performed after several years of storage or when the current IS is due for replacement. Acceptable data from both approaches increases confidence that the international standards have remained stable throughout their lifetime and the assigned values are valid for the direct calibration of replacement preparations.

Usage
For practical reasons the number of ampoules comprising a batch of material for an international standard has in the past been limited to around 4000. Therefore it is impractical to use international standards as working standards in laboratories, as the whole batch would be used very quickly. It is desirable to avoid too frequent replacements of international standards, as the replacement process is time-consuming; hence the main use of international

standards is to calibrate national, regional, or local standards. For plasma assays most reagent manufacturers issue commercial plasma standards that are calibrated in IUs against the appropriate IS. The considerable QC requirements for manufacturers of plasma standards could lead to excessive demand on the supply of WHO standards, and in order to mitigate this secondary plasma standard, calibrated for a multiple analytes and available in large quantities, has been developed under the auspices of the ISTH.

For assays of therapeutic concentrates, working standards are issued in the United States by the Food & Drug Administration's Center for Biologics Evaluation & Research (FDA/CBER), and in Europe, European Pharmacopeia (EP) standards by the European Directorate for the Quality of Medicines and Healthcare (EDQM). These are calibrated against the appropriate IS in multicenter studies. However, as the number of manufacturers is not large it is feasible for manufacturers to calibrate their in-house standards directly against WHO standards—this is preferable to using an intermediate working standard as it shortens the pathway between the international standard and the product.

Heparin and LMW heparin

The first international standard for UFH was established by WHO in 1942, and has been replaced at regular intervals; the current WHO standard, which was established in 2009, is the sixth. The EP and the US Pharmacopoeia (USP) both issue working standards; the EP standard is calibrated in IUs against the WHO standard, but the USP standard is calibrated in USP units, which previously differed from the IU by approximately 7% [13]. Harmonization of the USP unit with the IU was achieved in 2009 when the replacement USP standard was calibrated in the same exercise used to value assign the WHO sixth IS [14].

Despite the considerable technical differences, when different methods have been compared in international collaborative studies of UFH, the potencies given by the various methods have agreed to within a few percent [15]. This is a corroboration of the principle of "like versus like," in that the potencies are largely independent of the method used. However, when the first samples of LMW heparin were assayed against the UFH standard this was clearly not the case—there was large variability among laboratories, even when ostensibly using the same method. For instance, the CV among seven laboratories carrying out a chromogenic method on the same LMW heparin sample was 43% [16]. There was also a tendency toward nonparallelism between the log dose–response lines of the LMW heparin and the UFH standard, rendering many of the assays statistically invalid. In addition, as expected from the known properties of LMW heparin, there was a large difference in potency among methods based on inhibition of FXa, and those based in thrombin inhibition or delay of clotting times. The anti-Xa/anti-IIa ratio differed widely among the various LMW heparin products, and continues to do so.

Because of all these problems it became clear that the UFH standard was unsuitable for measurement of the anticoagulant activities of LMW heparins. It was therefore decided to establish a separate standard for LMW heparin, on the basis that "like versus like" would give better reproducibility. It was recognized that LMW heparins as a group were not identical to each other, and so the appropriate material for a standard had to be carefully chosen to be "in the middle" of the group with regard to its molecular weight and anticoagulant properties.

Following a preliminary study, two of eight LMW heparins were identified as giving the least interlaboratory variability when used as a standard for assay of the other preparations, with CVs in the range of 4–14% [16]. These two preparations were then subjected to a large international collaborative study, and one of the materials was established by WHO as the first international standard for LMW heparin in 1986 [17]. Although WHO standards are traditionally assigned a single potency, this would have been inappropriate in the case of LMW heparin, because of the large difference between potencies by anti-Xa and anti-IIa assays (around 2.5-fold). Accordingly, the LMW heparin standard was assigned two values, one for anti-Xa assays and another for anti-IIa assays (including aPTT).

The WHO first international standard has been used by manufacturers of all LMW heparins to calibrate their products, and was replaced in 2007 by the second IS, following an extensive international collaborative study [18].

It is important to recognize that, although the IUs for UFH and LMW heparin were identical in the international collaborative study to establish the first IS for LMW heparin, this was the only case for the mean of all the laboratories' results. Because of the nonparallelism and wide interlab variability in assays of LMW heparin versus the UFH standard, many individual laboratories would obtain different results if assaying a LMW heparin sample against both UFH and LMW heparin standards. Thus it is important that all LMW heparin samples, whether therapeutic products or patients' samples, should be assayed against a LMW heparin standard and not a UFH standard.

Thromboplastins

The prothrombin time (PT), first described in 1938, remains the most widely performed of all coagulation tests. Despite its simplicity, standardization of the measurements on a global basis has proved surprisingly difficult, and efforts are still continuing. One of the main uses of the PT is for monitoring anticoagulant therapy, and a detailed account of this is given in Chapter 23.

Two major steps forward in standardization of the PT were the establishment of International Reference Preparations (IRP) by the WHO, and the development of a method of conversion of locally measured PTs to a standardized value, the "international normalized ratio" (INR) [19, 20]. The first IRP for thromboplastin was a human brain combined preparation, chosen because human brain preparations were widely used at that time, and were the most sensitive to the reduced levels of vitamin K-dependent clotting factors induced by oral anticoagulants. In the absence of a previously defined "unitage" for thromboplastin reagents the first IRP was arbitrarily assigned an "international sensitivity index" of 1 [3]. The system of measurement described originally by Kirkwood [20] was for batches of thromboplastin reagents to be given an International Sensitivity Index (ISI) value by calibration against the IRP, or against a substandard calibrated against the IRP. The INR could then be calculated from the local PT ratio (PTR—patient's PT divided by normal PT) as follows:

$$INR = local\ PTR^{ISI}$$

On the whole this system has worked well, but discrepancies between results with different reagents can still occur, as indicated in Chapters 7 and 23. At the time of establishment of the first IRP, reagents prepared from rabbit brain and bovine brain were in common use, and IRPs were also established for rabbit and bovine thromboplastin. These were intended for calibration of reagents of the appropriate species, in an endorsement of the "like versus like" principle. The original IRPs, which were established in the 1970s, have been replaced, and the currently available IRPs (now named International Standards (IS)) are:

Human—fourth IS, rTF/09, established 2009 [21]
Rabbit—fourth IS, RBT/05, established 2005 [22]

The IRP for bovine thromboplastin has since been discontinued with the recommendation that manufacturers use the fourth IS rabbit thromboplastin, RBT/05, for the calibration of bovine combined thromboplastins [23].

Recently it has been recognized that calibration of the ISI of thromboplastin reagents may vary depending on the instrumentation used, and plasmas with defined INRs have been developed to overcome this. The ISTH/SSC has developed guidelines on the calibration and use of such plasmas [24], but as yet no international standards have been established for plasmas with defined INRs.

See also Chapter 23.

Coagulation factors and inhibitors

This is the largest group of international standards in the hemostasis field, and as indicated in Tables 4.1 and 4.2 standards for most factors are available in both plasma and concentrate forms.

Factor VIII

The first international standard for FVIII, established in 1971 [4], was a concentrate of low purity, typical of the relatively few products available at that time; it was calibrated against pools of fresh normal plasma in the 20 participating laboratories. The variability among laboratories in this first international collaborative study was extremely high, with potencies covering a tenfold range. Variability was somewhat lower in assays of lyophilized plasma, but this was not stable enough to qualify as an international standard. The first IS for FVIII was used successfully to calibrate manufacturers' concentrate standards, but its use to calibrate plasma standards such as the British Plasma Standards for FVIII was less satisfactory, because of high interlaboratory variability and a 20% difference between the results of one-stage and two-stage assays [25]. This is another example of the "like versus like" principle, and it became clear that a separate international plasma standard for FVIII would be desirable to calibrate local and commercial plasma standards. Changes in the method of collection and handling of plasma and in freeze-drying techniques led to improved stability of FVIII in lyophilized plasma, and eventually the first IS for FVIII plasma was established in 1981 [26], by assay against normal plasma pools in participants' laboratories; it was calibrated also for FVIII:Ag (previously named FVIII C:Ag) and for von Willebrand factor antigen and activity.

Both of these standards have been replaced at fairly frequent intervals because of high usage, and there have been three main issues in the last 25 years of FVIII standardization.

Different types of FVIII concentrate

Continuing developments of plasma-derived concentrates, due to requirements of viral inactivation and improved purification methods, as well as the introduction of recombinant products, have considerably broadened the range of FVIII products available. This makes the choice of material for the international standard important, since it has been shown that some concentrates give discrepancies between one-stage and chromogenic or two-stage methods [27].

Early attempts to measure FVIII:C in full-length recombinant FVIII concentrates, relative to the WHO third IS FVIII concentrate (plasma-derived), were associated with extremely large interlaboratory variability, with geometric coefficient of variation (GCVs) ranging from 39% to 137% depending on method [27, 28]. Initially, it was considered that a separate IS recombinant FVIII concentrate might be necessary to improve agreement among laboratories. However, subsequent studies revealed that the high variability could be overcome by the following specifications of assay methodology:

FVIII-deficient plasma
The use of hemophilic plasma or deficient plasma with a normal VWF level was found to be essential to give full potency in one-stage assays.

Assay buffers It was found that albumin at a concentration of 1% w/v (10 mg/mL) was necessary in all assay buffers in order to obtain reproducible results.

Predilution Predilution of both test and standard with hemophilic plasma, or its equivalent, was necessary for assay of all recombinant and high-purity plasma-derived products, whichever assay method was used.

These specifications precluded the need for a dedicated recombinant standard and were published as recommendations by SSC/ISTH [29] and also incorporated into the EP monograph for the assay of FVIII [30].

The sixth international standard was composed of recombinant FVIII, in recognition of the widespread use of recombinant products, and in anticipation that plasma-derived concentrates would suffer a rapid decline in production and use. However, in the event most manufacturers have continued to produce plasma-derived products, and since there are still more plasma-derived products than recombinant ones, the seventh IS and current eighth IS reverted to plasma-derived products. In the calibration of these standards there has been good agreement among laboratories; discrepancies between one-stage and chromogenic or two-stage methods were less than 10% for the sixth and seventh IS [31, 32] and there was absolute agreement for the eighth IS. However, this is not always the case—several concentrates have shown larger discrepancies when assayed against the IS, including the EP standard and the Mega 2 standard [33]; in the latter case the difference between one-stage and chromogenic potencies was over 30% and it was decided to label this standard with a different potency for each method. The B-domain-deleted recombinant concentrate also has a large discrepancy among methods, and even between different types of chromogenic or one-stage method [34]. These differences appear to be an inherent property of the materials and as far as possible it is best not to use such materials for standards—fortunately the majority of FVIII concentrates do not give discrepancies among methods when assayed against the IS using the ISTH/SSC recommendations.

International unit versus normal plasma

As already indicated, after establishment of the first International Standard for FVIII in plasma against the existing unit, that is, normal plasma pools, subsequent international standards have been calibrated against the previous one. However, although FVIII has been found to be very stable in these plasma standards, there is a slight risk that the IUs could drift from "normal plasma" over several calibrations during a long period of time. Hence in each collaborative study, normal plasma pools have been included to check the relationship between the IU and normal plasma.

For the first two replacements (second and third IS) the values against the previous standard were very similar to those against the mean of the plasma pools. However, for the calibration of the fourth versus the third standard, there was a discrepancy of about 15% between the two values, and it was decided to take the mean value as the potency of the fourth IS, in order to minimize the gap between the IU and normal plasma. The stability of FVIII in the plasma standards has been confirmed by real-time studies [35], and it seems likely that the apparent drift in the ratio of the IU to normal plasma is due to differences in donor population, and in methods of collection of the blood. When the first IS was established most blood was collected by syringes, whereas more recently Vacutainers are almost universally used—there is some evidence that these can lead to higher FVIII values in the plasma.

Despite the attempt to realign the IU in the fourth IS the discrepancy recurred with the fifth IS where there was a difference of around 10% between the values against the fourth IS and against the mean of the plasma pools [36]. Similarly, the value assignment of the current sixth IS was associated with a discrepancy of around 15%. However, it was decided not to make further adjustments to the IU, in view of the good stability data for both the fourth and fifth IS, and also because too frequent changes in the IU cause difficulties for manufacturers of secondary standards.

Plasma and concentrate units and in vivo recovery

The assay of FVIII concentrates against plasma standards has been a long-standing problem because of wide variability among laboratories and a basic difference among assay methods, and for these reasons two separate WHO standards for plasma and concentrates were developed. However, although such comparisons are avoided in routine assays, they are relevant to manufacturers of plasma-derived concentrates, and especially to clinicians measuring *in vivo* recovery. In the latter situation, patients' postinfusion samples, which essentially consist of concentrates "diluted" in the patient's hemophilic plasma, are usually assayed against a plasma standard.

It was first found in 1978 [37] that when concentrates were assayed against plasma the potencies were higher by the two-stage method than by one-stage assays—the average discrepancy from a number of collaborative studies at this time was 20%. Since then the same trend has been found in almost every collaborative study, although the size of the discrepancy varies from study to study, and possibly with different types of concentrates.

In recent years the chromogenic method has largely replaced the two-stage clotting method for assay of concentrates, and not surprisingly it also gives higher results than the one-stage method, being based on the same principles as the two-stage method. Despite considerable investigation the basic causes of this discrepancy remain unknown, although it is thought that the extensive processing applied to both plasma-derived and recombinant concentrates could lead to differences in their rates of activation and inactivation in the two method types from the FVIII in normal plasma, and there is some evidence for this from recent studies [38]. For largely historical reasons, when the WHO concentrate and plasma FVIII standards are compared against each other, the values are approximately equivalent by one-stage assays but not by two-stage or chromogenic methods.

There is some evidence that the discrepancy is greater for recombinant concentrates than for plasma-derived products. In the collaborative study to calibrate the fifth IS FVIII concentrate, which included both the WHO plasma standard and a recombinant concentrate, the ratio of chromogenic to one-stage potencies was 1.48, and in the sixth IS study [31] it was 1.26. These figures help to explain the large discrepancies between chromogenic and one-stage potencies found in patients' samples after infusion of recombinant concentrates [39]. It appears that after infusion, the recombinant products behave in an essentially similar manner in these assays to samples produced by diluting them *in vitro* in hemophilic plasma.

The situation with plasma-derived products is variable, dependent on the nature of the product and the test systems used. For instance, in a study by Lee et al. [40], Hemofil M was found to give a 20% discrepancy in postinfusion plasmas between one-stage and chromogenic methods, whereas in a study of a similar product performed at Central Laboratory of the Netherlands Red Cross Blood Transfusion Service (CLB), there was no difference between the methods (K. Mertens, personal communication). Equivalence between the methods was also found in a UK NEQAS study on a postinfusion sample from a different type of plasma-derived concentrate.

A resolution of this problem is only possible when the exact causes of the discrepancy are discovered; it may then be possible to adjust one or both of the methods to give similar values. In the meantime, a practical solution that has been discussed by the FVIII/FIX subcommittee of ISTH/SSC is to regard the postinfusion samples as concentrates, "diluted" in a patient's plasma, which is essentially what they are, and use a concentrate standard, diluted in hemophilic plasma, instead of a plasma standard, to construct the standard curve. Considering the close agreement among assay methods on recombinant concentrates when concentrate standards are used (see previous section), this should provide good agreement on *in vivo* recoveries of recombinant concentrates when measured by chromogenic and one-stage methods. However, the nature of the concentrate standard needs to be carefully considered; it should be as similar as possible to the injected product. Thus, whereas either of the full-length recombinant concentrates could serve as a standard for the other, plasma samples following infusion of the B-domain-deleted product, ReFacto, would need a ReFacto concentrate standard.

This approach has recently been tested in *in vivo* recovery studies, in which patients' samples after infusion of Recombinate, Kogenate, and Alphanate were assayed against both a plasma standard and a concentrate standard. As shown in Table 4.4, for

Table 4.4 Comparison of plasma and concentrate standards on postinfusion samples

| Concentrate infused | Ratio chromogenic: one-stage | | Concentrate standard |
	Plasma standard	Concentrate standard	
Recombinate	1.24	1.02	Recombinate
Kogenate	1.20	0.99	Kogenate
Alphanate	1.00	0.86	Kogenate

Recombinate and Kogenate the discrepancy between one-stage and chromogenic methods using the plasma standard was completely abolished with the appropriate concentrate standard. However, in the case of Alphanate the use of a concentrate standard, in this case not the same as the product infused, made the situation worse. Therefore the use of concentrate standards needs to be product specific, and should probably be restricted to recombinant and very high-purity plasma-derived products.

Factor IX

Standardization of FIX assays has presented fewer problems than that of FVIII. This is because there is predominantly a single assay method, the one-stage clotting assay, used for both plasma and concentrates. As for FVIII, a concentrate standard was the first to be established by WHO, for therapeutic materials, and this consisted of a prothrombin complex concentrate (PCC) [41]. During the late 1990s there was a switch to high-purity single FIX concentrates as the mainstay of therapy; this did not appear to cause any problems in assay standardization and it was found that PCCs and single FIX concentrates could be assayed satisfactorily against each other. The WHO third IS was a single FIX concentrate and was shared among WHO, FDA/CBER, and the EP/EDQM, thus avoiding the need for calibration of separate working standards and thereby harmonizing the labeling of FIX concentrates on a worldwide basis. This example was followed for the current WHO fourth IS, which also serves as the EP/EDQM and FDA/CBER standards.

As for FVIII, it was found that predilution of concentrates in FIX-deficient plasma was necessary to obtain optimum and reproducible potency when assaying concentrates against a concentrate standard, and also when comparing concentrates against plasma [42]. An international plasma standard for FIX, together with the other vitamin K-dependent factors II, VII, and X, was established by the WHO in 1987 [43], and most local and commercial plasma standards are now calibrated in IU. However, UK NEQAS surveys continue to show wide variability among laboratories, probably due to the multiplicity of aPTT reagents and deficient plasmas used (see Chapter 6). As with FVIII, artificially depleted plasmas have become the main type of FIX-deficient

reagent used, but there has been no systematic study of their performance compared with hemophilia B plasma.

von Willebrand factor

Development of the von Willebrand factor standard differed from FVIII and FIX, in that a plasma standard was established first—as mentioned this was the same plasma as that calibrated for FVIII. The first IS was calibrated for both VWF antigen and ristocetin cofactor activity, against the mean of the plasma pools, comprising over 200 donors [26]. As in established WHO practice, subsequent standards were calibrated against the previous one, but, as for FVIII, comparisons were also made against normal pools. In the collaborative study to calibrate the fourth IS there were significant differences between the values against the third IS and against the mean of the normal pools—14% for VWF:Ag and 20% for VWF:RCo and, as for FVIII, it was decided to take the mean of the two values as the potency of the fourth IS. In the calibration of the fifth IS there was no significant difference in the values against the previous standard (fourth IS) and against the mean of the plasma pools. Calibration of the current sixth IS was associated with no significant difference in VWF:RCo values against the fifth IS and the plasma pools but there was a significant discrepancy for VWF:Ag. In consideration of the good stability of the previous standards and in the interests of continuity of the IU it was decided to assign the mean values estimated relative to the previous WHO IS for both the fifth and sixth IS. Following the introduction of the collagen-binding assay as an alternative to the ristocetin cofactor method this analyte was introduced as a new value assignment to the fifth IS [36].

The increasing use of concentrates containing VWF for treatment of von Willebrand disease led to the need for a VWF concentrate standard—as is generally the case, assays of VWF concentrates against the plasma standard were found to be highly variable. Following an international collaborative study the first IS for VWF concentrate was established with assigned values for VWF antigen and VWF:RCo. However, estimates of collagen-binding activity were too variable to allow an assignment of mean potency, with major differences in potency according to the different collagen reagents used [44, 45]. More recently, the collaborative study for the replacement of the first IS by the second IS, in 2010, yielded much lower interlaboratory variability for estimates of collagen-binding activity with no significant difference among collagen reagents. This allowed the assignment of a mean value for collagen binding to the second IS [46].

Fibrinogen

Fibrinogen is the only coagulation factor to be assigned a potency in milligrams rather than units of activity. This relates back to early methods of measurement, where because of its unique clottability the amount of protein in a clot, which could be measured in milligrams, was assumed to be equivalent to the fibrinogen content of a plasma or purified sample. However, in practice this method proved difficult to standardize because of variable conditions of formation of the clot and different amounts of other proteins absorbed. Most clinical laboratories use the Clauss method, based on comparative measurement of thrombin clotting times of dilutions of plasma, against a plasma standard. Accordingly, a WHO standard for fibrinogen, plasma was established in 1992 [47], and to maintain continuity with established clinical practice, this was calibrated in milligrams using clot weight methods. The second IS for fibrinogen was calibrated against the first IS, using mostly Clauss methods [48].

Although fibrinogen concentrates are rarely used as therapeutic materials in themselves, they are an essential component of fibrin sealant preparations that are being used more frequently. The fibrinogen content of these preparations is measured as total protein and clottable protein and these measurements do not have an absolute requirement for a standard. However, in a collaborative study high variability was found for both of these measurements and it was shown that variability could be considerably reduced by comparison against a fibrinogen standard. Accordingly the first IS for fibrinogen concentrate was established by WHO in 1999, calibrated in milligrams for total and clottable protein [49].

Thrombin

Thrombin was one of the earliest components of the coagulation system to be standardized; the National Institutes of Health (NIH) originally defined the unit of activity as the amount required to clot a fibrinogen preparation in 15 seconds, and NIH established a standard based on this unitage before the WHO standard was prepared. When the first IS for thrombin was established by WHO in 1970, attempts were made to link the unitage to the NIH unit. However, it subsequently became apparent that there was a discrepancy between NIH units and IUs, the degree of difference depending on the assay methods used. This discrepancy was resolved a few years ago by establishment of a joint WHO/NIH standard with a common unitage [50].

Other coagulation factors and inhibitors

The establishment of international standards for the other coagulation factors and inhibitors has followed the same pattern as for FVIII and FIX, with separate standards for plasma and concentrates where the latter exist (see Tables 4.1 and 4.2).

Prothrombin complex factors
The WHO standard for FIX plasma was also calibrated for factors II, VII, and X. In addition to the IS for FIX concentrate a separate international standard was established for factors II and X concentrate, to be used by manufacturers of PCCs. A further separate international standard was established for FVII concentrate, and since this was found to be unsuitable for assay of the recombinant FVIIa product, a different IS was established for the latter preparation.

Inhibitors
Antithrombin was the first plasma inhibitor to be standardized, with the establishment of an international standard for plasma, followed by establishment of a separate standard for concentrate. In both these standards different values were assigned for activity and antigen, though the values are very similar. Plasma standards have been established for protein C and protein S, and most recently an international standard for protein C concentrate has been added.

Other plasma clotting factors
International plasma standards have been established for factors V, XI, and XIII. Although therapeutic concentrates are available for factors XI and XIII, these are used rarely and the number of manufacturers is small; hence the establishment of separate concentrate standards for these two factors has been of low priority.

Table 4.5 Standards in fibrinolysis

Material	2011 WHO standard or reference reagent
Plasmin	3rd
PAI-1	1st
Streptokinase	3rd
Streptodornase	1st
tPA activity	3rd
tPA antigen	1st
Urokinase	1st

Fibrinolysis standards

The absence of genetic deficiency states for fibrinolysis components in plasma has meant that assays of these components are carried out much less frequently in plasma samples than those of coagulation factors. As shown in Table 4.5, attention has focused on development of international standards for therapeutic materials, for use by manufacturers of these products, as well as standards for some of the main components of the fibrinolytic system, that is, plasmin and plasminogen activator inhibitor-1. The first IS to be established in this area was Streptokinase, in the 1960s, and this was followed by the plasmin Urokinase and the tissue plasminogen activator tPA. Recently the need for plasma standards for diagnostic purposes has been recognized, and work is in progress on development of international plasma standards for some of the fibrinolytic components. However, the most clinically useful measurement in this area, the D-dimer, has proved difficult to standardize, as described in detail in Chapter 13.

References

1. Jeffcoate SL. From insulin to amylin: 75 years of biological standardisation in endocrinology. *Dev Biol Stand.* 1999;100:39–47.
2. Brozovic M, Bangham DR. Standards for heparin. *Adv Exp Med Biol.* 1975;52:163–179.
3. Biggs R, Bangham DR. Standardisation of the one-stage prothrombin time test for the control of anticoagulant therapy. The availability and use of thromboplastin reference preparations. *Thromb Diath Haemorrh.* 1971;26(1):203–204.
4. Bangham DR, Biggs R, Brozovic M, Denson KWE, Skegg JL. A biological standard for measurement of blood coagulation factor VIII activity. *Bull World Health Organ.* 1971;45:337–351.
5. Jaques LB. The heparins of various mammalian species and their relative anti-coagulant potency. *Science.* 1940;92(2395):488–489.
6. Seegers WH, Brinkhous KM, Smith HP, Warner ED. The purification of thrombin. *J Biol Chem.* 1938;126:91–95.
7. Recommendations for the preparation, characterisation and establishment of international and other biological reference standards (revised 2004). WHO Technical Report Series 2007. Geneva, Switzerland: WHO 2007;932:73–131.
8. Campbell PJ. International biological standards and reference preparations. I. Preparation and presentation of materials to serve as standards and reference preparations. *J Biol Stand.* 1974;2:249–258.
9. Campbell PJ. International biological standards and reference preparations. II. Procedures used for the production of biological standards and reference preparations. *J Biol Stand.* 1974;2(4):259–267.
10. Kirkwood TBL. Predicting the stability of biological standards and products. *Biometrics.* 1977;33:736–742.
11. Kirkwood TBL, Tydeman MS. Design and analysis of accelerated degradation tests for the stability of biological standards II. A flexible computer program for data analysis. *J Biol Stand.* 1984;12:207–214.
12. Barrowcliffe TW, Matthews KB. Standards and quality control in the blood coagulation laboratory. In: Rizza C, Lowe G, eds. *Haemophilia and Other Inherited Bleeding Disorders.* Philadelphia, PA: WB Saunders, 1997:115–149.
13. Barrowcliffe TW, Mulloy B, Johnson EA, Thomas DP. The anticoagulant activity of heparin: measurement and relationship to chemical structure. *J Pharm Biomed Anal.* 1989;7(2):217–226.
14. Gray E, Mulloy B. International collaborative study to establish the 6th International Standard for unfractionated heparin. Unpublished WHO report, 2008.
15. Gray E, Walker AD, Mulloy B, Barrowcliffe TW. A collaborative study to establish the 5th International Standard for unfractionated heparin. *Thromb Haemost.* 2000;84(6):1017–1022.
16. Barrowcliffe TW, Curtis AD, Tomlinson TP, Hubbard AR, Johnson EA, Thomas DP. Standardisation of low molecular weight heparins: a collaborative study. *Thromb Haemost.* 1985;54(3):675–679.
17. Barrowcliffe TW, Curtis AD, Johnson EA, Thomas DP. An international standard for low molecular weight heparin. *Thromb Haemost.* 1988;60(1):1–7.

18. Gray E, Rigsby P, Mulloy B. Establishment of the 2nd International Standard for low molecular weight heparin. NIBSC unpublished report, 2005.

19. Bangham DR, Biggs R, Brozović M, Denson KW. Calibration of five different thromboplastins, using fresh and freeze-dried plasma. *Thromb Diath Haemorrh.* 1973;29(2):228–239.

20. Kirkwood TB. Calibration of reference thromboplastins and standardisation of the prothrombin time ratio. *Thromb Haemost.* 1983;49(3):238–244.

21. Tripodi A, Chantarangkul V, van den Besselaar AMHP, Witteveen E, Hubbard AR. International collaborative study for the calibration of a proposed International Standard for thromboplastin, human, plain. *J Thromb Haemost.* 2010;8:2066–2068.

22. Chantarangkul V, van den Besselaar AMHP, Witteveen E, Tripodi A. International collaborative study for the calibration of a proposed International Standard for thromboplastin, rabbit, plain. *J Thromb Haemost.* 2006;4:1339–1345.

23. van den Besselaar AMHP, Witteveen E, Tripodi A. Calibration of combined thromboplastins with the International Standard for thromboplastin, rabbit, plain. *J Thromb Haemost.* 2011;9:881–882.

24. van den Besselaar AM, Barrowcliffe TW, Houbouyan-Reveillard LL, et al. Subcommittee on Control of Anticoagulation of the Scientific and Standardisation Committee of the ISTH. Guidelines on preparation, certification, and use of certified plasmas for ISI calibration and INR determination. *J Thromb Haemost.* 2004;2(11):1946–1953.

25. Barrowcliffe TW, Kirkwood TBL. Standardisation of Factor VIII. I: calibration of British Standards for Factor VIII clotting activity. *Br J Haematol.* 1980;46:471–481.

26. Barrowcliffe TW, Tydeman MS, Kirkwood TBL, Thomas DP. Standardisation of factor VIII. III: establishment of a stable reference plasma for factor VIII-related activities. *Thromb Haemost.* 1983;50:690–696.

27. Barrowcliffe TW, Raut S, Sands D, Hubbard AR. Coagulation and chromogenic assays of factor VIII activity: general aspects, standardization, and recommendations. *Semin Thromb Hemost.* 2002;28(3):247–256.

28. Barrowcliffe TW. Standardization of FVIII & FIX assays. *Haemophilia.* 2003;9(4):397–402.

29. Barrowcliffe TW. Recommendations for the assay of high-purity factor VIII concentrates. *Thromb Haemost.* 1993;70(5):876–877.

30. Assay of human coagulation factor VIII (2.7.4). In: *European Pharmacopoeia.* 5th ed. Strasbourg, France: Council of Europe; 2005:194–195.

31. Raut S, Heath AB, Barrowcliffe TW. A collaborative study to establish the 6th international standard for factor VIII concentrate. *Thromb Haemost.* 2001; 85(6):1071–1078.

32. Raut S, Bevan S, Hubbard AR, Sands D, Barrowcliffe TW. A collaborative study to establish the 7th international standard for factor viii concentrate. *J Thromb Haemost.* 2005;3(1):119–126.

33. Kirschbaum N, Wood L, Lachenbruch P, et al. Calibration of the Ph. Eur. BRP Batch 3/Mega 2 (US/FDA) standard for human coagulation factor VIII concentrate for use in the potency assay. *Pharmeuropa Spec Issue Biol.* 2002;1:31–64.

34. Hubbard AR, Sands D, Sandberg E, Seitz R, Barrowcliffe TW. A multi-centre collaborative study on the potency estimation of ReFacto. *Thromb Haemost.* 2003;90:1088–1093.

35. Hubbard AR. International biological standards for coagulation factors and inhibitors. *Semin Thromb Haemost.* 2007;33:283–289.

36. Hubbard AR, Heath AB. Standardization of factor VIII and von Willebrand factor in plasma: calibration of the WHO 5th International Standard (02/150). *J Thromb Haemost.* 2004;2:1380–1384.

37. Kirkwood TBL, Barrowcliffe TW. Discrepancy between 1-stage and 2-stage assay for factor VIII:C. *Br J Haematol.* 1978;40:333–338.

38. Hubbard AR, Weller LJ, Bevan SA. Activation profiles of FVIII in concentrates reflect one-stage/chromogenic potency discrepancies. *Br J Haematol.* 2002;117:957–960.

39. Lee CA, Owens D, Bray G, et al. Pharmacokinetics of recombinant factor VIII (recombinate) using one-stage clotting and chromogenic factor VIII assay. *Thromb Haemost.* 1999;82(6):1644–1647.

40. Lee C, Barrowcliffe TW, Bray G, et al. Pharmacokinetic in vivo comparison using 1-stage and chromogenic substrate assays with two formulations of hemofil-M. *Thromb Haemost.* 1996;76:950–956.

41. Brozovic M, Bangham DR. Study of a proposed international standard for factor IX. *Thromb Haemost.* 1976;35:222–236.

42. Barrowcliffe TW, Tydeman MS, Kirkwood TBL. Major effect of prediluent in factor IX clotting assay. *Lancet.* 1979;2:192.

43. Barrowcliffe TW. Standardisation http://www.blackwell-synergy.com/doi/ref/10.1046/j.1365-2516.2003.00773.x—q20#q20of Factors II, VII, IX, and X in plasma and concentrates. *Thromb Haemost.* 1987;59:334.

44. Hubbard AR, Sands D, Chang AC, Mazurier C. Standardisation of von Willebrand factor in therapeutic concentrates: calibration of the 1st international standard for von Willebrand factor concentrate (00/514). *Thromb Haemost.* 2002;88:380–386.

45. Hubbard AR. von Willebrand factor standards for plasma and concentrate testing. *Semin Thromb Hemost.* 2006;32:522–528.

46. Hubbard AR, Hamill M, Beeharry M, Bevan SA, Heath AB. Value assignment of the WHO 2nd international standard von Willebrand factor, concentrate (09/182). *J Thromb Haemost.* 2011;9:1638–1640.

47. Gaffney PJ, Wong MY. Collaborative study of a proposed international standard for plasma fibrinogen measurement. *Thromb Haemost.* 1992;68:428–432.

48. Whitton CM, Sands D, Hubbard AR, Gaffney PJ. A collaborative study to establish the 2nd international standard for fibrinogen plasma. *Thromb Haemost.* 2000;84:258–262.

49. Whitton C, Sands D, Barrowcliffe TW. Establishment of the 1st international standard for fibrinogen, concentrate. NIBSC unpublished report, 2003.

50. Whitton C, Sands D, Lee T, Chang A, Longstaff C. A reunification of the US ("NIH") and international unit into a single standard for thrombin. *Thromb Haemost.* 2005;93(2):261–266.

5 Sample integrity and preanalytical variables

Dorothy (Adcock) Funk

Colorado Coagulation, a business unit of Esoterix, Inc., Englewood, CO, USA

Introduction

Laboratory testing is an integral component of clinical decision making as it aids in the determination of patient diagnosis and treatment. The ability to provide optimal clinical care is highly dependent on accurate and reliable laboratory results. Error leading to the reporting of an erroneous result can be introduced at any point of the testing process, from sample collection to result reporting. Due to the advances in instrument technology and informatics, analytical variability no longer represents the major cause of laboratory inaccuracy. Today the preanalytical phase of testing is the source of many, if not the majority of inaccurate laboratory results [1–3]. The preanalytical phase of testing refers specifically to the period of time beginning with patient identification and ending with specimen analysis. Errors in the preanalytical phase are generally a reflection of improper specimen collection, processing, or unsuitable conditions during sample transportation and/or storage. Samples for hemostasis testing are particularly susceptible to conditions that may impair sample integrity due to a number of factors including the *in vitro* lability of platelets and coagulation factors, the complex nature of the reactions commonly measured in the hemostasis laboratory, and because clot formation is naturally initiated with sample collection and therefore must be completely inhibited for analysis of many of the hemostatic factors. In the coagulation laboratory, knowledge of preanalytical variables and their impact on the accuracy of test results is crucial. Patient-related conditions such as intravascular hemolysis, lipemia, icterus, as well as certain medications, may also interfere with accurate result reporting. Although these patient conditions must be recognized and acknowledged, they are largely out of the control of the laboratory and will not be emphasized in this chapter.

In every step of this process, from sample procurement to analysis, the potential exists for sample integrity to be compromised. Improper sample collection, processing, and/or handling can have a critical impact on both the platelets and plasma factors involved in hemostasis. The effect of improper preanalytical conditions can be to reduce some platelet-related and plasma factor activities and, surprisingly, elevate others. For example, activation of a sample due to exposure to cold may cause an elevation of factor VII activity and a drastic drop in factor VIII activity levels [4, 5]. A spurious decrease in factor VIII activity due to improper sample storage, for example, may lead to an inappropriate diagnosis of hemophilia A or von Willebrand disease. Compromise of sample integrity leading to erroneous result reporting may lead not only to patient misdiagnosis but also to improper medication dosing and overall patient mismanagement, which may end in life-threatening therapeutic misadventures.

In order to assure the highest quality of laboratory testing results, it is imperative that sample integrity

Quality in Laboratory Hemostasis and Thrombosis, Second Edition. Edited by Steve Kitchen, John D. Olson and F. Eric Preston.

be preserved at every step of the process. Guidelines for sample handling should be strictly followed and deviations avoided unless their impact, or lack thereof, on coagulation testing is known.

Sample acquisition (specimen collection)

The importance of positive patient identification cannot be overemphasized. The conscious patient should be asked to identify him- or herself and asked for a form of identification. In the case of the hospitalized patient, the positive identification provided for patients by the institution must be verified. Positive identification of hospitalized patients using bedside electronic or bar-code methods reduces the risk of patient misidentification. Labels for the specimens to be collected must be prepared in advance, taken to the collection site or bedside and, after collection, the filled tubes labeled in the presence of the patient and before leaving the bedside. Each tube should be labeled with the patient's name and an additional identifier such as date of birth or medical record number.

Venipuncture is the most common and preferred method of sample collection for coagulation testing. Ideally, the patient should be made comfortable and at ease during the procedure. In situations of stress, for example, if a child is very tearful or upset at the time of the phlebotomy, certain hemostatic proteins such as von Willebrand factor (VWF), factor VIII, and fibrinogen may increase, as these are acute phase reactant proteins. This may cause spurious shortening of the activated partial thromboplastin time (aPTT) or bring low levels of these factors into the normal range resulting in a missed diagnosis, for example, of hemophilia or von Willebrand disease.

Blood samples should be procured in a relatively atraumatic fashion and during collection; the blood should flow freely into the collection container. When obtaining plasma for coagulation testing, it is imperative that clotting of the sample be avoided. Samples, for which the blood is slow to fill the collection container, where there is prolonged use of a tourniquet or considerable manipulation of the vein by the needle, may develop a clot *in vitro* [6]. These situations therefore must be avoided. The presence of clot in the collection container is cause for specimen rejection. Clot development may result in *in vitro* consumption of clotting factors, activation of clotting factors,

activation of platelets and platelet granule release, any of which may alter results of hemostasis assays. Integrity of the sample may be affected even if the clots are not visible to the naked eye.

Another important means to prevent *in vitro* clot formation is to adequately and promptly mix the sample following collection to insure complete distribution of anticoagulant. When using evacuated collection tubes, three to six complete end-over-end inversions are recommended [7]. Vigorous shaking is to be avoided so as not to induce hemolysis or activate platelets [6].

The specimen collection system
Each component of the specimen collection system may potentially impact the quality of the sample for coagulation testing. Knowledge regarding the impact of these various components, including needle gauge, composition of the specimen container, fill volume, and anticoagulant composition and concentration, on sample integrity is therefore imperative.

Needle gauge In general, needle gauge from 19 to 23 is optimal for blood collection. Gauge refers to the measure of the diameter of the needle bore. The larger the gauge, the smaller the needle bore. For collection of plasma samples, 21-gauge needles are most commonly used although 22-gauge needles provide adequate blood flow potentially with less discomfort [8]. While 19- to 21-gauge needles are often employed for large antecubital veins, 23-gauge needles are often used for smaller secondary veins. Very small needles, such as those greater than 25 gauge, should be avoided, if possible, as the slower rate of blood flow through the small bore may induce clotting or activation of the sample [2, 8]. Very large bore needles, such as those less than 16 gauge, may induce hemolysis of the sample due to turbulence of flow through the needle [9].

Collection container For hemostasis testing, the primary collection tube and all aliquot tubes must be composed of a nonactivating material such as polypropylene plastic or silicone-coated glass, in order to avoid initiation of clotting due to activation in the collection container [10]. Blood for hemostasis testing can be collected in either evacuated tubes or syringes as long as the composition of the container is

Table 5.1 Effect of sodium citrate concentration of the PT and aPTT in normal individuals and in the presence of anticoagulant therapy

| | Prothrombin time (s) using innovin[a] | | | Activated partial thromboplastin time (s) using actin FS[a] | | |
| | Citrate concentration | | | Citrate concentration | | |
Treatment	3.2%	3.8%	p value	3.2%	3.8%	p value
No anticoagulant	11.2 ± 2.5	11.8 ± 2.3	<0.0004	28.2 ± 4.0	30.3 ± 3.5	0.0006
UFH	16.4 ± 8.3	17.8 ± 9.9	<0.0005	44.0 ± 11.0	48.6 ± 14.0	0.0001
UFH plus AVK	25.1 ± 28.0	26.3 ± 28.0	<0.2	65.5 ± 16.0	69.0 ± 14.0	0.0109
AVK	27.6 ± 13.0	34.3 ± 17.0	<0.0001	40.2 ± 9.7	44.1 ± 13.0	0.0001

[a]Dade Behring, Marburg Germany.
UFH, unfractionated heparin; AVK, antivitamin K therapy.

nonactivating. It has been reported that variations in normal range and assay results may vary depending on whether the sample is collected in glass or plastic containers [11]. More recent published studies, however, have demonstrated no clinically significant differences in results when samples are collected in either glass- or plastic-evacuated tubes [12, 13]. To optimize standardization, facilities should harmonize their collection containers to one composition or another. Plastic-evacuated tubes may be preferred or required in certain regions as these carry a lower risk of breakage and therefore reduced potential for injury and exposure to infectious materials. If a syringe is used to collect the sample, a smaller size such as 20 mL or less is recommended to avoid *in vitro* clot formation. Blood and anticoagulant should be mixed within 30 seconds following the phlebotomy. In order to prevent clotting of the sample *in vitro*, all samples must be adequately and rapidly mixed (three to six complete inversions) to ensure complete distribution of anticoagulant.

Anticoagulant Samples for plasma-based hemostasis testing should be anticoagulated with sodium citrate. Some evacuated tube manufacturers standardize the color of the evacuated tube stopper and in this instance sodium citrate is the type of anticoagulant found in a light blue stopper tube from the majority of manufacturers. The World Health Organization (WHO) and Clinical Laboratory Standards Institute (CLSI) recommend 105 to 109 mmol/L, 3.13% to

3.2% (commonly described as 3.2%) of the dihydrate form of trisodium citrate ($Na_3C_6H_5O_7 \bullet 2H_2O$), buffered or nonbuffered as the anticoagulant of choice for hemostasis testing rather than 129 mmol/L, 3.8% (commonly described as 3.8%), although either is acceptable [7, 14].

In order to reduce result variability, it is important to standardize to only one anticoagulant concentration within a laboratory system. This is because clotting times, such as the aPTT and prothrombin time (PT), vary with different concentrations of sodium citrate, particularly if the clotting time is prolonged [15] (Table 5.1). Clotting times tend to be longer in 3.8% versus 3.2% sodium citrate because the higher concentration of citrate binds more assay-added calcium, making less available to promote clot formation. Significant error can be introduced in particular when determining the international normalized ratio (INR) if different concentrations of sodium citrate are used in the sample to be tested versus the concentration of anticoagulant used to determine mean normal PT and international sensitivity index (ISI) of the reagent.

Other anticoagulants such as ethylenediaminetetraacetic acid (EDTA) or heparin are not acceptable for hemostasis testing. Samples collected in purple or green stopper tubes or the use of serum for testing will lead to aberrant results. In serum, factors VII and IX are activated resulting in supranormal values while factors V and VIII are low such that PT and aPTT result in no clot. EDTA plasma, on the other hand, results in moderate prolongation of the PT and

Table 5.2 Effect of sample matrix on common hemostasis assays

Tube type assay	3.2% Citrate mean/range	EDTA mean/range	Sodium heparin mean/range	Serum mean/range
aPTT (s)	29/25–33	68/45–92	>180	>180
PT (s)	12.4/11.5–13.2	23/19–27	>60	>60
dRVVT (s)	34.6/27–43	55/45–64	>150	>150
FV Act (%)	113/84–142	71/39–103	81/59–103	23/13–33
FVII Act (%)	115/50–180	116/51–182	77/43–107	308/80–437
FVIII Act (%)	141/80–202	7.5/2–19	<1	4.5/1.3–7.7
FIX Act (%)	122/97–148	115/63–168	<1	350/135–565
VWF:Ag (%)	122/50–194	143/59–228	70/42–98	101/32–169
VWF:RCo (%)	114/41–188	131/46–215	37/13–60	74/25–124
PC Ag	97/60–134	115/97–159	125/94–156	120/71–169
PC Act (%)	111/66–155	152/100–205	<1	21.6/0–70
PS Act (%)	96/73–119	30/17–42	<1	15.3/0–39.5
Free PS Ag (%)	108/72–144	131/91–171	126/94–159	131/97–164
AT Act (%)	102/86–118	121/105–138	126/108–143	47/30–65
AT Ag (%)	110/832–138	121/92–150	100/83–118	114/79–148

Source: Unpublished data. Valcour A, Marshall T. 2007 Laboratory Corporation of America®.

aPTT with significant reduction of factor VIII activity. Plasma collected in EDTA, *importantly*, shows an *inhibitor effect* in mixing studies and may lead to spurious identification of a factor V or VIII inhibitor [16]. See Table 5.2 for the effect of incorrect sample type on common hemostasis assays. The receipt of serum or plasma other than that collected in sodium citrate for the performance of clot-based assays must result in specimen rejection. Reference laboratories that receive frozen plasma aliquot tubes rather than the primary collection tubes must be especially aware of the possibility that the sample is other than citrated plasma as the visual appearance of these samples is the same for all, once they have been aliquoted into a secondary tube.

Special sodium citrate collection tubes Sodium citrate collection tubes may contain additional special additives that are necessary or preferable in order to ensure optimum sample integrity for certain hemostasis assays. These tubes can be categorized as (1) tubes that prevent platelet activation, (2) tubes that are highly acidified to stabilize factors of the fibrinolytic system, and (3) tubes that contain protease inhibitors.

Citrate, theophylline, adenosine, and dypyridamole (CTAD) comprise a cocktail of additives that prevents *in vitro* platelet activation. These tubes afford more reliable measure of unfractionated heparin (UFH)

levels due to diminished effect of platelet factor 4 (PF4), a potent neutralizer of UFH that is released from platelets [17, 18]. Whole blood samples containing UFH must be processed within 1 hour of collection to allow separation of the cellular fraction from the plasma. Four-hour unprocessed stability has been demonstrated in samples collected into CTAD and stored at room temperature [17]. In general, CTAD tubes are recommended for the determination of markers of platelet activation such as ß-thromboglobulin or PF4. These tubes may also be useful when determining plasma levels of analytes that have significant platelet stores such as plasminogen activator inhibitor-1 (PAI-1). In this situation, CTAD prevents release of the analyte from the platelet store during collection and processing and allows more accurate measure of the plasma concentration.

Additionally, the use of sodium citrate with added protease inhibitor(s) such as D-phenylalanine–proline–arginine–chloromethylketone (PPACK) can protect the integrity of the plasma sample from protease activity prior to performing nonroutine coagulation assays [19]. The package insert associated with the special evacuated tube should be referenced to determine the assays for which these different anticoagulant tubes are recommended. If these special collection tubes are used for routine hemostasis assays, reference range must be determined based on samples collected in the same type of special collection tube in order to understand potential matrix effect.

Blood to anticoagulant ratio (fill volume) Sodium citrate is provided as a liquid anticoagulant and the recommended ratio of blood to sodium citrate anticoagulant in blood collection containers is 9:1. Anticoagulant effect of sodium citrate is attributed to its ability to bind calcium in the plasma, making the calcium unavailable to promote clot formation. Collection containers that are underfilled contain proportionally more sodium citrate per volume of plasma, which binds a greater amount of calcium, potentially leading to longer clotting times [20]. Dilutional effect of the plasma due to the liquid anticoagulant in underfilled tubes may also contribute to prolonged clotting times. The degree to which fill volume effects clotting time depends, in addition, on citrate concentration used, the size of the evacuated tube, assay to be measured, and the reagent used in testing. Samples drawn into 3.8% sodium citrate are more prone to prolongation of clotting time in underfilled tubes than those drawn into 3.2% sodium citrate. Underfilling the blue stopper tube causes greater prolongation of the aPTT than the PT. Small volume or "pediatric" tubes, such as those that draw in the range of 2 mL or less, may show statistically significant elevations in INR when sample tube fill volumes are less than 90% [21]. Unless local studies have been performed to demonstrate acceptability of reduced fill volumes, or package inserts state differently, blue stopper evacuated tubes that are less than 90% filled are considered unacceptable for testing. Overfilling of evacuated tubes may occur if the rubber stopper is removed and additional sample added. This should be avoided as it may lead to inadequate volume of anticoagulant and limited sample mixing potential with resultant *in vitro* clot formation.

Combining samples from different evacuated collection tubes into a sodium citrate tube is *prohibited*, even if contents of two underfilled sodium citrate tubes are combined. Adding specimen from one blue stopper tube to another alters the blood to anticoagulant ratio, potentially prolonging the clotting time. The addition of blood from a red stopper tube to an incompletely filled blue stopper tube may cause activation of the plasma sample and spuriously shorten the plasma clotting time. This could bring a prolonged result erroneously into the normal range.

Hematocrit Samples from patients with hematocrits greater than 55% may demonstrate spuriously prolonged PT and PTT results, particularly if the sample is drawn into 3.8% rather than 3.2% sodium citrate [22, 23]. Samples with elevated hematocrits mimic the effect of an underfilled tube because the volume of packed cells is increased and the volume of plasma reduced. Prolongation of clotting times is due to the dilutional effect of the liquid anticoagulant and the excess citrate concentration [23]. Samples with hematocrits above 55% should have the volume of sodium citrate adjusted (decreased) using the following formula:

$$C = (1.85 \times 10^{-3})(100 - \text{Hct})(V_{\text{Blood}})$$

Where C is the volume of citrate remaining in the tube; Hct is the hematocrit of the patient; V is the volume of blood to be added; and (1.85×10^{-3}) is a constant [7].

A simplified method to overcome citrate effect in most samples with elevated hematocrit is to remove 0.1 mL of sodium citrate from a 5-mL evacuated tube. Removing this constant volume of anticoagulant is generally sufficient, since most samples with an elevated hematocrit have values that fall between 0.55 (55%) and 0.65 (65%) [7]. It is not necessary to adjust the volume of sodium citrate concentration for anemic samples, as low hematocrit values do not affect aPTT and PT test results [24].

Tourniquet use
Tourniquets are often used during phlebotomy to assist in localization of the vein. Application should be tight enough such that venous, but not arterial flow, is obstructed. The tourniquet should be applied for the minimum period of time necessary to identify the vein and should be removed when the needle is safely in the vein [25]. In general, tourniquets should not remain in place for greater than 1 minute. Tourniquets are often incorrectly left in place not just to localize the vein, but until sample collection is complete. This may not only promote *in vitro* clot formation but also cause a spurious change in test results as venous stasis induced by the tourniquet causes local hemoconcentration [26]. This can cause clinically significant variations in a variety of assays such as the aPTT, PT, fibrinogen, D-dimer, and select factor activities. While an effect

Table 5.3 Effect of preanalytical variables on markers of thrombin generation

	Thrombin antithrombin complex (ng/mL)	Prothrombin fragment 1.2 (nmol/L)
Reference range	<5.1	0.4–0.8
Reference	1.75	0.59
Inadequate mix	4.18	0.7
Tourniquet 3 min	47.4	1.5

on assay parameters may be evident after as little as 1 minute of tourniquet use, application of a tourniquet for 3 minutes may cause significant variation in results. Comparing application of a tourniquet for 3 minutes versus 1 minute, Lippi et al. demonstrated a 3.1% shortening of the PT, a 10.1% increase in fibrinogen, 13.4% increase in D-dimer, 10.6% increase in FVII activity, and 10.2% increase in factor VIII activity [26].

Certain special coagulation assays, such as those that measure thrombin generation markers (e.g., thrombin antithrombin complex [TAT] and prothrombin fragment 1.2 [PF1.2]), should be drawn without the use of a tourniquet. Tourniquet application during sample procurement may lead to spurious elevation of these markers, particularly if the tourniquet is left in place for more than 1 minute. To demonstrate the potential of improper specimen collection handling, three blue stopper tubes were collected from a healthy volunteer and tested in the author's laboratory. Sample-designated "reference" was drawn according to proper technique, specifically with minimal use of a tourniquet and adequate mixing of the evacuated collection tube. The sample designated "inadequate mix" was collected without use of a tourniquet and was subjected to only one inversion of the evacuated tube post collection versus the recommended three to six inversions of the sample. The sample designated "tourniquet three minutes" was collected following the application of a tourniquet for 3 minutes and was adequately mixed by five end-over-end inversions of the evacuated tube. Results are shown in Table 5.3. Although an effect of improper sample handling can be seen in both assays, TAT results demonstrate exquisite susceptibility to preanalytical variables.

Order of draw and use of a discard tube

For many years it was standard practice to draw a discard tube or nonadditive tube before filling a coagulation tube, in order to minimize contamination by "tissue juice" (tissue thromboplastin) [27]. In the 1940s, Armand Quick, the originator of the PT assay, cited "tissue juice" as the most important external substance that could influence the coagulation reaction, suggesting that it was of "utmost importance to exclude all traces from the specimen to be tested" [28]. To avoid tissue thromboplastin contamination, a "two-syringe" technique was introduced and is still practiced in some laboratories. For the "two-syringe" technique, a needle and attached syringe containing no additive is used to draw (and discard) a small quantity of blood, (e.g., 2 to 5 mL). With the needle left in place, the first syringe is removed and a second syringe attached and additional sample drawn. Following collection of blood into the second syringe, the appropriate volume of anticoagulant is added and the sample is properly mixed. Coagulation testing is performed on blood collected into the second syringe. This technique was extrapolated to an evacuated tube system, giving rise to the use of a discard tube.

A number of published studies have refuted the need for a discard tube and have consistently demonstrated no significant difference in the aPTT and PT results between the first and second tubes drawn [29–31]. For routine coagulation testing, therefore, the use of a discard tube is no longer required. When using a winged collection set to draw either routine or specialized hemostasis assays, a discard tube is required (see below). It is currently recommended that specimens for routine coagulation testing be the first tube drawn if a series of tubes are being collected [32]. Discontinuation of the use of a discard tube for routine coagulation testing not only minimizes the amount of blood withdrawn from a patient but also reduces the amount of medical waste, without compromising quality of results.

There are a number of published studies that demonstrate that a discard tube for special coagulation studies is not needed. Raijmakers et al. have demonstrated that the use of a discard tube makes little, if any, clinically significant difference in the results of protein C, antithrombin, FII, FV, FVIII, FIX, and FX assays [33, 34].

If a discard tube is used *prior to* collecting blood for coagulation testing or if the blue stopper tube is collected with a series of tubes, the coagulation tube must be filled after a nonadditive tube. This recommendation is based on potential contamination of the sample for coagulation testing by additive adherent to the plunger of the evacuated tube holder if the coagulation tube is drawn following an additive tube [35]. A red stopper serum collection tube containing clot activator is considered an additive tube and should not be used as a discard tube for coagulation studies.

A discard tube is recommended if citrated plasma is obtained using a winged (butterfly needle) collection system [7]. The volume of blood that is drawn and discarded should equal at a minimum the amount of air that fills the tubing of the winged collection set. Failure to use a discard tube may lead to underfilling of the evacuated tube due to the volume of air in the tubing.

The general recommendations for order of draw when collecting a sample for routine coagulation testing are as follows:
• If multiple evacuated tubes will be collected, the coagulation tube should be the first tube drawn.
• If only one evacuated tube will be collected, the blue stopper tube can be the only tube drawn and a discard tube is not necessary.
• There are no data to support the need for a discard tube for specialty coagulation testing.
• If using an evacuated tube collection system, the tube for hemostasis testing should not be collected following collection of an additive tube.
• When using a winged collection system, a discard tube is recommended to account for the volume of air in the flexible tubing.

Collecting samples from a vascular access device
Blood for hemostasis testing should ideally be collected directly from a peripheral vein. It may be necessary, on occasion, to obtain blood from an existing vascular access device (VAD) such as an intravenous (IV) line, a central line, or saline lock. When drawing a sample from a VAD, the potential exists for heparin contamination and sample dilution due to contamination of the specimen with IV fluids. In order to collect samples for coagulation testing, it is recommended that the line is flushed be saline and that six dead space volumes of the VAD be discarded [7, 36]. If the sample is drawn from a capped IV port such as

a saline lock, two dead space volumes of the catheter extension set should be discarded [37].

Transportation of whole blood specimens to the laboratory

Following collection, samples should be transported to the laboratory at room temperature in a manner consistent with the institutional policy to prevent infectious exposure. The practice of transporting samples on ice for coagulation testing is no longer recommended. This is due to the potential for cold activation of the sample (see paragraph below) [4, 5]. In order to prevent sample deterioration, samples should preferably be transported to the laboratory and processed within 1 hour of collection. During transportation and storage, samples should remain capped both for safety reasons and to maintain proper pH of the sample. Transportation using a pneumatic tube system is generally acceptable for hemostasis testing, as long as the pneumatic system does not induce excessive vibration and shock that may denature proteins and activate platelets [38]. Samples for platelet function testing should not be transported in a pneumatic tube as this method of transportation may activate platelets. During sample transportation, extremes of temperature must be avoided in order to maintain sample integrity [39].

Refrigerated storage of whole blood—adverse effects
Cold storage of citrated whole blood prior to centrifugation, by placing samples either in an ice bath or in refrigerated (2–8°C) storage, may lead to platelet activation, activation of factor VII, and significant time-dependent loss of both factor VIII and VWF [40]. Bohm et al. demonstrated that whole blood samples stored on crushed ice resulted in significant loss of VWF antigen, VWF activity, and factor VIII activity after 3 hours storage with up to 50% loss from baseline at 6 hours. Refaii demonstrated that levels could be restored if the whole blood sample was rewarmed prior to centrifugation [41]. The effect of cold storage may be greater on VWF function than protein concentration. The VWF activity assay tends to decrease to a greater extent than the antigen assay in response to cold whole blood storage [5]. Improper storage of whole blood at cold temperatures may cause VWF and factor VIII values to fall into the abnormal range

and result in the misdiagnosis of hemophilia A or von Willebrand disease. As VWF activity tends to fall to a greater degree than VWF antigen, cold storage may simulate a type 2 pattern of von Willebrand disease.

Loss of VWF antigen and activity may be due to cold-induced activation of platelets or release of VWF-cleaving proteases or reductases that degrade VWF in the sample [40–42]. Details regarding preanalytic issues and VWF are discussed in Chapter 17.

Specimen Processing

To maintain the highest level of specimen integrity, all samples should be processed as quickly as possible—ideally within the first hour after collection. In order to maintain the highest integrity, samples should remain capped and at room temperature until centrifugation. Prior to processing, samples should be examined for the presence of a clot. This is often accomplished by observation with tilting of the tube or by inserting and removing two wooden applicator sticks. The identification of a clot demands specimen rejection.

Centrifugation

Plasma is generally prepared by centrifugation of the whole blood sample. Centrifugation should take place at room temperature in a centrifuge that has a rotor with swing out buckets to facilitate the separation of plasma from the cellular components [43]. It is generally recommended that the primary tube for coagulation testing be centrifuged at $1500 \times g$ for no less than 15 minutes [7]. A temperature-controlled centrifuge is not strictly required for processing routine coagulation assays because whole blood centrifugation at different temperatures does not introduce significant analytical or clinical bias [44].

The generation of platelet poor plasma (post centrifugation platelet count $<10 \times 10^9$/L) is especially important if the sample is subjected to certain assays such as lupus anticoagulant testing, antiphospholipid antibody testing, or monitoring of UFH therapy, or if the sample is frozen prior to analysis. Double centrifugation can be performed to ensure the plasma is platelet-poor. Following initial centrifugation, the plasma is transferred to a nonactivating plastic centrifuge tube using a plastic pipette, then centrifuged again for about 10 minutes. The plasma is aliquoted

to a secondary tube, taking care not to include the residual platelets that may have collected at the bottom of the centrifuge tube. It has been demonstrated that platelet counts of at least 199×10^9/L or greater do not compromise results of PT and aPTT assays, when the samples are tested fresh [45]. In general, centrifugation should occur at a determined G force to produce platelet-poor plasma such that the postcentrifugation plasma platelet count is less than or equal to 10×10^9/L. Using relative centrifugal forces (RCFs) greater than $1500 \times g$ is not recommended as this may induce platelet activation and lysis of red blood cells [46].

Lippi et al. have demonstrated that centrifugation of samples at $1500 \times g$ for either 5 or 10 minutes yields PT, aPTT, and fibrinogen results essentially identical to those samples centrifuged for 15 minutes. In this study, samples spun for 2 minutes or less resulted in an increased bias in aPTT in seconds with no significant bias in PT [44]. Marlar has reported that STAT centrifuges or those that spin at a greater speed over a shorter period of time are acceptable as long as the plasma is made platelet poor by the process [47].

Filtration of plasma to reduce platelet contamination

Micropore filters such as a 0.2-μm Millipore filter have been used to prepare platelet-poor plasma and therefore remove platelet phospholipid that may interfere with tests for antiphospholipid antibodies [48]. Filtered plasmas, however, may demonstrate falsely prolonged aPTT and PT results and plasma prepared in this manner should not be used for factor analysis and VWF testing. It has been shown that filtration of plasma through a micropore filter selectively removes a number of plasma factors including factors V, VIII, IX, XII, and VWF. Loss of factor VIII and VWF through a micropore filter is especially striking and may lead to an erroneous diagnosis of hemophilia A or von Willebrand disease [49].

Hemolyzed, lipemic, and icteric samples

Plasmas that are lipemic or icteric may show interference with light transmission when a coagulation analyzer with an optical end point determination is used unless the instrument uses a wavelength that does not show interference. Ultracentrifugation to clear lipemia is used in some centers; however, there have been no published studies that validate this procedure. The concern is that ultracentrifugation may result in spuriously low fibrinogen values. Mechanical and/or electromechanical methods for clot detection should be utilized when possible for plasma samples that are icteric, lipemic, or contain substances that interfere with light transmission. While hemolysis may interfere with light transmission, the greater concern is that lysis of the red cell membranes and release of red cell contents into plasma may lead to activation of the plasma sample altering coagulation parameters [50]. Lippi reported that hemolysis may lead to statistically significant increases in PT and D-dimer and significant decreases in aPTT and fibrinogen while others have reported that hemolysis has no significant effect on aPTT and PT [50, 51]. Until further studies are published, it is recommended that hemolyzed samples are not analyzed. Samples that appear hemolyzed due to the presence of a hemoglobin substitute are not a cause of specimen rejection and these samples should be evaluated using a mechanical or electromechanical method for clot detection.

Stability and storage of plasma samples

Once the whole blood sample is centrifuged, plasma can remain on the cells in a capped primary tube until testing or it can be aliquoted and stored in a secondary tube. When aliquoting the plasma, care must be taken to not disturb the buffy coat (layer of cells between the red cells and plasma) or introduce this cellular component back into the plasma. During storage, samples should remain capped.

Stability of plasma samples depends on which assay(s) will be performed as well as the temperature and conditions of storage. The following sample stabilities are provided as a guideline and generally represent a very conservative approach to specimen handling. Laboratories may choose to perform their own studies and validate sample stabilities that are different than those listed.

• Samples for platelet function testing should remain at room temperature and testing completed within 3 to 4 hours of collection.
• Samples for PT/INR evaluation are stable at room temperature for 24 hours [18]. Samples can be stored as whole blood or centrifuged.

• Samples for aPTT testing that *do not contain UFH* should be maintained at room temperature if testing will be completed within 4 hours [18]. Limited stability is due largely to time-dependent degeneration or loss of labile factors, particularly factor VIII and possibly factor V [52, 53]. Samples that cannot be tested within 4 hours should be centrifuged and the plasma aliquot frozen.
• Samples containing UFH must be processed within 1 hour of collection due to the release of PF4 from platelets *in vitro* and subsequent neutralization of heparin, resulting in a spuriously low heparin level as measured by an aPTT and/or anti-FXa assay. If the whole blood sample is centrifuged within 1 hour of collection, the plasma can be left on top of the cells in a capped primary tube at room temperature for up to 4 hours before testing [18].
• Stability of plasma samples for special coagulation assays (except FVIII, anti-FXa for UFH as described above) is largely unknown. It has been demonstrated that protein S activity is labile with statistically significant loss of activity demonstrated at 8 hours— while fibrinogen, protein C, and antithrombin activity remain relatively constant for up to 7 days [53]. Stability of the vitamin K-dependent factors has been reported to be 24 hours at room temperature [54]. This is consistent with other studies that report 24-hour stability of PT/INR determination.

If samples for coagulation testing are stored frozen, they should not be maintained in freezer that has automatic defrost cycles. The use of frost-free freezers for patient samples is acceptable provided that freezers are monitored by a continuous-monitoring temperature-recording device, or a minimum–maximum thermometer, enabling the laboratory to show that the acceptable temperature range is never exceeded. For long-term storage of plasma samples, samples should remain at −20°C for no more than 2 weeks. Storage for longer periods of time can be accomplished by maintaining samples at −70°C or colder. Stability of many common plasma coagulation factors at ultracold (<−70°C) temperatures has been published by Woodhams et al. [55].

Controlled thawing of frozen plasma samples

Prior to testing, previously frozen plasma samples should be thawed in a 37°C water bath for approximately 5 minutes or until completely thawed. Samples should be monitored closely to avoid inadequate or excessive incubation in the heated water bath. Plasma samples that are inadequately thawed may have spuriously low factor VIII, VWF, and fibrinogen levels due to the presence of cryoprecipitate. Likewise, plasma that is subjected to prolonged heating or excessive temperature during thawing may be compromised. In our laboratory we demonstrated that VWF antigen levels may decrease by 50% and activity levels by 80% when samples are subjected to excessive temperatures (e.g., 60°C for 10 minutes). Once thawed, samples must be thoroughly mixed prior to testing.

Conclusion

Attention to the preanalytical phase of hemostasis testing is crucial in order to provide the highest quality of laboratory results. Deviations from published guidelines may significantly impact sample integrity leading to the potential for patient misdiagnosis and mismanagement. Unless local validation is performed, guidelines for proper sample collection, handling, and transport should be made widely available and strictly followed.

Common sources of error

- Anticoagulant other than sodium citrate
- Incomplete filling of evacuated tube
- Inadequate mixing of evacuated tube
- Storage of the whole blood sample on ice or in a refrigerated setting

The ideal sample for hemostasis testing

- Atraumatic phlebotomy with minimal tourniquet use
- Draw 3.2% blue stopper tube first or only after a nonadditive tube
- Fill tube adequately (no less than 90% fill)
- Adequately and thoroughly mix with anticoagulant
- Transport promptly at room temperature
- Centrifuge within 1 hour of phlebotomy to obtain platelet poor plasma
- Test plasma or aliquot into a nonactivating secondary tube immediately following centrifugation

Causes for specimen rejection

- Specimen collected into tube containing other than sodium citrate anticoagulant
- Samples that contain a clot
- Samples with other than a 9:1 blood to anticoagulant ratio
  - Samples less than 90% filled
  - Samples that are overfilled
  - Samples with hematocrit >55%
- Samples that are hemolyzed

References

1. Lippi G, Mattiuzzi C, Guidi GC. Laboratory quality improvement by implementation of phlebotomy guidelines. Letter to the Editor. *Med Lab Observer*. 2006;6–7.
2. Lippi G, Salvagno G, Montagnana M, Franchini M, Guidi GC. Phlebotomy issues and quality improvement in results of laboratory testing. *Clin Lab*. 2006;52:217–30.
3. Kalra J. Medical errors: impact on clinical laboratories and other critical areas. *Clin Biochem*. 2004;37:1052–1062.
4. Morrissey JH, Macik BG, Neuenschwander PF, Comp PC. Quantitation of activated factor VII levels in plasma using tissue factor mutant selectively deficient in promoting factor VII activation. *Blood*. 1993;81:734–744.
5. Favaloro EJ, Soltani S, McDonald J. Potential laboratory misdiagnosis of hemophilia and von Willebrand disorder owing to cold activation of blood samples for testing. *Am J Clin Pathol*. 2004;122:686–692.
6. Ernst DJ, Ernst C. Phlebotomy tools of the trade: Part 4. Proper handling and storage of blood samples. *Home Healthcare Nurse*. 2003;21:266–270.
7. Clinical and Laboratory Standards Institute. *H21-A5, Collection, transport and processing of blood specimens for testing plasma-based coagulation assays and molecular hemostasis assays*; Approved Guidelines–5th Edition. CLSI, 2008.
8. Ernst DJ, Ernst C. Phlebotomy tools of the trade. *Home Healthcare Nurse*. 2002;20:151–153.
9. Sharp Mk, Mohammad SF. Scaling of hemolysis in needles and catheters. *Ann Biomed Engin*. 1998;26:788–797.
10. Jaques LB, Fidlar E, Felsted ET, Macdonald AG. Silicones and blood coagulation. *Canad M A J*. 1946;56:26–31.
11. Fiebig EW, Etzell JE, Ng VL. Clinically relevant differences in prothrombin and INR values related to blood sample collection in plastic vs glass tubes. *Am J Clin Pathol*. 2005;124:902–909.

12. Tripodi A, Chantarangkul V, Bressi C, Manucci PM. How to evaluate the influence of blood collection systems on the international sensitivity index. Protocol applied to two new evacuated tubes and eight coagulometer/thromboplastin combinations. *Thromb Res.* 2002;108:85–89.

13. Kratz A, Stanganelli N, van Cott EM. A comparison of glass and plastic blood collection tubes for routine and specialized assays: a comprehensive study. *Arch Pathol Lab Med.* 2006;130:39–44.

14. WHO Expert Committee on Biological Standardization. Guidelines for thromboplastins and plasma used to control oral anticoagulant therapy. WHO Technical Report series. No 880, Geneva: World Health Organization; 1999.

15. Adcock DM, Kressin DC, Marlar RA. Effect of 3.2% vs 3.8% sodium citrate concentration on routine coagulation testing. *Am J Clin Pathol.* 1997;107:105–110.

16. Favaloro EJ, Bonar R, Duncan E, Earl G, Low J, Aboud M, et al. Identification of factor inhibitors by diagnostic hemostasis laboratories. A large multi-centre evaluation. *Thromb Haemost.* 2006;96:73–78.

17. van den Besselaar AMHP, Meeuwisse-Braun J, Jansen-Gruter R, Bertina RM. Monitoring heparin by the activated partial thromboplastin time—the effect of preanalytical conditions. *Thromb Haemost.* 1987;57:226–231.

18. Adcock DA, Kressin DC, Marlar RA. The effect of time and temperature variables on routine coagulation tests. *Blood Coagul Fibrinolysis.* 1998;9:463–470.

19. Rahr HB, Sorenson JV, Danielsen D. Markers of coagulation and fibrinolysis in blood drawn into citrate with and without D-Phe-Pro-Arg-chloromethylketone (PPACK). *Thromb Res.* 1994;73:279–284.

20. Adcock DM, Kressin DC, Marlar RA. Minimum specimen volume requirements for routine coagulation testing. Dependence on citrate concentration. *Am J Clin Pathol.* 1998;109:595–599.

21. Chuang J, Sadler MA, Witt DM. Impact of evacuated collection tube fill volume and mixing on routine coagulation testing using 2.5 mL (pediatric) tubes. *Chest.* 2004;126:1262–1266.

22. Koepke JA, Rodgers JL, Ollivier MJ. Pre-instrument variables in coagulation testing. *Am J Clin Pathol.* 1975;64:591–596.

23. Marlar RA, Potts RM, Marlar AA. Effect on routine and special coagulation testing values of citrate anticoagulant adjustment in patients with high hematocrit values. *Am J Clin Pathol.* 2006;126:400–405.

24. Siegel JE, Swami VK, Glenn P, et al. Effect (or lack of it) of severe anemia on PT and aPTT Results. *Am J Clin Pathol.* 1998;110:106–110.

25. Kiechle FL, Adcock DM, Calam RR, Davis C, Schwartz JG. *So you're Going to Collect a Blood Specimen. An Introduction to Phlebotomy.* 12th ed. Northfield, IL: College of American Pathologists; 2007.

26. Lippi G, Savagno GL, Montagnana M, Guidi GC. Short-term stasis influences routine coagulation testing. *Blood Coagul Fibrinolysis.* 2005;16:453–458.

27. McPhedran P, Clyne LP, Ortoli NA, Gagnon PG, Sanders FJ. *Am J Clin Pathol.* 1974;62:16–20.

28. Quick AJ, Honorato R, Stafanini M. The value and limitations of the coagulation time in the study of hemorrhagic diseases. *Blood.* 1948;3:1120–1129.

29. Brigden ML, Graydon C, Mcleod B, Lesperance M. Prothrombin time determination. The lack of need for a discard tube and 24-hour stability. *Am J Clin Pathol.* 1997;108:422–426.

30. Yawn BP, Loge C, Dale J. Prothrombin time one tube or two. *Am J Clin Pathol.* 1996;105:794–797.

31. Adcock DM, Kressin DC, Marlar RA. Are discard tubes necessary in coagulation studies? *Lab Med.* 1997;28:530–533.

32. CLSI *H3-A5, Procedures for the collection of diagnostic blood specimens by venipuncture: Approved Standard.* 5th ed. Wayne, PA: Clinical and Laboratory Standards Institute; 2003.

33. Raijmakers MTM, Menting CHF, Vader HL, et al. Collection of blood specimens by venipuncture for plasma-based coagulation assays: necessity of a discard tube. *Am J Clin Pathol.* 2010;133:331–335.

34. Smock KJ, Crist RA, Hansen SJ, et al. Discard tubes are not necessary when drawing samples for specialized coagulation testing. *Blood Coagul Fibrinolysis.* 210(21):279–282.

35. Calam RR, Cooper MH. Recommended "order of draw" for collecting blood specimens into additive-containing tubes. *Clin Chem.* 1982;28:1399.

36. Laxson CJ, Titler MG. Drawing coagulation studies from arterial lines: an integrative literature review. *Am J Critical Care.* 1994;1:16–24.

37. Powers JM. Obtaining blood samples for coagulation studies from a normal saline lock. *Am J Critical Care.* 1999;8:250–253.

38. Dyszkiewicz-Korpanty A, Quinton R, Jassine J, Sarode R. The effect of pneumatic tube transport on PFA-100™ closure time and whole blood aggregation. *J Thromb Haemost.* 2004;2:354–356.

39. van Geest-Daalderop JH, Mulder AB, Boonman-deWinter LJ, Hoekstra MM, van den Besselaar AM. Preanalytical variables and off-site blood collection: influences on the results of the prothrombin time/international normalized ratio test and implications for monitoring oral anticoagulant therapy. *Clin Chem.* 2005;51:561–568.

55

40. Bohm M, Teaschner S, Kretzschmar E, Gerlach R, Favaloro EJ, Scharrer I. Cold storage of citrated whole blood induces drastic time-dependent losses of factor VIII and von Willebrand factor: potential for misdiagnosis of haemophilia and von Willebrand disease. *Blood Coagul Fibrinolysis*. 2006;17:39–45.

41. Refaii MA, van Cott EM, Lukoszyk M, Hughes J, Eby CS. Loss of factor VIII and von Willebrand activities during cold storage of whole blood is reversed by rewarming. *Lab Hematol*. 2006;12:99–102.

42. Favaloro E, Nair SC, Forsyth CJ. Collection and transport of samples for laboratory testing in von Willbrand's disease (VWD): time for a reappraisal? *Thromb Haem*. 2001;86:1589–1590.

43. Lippi G, Salvagno GL, Montagnana M, Monzato F, Guidi GC. Influence of the centrifuge time of primary plasma tubes on routine coagulation testing. *Blood Coagul Fibrinolysis*. 2007;18:525–528.

44. Lippi G, Franchini M, Montagnana M, Salvagno GL, Poli G, Guidi GC. Quality and reliability of routine coagulation testing: can we trust the sample? *Blood Coagul Fibrinolysis*. 2006;17:513–519.

45. Carroll WE, Wolitzer AO, Harris L, Ling MC, Whitaker ML, Jackson RD. The significance of platelet counts in coagulation studies. *J Med*. 2001;32:83–96.

46. Aursnes I, Vikholm V. On possible interaction between ADP and mechanical stimulation in platelet activation. *Thromb Haemost*. 1984;51:54–56.

47. Nelson S, Pratt A, Marlar RA. Rapid preparation of plasma for "stat" coagulation testing. *Arch Pathol Lab Med*. 1994;118:175–176.

48. Sheppard CA, Channell C, Ritchie JC, Duncan A. Preanalytical variables in coagulation testing. Letter to the editor. *Blood Coagul Fibrinolysis*. 2006;17:425–428.

49. Favaloro EJ. Preanalytical variables in coagulation testing. Letter to the editor. *Blood Coagul Fibrinolysis*. 2007;18:86–89.

50. Lippi G, Montagnana M, Salvagno L, Guidi GS. Interference of blood cell lysis in routine coagulation testing. *Arch Pathol Lab Med*. 2006;130:181–184.

51. Laga AC, Cheves TA, Sweeney JD. The effect of specimen hemolysis on coagulation test results. *Am J Clin Pathol*. 2006;126:748–755.

52. O'Neill EM, Rowley J, Hanson-Wicher H, McCarter S, Ragno G, Valeri CR. Effect of 24-hour whole-blood storage on plasma clotting factors. *Transfusion*. 1999;39:488–491.

53. Heil W, Grunewals R, Amnd M, Heins M. Influence of time and temperature on coagulation analysis in stored plasma. *Clin Chem Lab Med*. 1998;36:459–452.

54. Awad MA, Selim TE, Al-Sabbagh FA. Influence of storage time and temperature on international normalized ratio (INR) levels and plasma activities of vitamin K dependent clotting factors. *Hematology*. 2004;9:333–337.

55. Woodhams B, Giradot O, Blanco M, Collesse G, Gourmelin Y. Stability of coagulation proteins in frozen plasma. *Blood Coagul Fibrinolysis*. 2001;12:229–236.

6

Internal quality control in the hemostasis laboratory

Steve Kitchen[1,2,3], F. Eric Preston[3,4], & John D. Olson[5,6]

[1]Sheffield Hemophilia and Thrombosis Centre, Royal Hallamshire Hospital, Sheffield, UK
[2]UK National External Quality Assessment Scheme (NEQAS) for Blood Coagulation
[3]WHO and WFH International External Quality Assessment Programs for Blood Coagulation, Sheffield, UK
[4]University of Sheffield, Sheffield, UK
[5]Department of Pathology, University of Texas Health Science Center
[6]University Health System, San Antonio, TX, USA

Introduction

Many tests performed in coagulation laboratories are vital for the accurate diagnosis and safe management of patients with familial and acquired bleeding and thrombotic disorders. There are many examples where an inaccurate result could have very serious consequences for patients. Safe use of dangerous drugs such as the anticoagulants used in the treatment of approximately 1% of the population in the developed Western world is only possible with well-controlled laboratory methods.

There are many other instances where treatment is highly dependent on the results of coagulation rests. In relation to diagnosis it is particularly important that results are accurate and reliable when investigations are undertaken to determine possible familial disorders of hemostasis. A laboratory error may lead to misdiagnosis, and whether an error leads to a subject being misdiagnosed as having, or not having, a familial defect, there could be serious clinical consequences.

The scope and volume of testing in coagulation laboratories has continued to increase over recent years. Workload increases and major expansion in the regulatory requirements in terms of documentation have not always been fully matched by increases in staffing. Furthermore, automated analyzers in hemostasis laboratories are increasingly complex requiring a higher level of understanding and vigilance than might not have previously been the case. Taking all these factors together the potential for laboratory error in hemostasis laboratories has increased substantially. The purpose of quality control is to provide the documentary evidence that test results are correct and safe to be released to clinicians for patient management.

The following text deals with all aspects of internal quality control (IQC) in relation to laboratory tests of hemostasis for the benefit of patient care. This is only one component of quality management (see Chapter 1). Issues related to quality control of near-patient testing or point-of-care tests of hemostasis are dealt with elsewhere in this publication (Chapter 8).

IQC materials

Materials used for IQC should be similar in properties to test samples. Wherever possible quality control materials of human origin should closely resemble human test samples. Preparation of all vials or aliquots of the control material should be identical so that any variation in test results is not a consequence of vial to vial variation. The IQC material should also be stable for its intended period of use. In respect of hemostatic tests and assays, IQC materials are stable over a restricted time period, often dependent on the storage conditions. For IQC materials it is advantageous for the same batch or lot number of material to be used over a period of months. This limits the frequency with which the batch number is changed and facilitates detection of drift in the assay system under assessment (see later in this text). Stability of plasma for many coagulation test measurements is restricted to several hours, although for some tests plasma is stable for 24 hours or more. In order to extend this stability, IQC materials should be deep frozen (preferably at −35°C or lower) or lyophilized in order to ensure adequate stability over time. If deep-frozen QC material is used, it should be thawed rapidly at 37°C for 5 minutes and the vial inverted several times to ensure full dissolution of any precipitated protein such as fibrinogen or von Willebrand factor (with associated FVIII:C). Frozen IQC material has the advantage that reconstitution is not required and therefore precludes the necessity of adding distilled water, a potential source of pipetting error. Use of contaminated or impure distilled water for reconstitution can also adversely affect the results of coagulation tests, and again this is avoided if frozen material is employed. The use of deep-frozen material can result in some longer-term instability leading to prolongation of screening tests and/or loss of activity. This can be avoided by rapid freezing of the IQC material during preparation and use of lower storage temperatures.

Domestic grade −20°C freezers are inadequate for storage of frozen plasma for coagulation tests, particularly where auto-defrosting cycles lead to temperatures fluctuating above −20°C where partial defrosting of stored material can occur. Such plasma samples are especially susceptible to cryoprecipitation and cold activation.

Poorly handled frozen material may suffer from gain of function through cold activation of FVII and FXII/FXI that, in addition to affecting assays of these two procoagulants, also causes shortening of activated partial thromboplastin times (aPTT) or prothrombin times (PT). Artifactual loss of some clotting proteins can occur in partially thawed samples leading to misdiagnosis. We recently noted apparent deficiency of antithrombin (AT) in several samples that had been referred from another center, where storage in a domestic grade −20°C freezer was associated with partial thaw and loss of activity. Despite these potential disadvantages, the use of deep-frozen material remains an attractive option. In this regard Woodhams et al. [1] have demonstrated that many tests of hemostasis, including PT, aPTT, thrombin time (TT), fibrinogen, factors II, V, VII, VIII, IX, XI, XII, D-dimer, protein C (PC), protein S (PS), AT activity are stable for up to 3 months in plasma frozen at −24°C and for at least 18 months at −74°C where stability was defined as <10% change from the baseline result immediately after freezing. Intermediate storage temperatures of around −35°C to −40°C as used in many centers are suitable for storage of frozen IQC plasma for at least 3 months. It should not be assumed that these findings are applicable to all test systems. Results may be reagent dependent, particularly for screening tests. The authors have seen minor shortening or minor lengthening of screening tests (PT and aPTT) with different measurement systems.

The majority of manufacturers of commercial IQC material prefer lyophilization as a means to extend the stability of plasma, mainly because such plasmas are normally stable for several weeks at ambient temperatures (at least in temperate climates) and this allows material to be transported inexpensively between sites without special measures. Lyophilized IQC plasma material normally requires buffering to ensure that the reconstituted plasma will be stable. Manufacturers of commercial materials may not state the nature of buffering used but will normally give an indication of the period of time over which the IQC will be stable. Lyophilization increases the pH of plasma as a consequence of loss of dissolved gasses. Buffering of plasma prior to lyophilization reduces this effect but does not abolish it completely. Unbuffered lyophilized plasma normally suffers more from postreconstitution instability with a gradual increase in pH. This may be accompanied by altered results in coagulation tests. This is particularly apparent for screening tests such as aPTT and changes in results may be less marked in tests where the reagents are well-buffered, such as coagulation factor assays. If buffering is inadequate the aPTT may prolong by 10–20% within 1 hour of reconstitution, depending on the reagent. For reconstitution of lyophilized samples it is important to use distilled water with pH 6.8–7.2 and to allow at least 10 minutes for reconstitution. If commercial QC material is used this should be reconstituted according to manufacturers' instructions using an accurate pipetting system.

It is extremely useful to test at least two QC samples with different levels of abnormality as recommended in some relevant guidelines [2, 3]. The most suitable levels will depend on the nature of the test sample population. For screening tests, centers should analyze QC samples with normal levels and at least one further level where the result is outside the reference range. This means that within limits QC results can confirm that the method is under control for both normal and abnormal sample analysis. If control of oral anticoagulant (OAC; e.g., coumarin) therapy is an important component of the workload then the second level of IQC for the PT/INR test system could have an INR in the midtherapeutic range. If a center is involved in the diagnosis of bleeding disorders then an IQC with a level of FVIII:C, FIX, and von Willebrand factor (VWF) in the range 30–50 IU/dL is particularly appropriate since this is a critical area for establishing a diagnosis or for monitoring response to therapy. For thrombophilia work IQC samples with results around the interface between normal and abnormal are useful since once again this is a critical area where good evidence that the method is under control is helpful.

In the selection of QC material the risk of transmission of blood-borne viruses should be considered and high-risk material should not be used.

Frequency of IQC testing

There are number of issues to take into account when considering the frequency of IQC testing including the number of patient samples being analyzed and the way in which these samples are processed. For tests that are performed in discrete batches at least one level of QC material should be included with each batch. Where there is continuous processing, for example, when using many types of modern auto analyzers, then a QC sample should be included at regular intervals. There is some evidence that a combination of IQC testing at fixed time intervals with further IQC testing performed randomly at additional times may be better for detection of error conditions [4].

When large numbers of samples are processed then QC testing can be fixed at timed intervals or after a certain number of test samples have been analyzed. Such decisions should also take account of the consequences of releasing incorrect results. The frequency should be set so that recall of erroneous patient results is avoided. For screening tests such as PT/INR or aPTT in departments processing more than 100 samples per day testing every 2 hours does not represent too large a financial burden in relation to the cost, and is easily achieved.

There are published recommendations in relation to the frequency of testing IQC material for some coagulation tests. The Clinical Laboratory Standards Institute (CLSI, formerly NCCLS) have recently updated their guideline document dealing with PT and aPTT [2]. This recommends testing at least two levels of control material every 8 hours for all nonmanual PT and aPTT coagulation test systems, but recognizes that if the volume of testing is high, more frequent QC testing should be performed. This document also recommends that when continuous sample processing occurs, as in many large laboratories in established centers, then at least one from the two or three levels of IQC should be alternately tested at least every 4 hours. In our experience the frequency should be increased to every 2 hours during periods of testing when more than 20 samples per hour are being analyzed. This CLSI document also reminds us that the first test performed after reagent addition or important instrument change should be the QC sample. This is of particular importance after daily instrument maintenance. Some analyzers now allow several different positions to be occupied by the same reagent. The instrument is then programmed to automatically switch to a new vial of reagent when the first has been consumed. When this occurs it is important that an IQC sample is tested from each reagent reservoir before patient samples are analyzed. Only after an IQC result within the target range has been obtained is it safe to proceed with patient testing.

In relation to fibrinogen testing the inclusion of at least one abnormal control with a decreased fibrinogen level of 0.8–1.2 g/L with each batch of samples has been recommended [5] although in practice any abnormal control with a level between 0.3 and 1.4 g/L is probably suitable. The same authors recommend testing normal and abnormal samples at a minimum of every 20 samples in laboratories where many fibrinogen determinations are performed. For current autoanalyzers a single normal IQC every 20 samples is acceptable for routine purposes. The inclusion of an abnormal control at least daily gives additional confidence that the method is under control for measurement at a level where inaccurate results are of particular importance for patient management. When performing coagulation factor assays there is a recommendation to include both an abnormal and normal IQC with each batch of tests [6]. A UK guideline [3] also recommends that at least two QC samples (with different levels) be used. In contrast, the UK Haemophilia Centre Doctors Organization (HCDO)

[7] and the World Federation of Hemophilia (WFH) recommend a single level of IQC in some settings [8].

The extra information provided by testing two levels of IQC has to be balanced against the additional costs incurred. When tests are performed in batches of less than ten then a single level of IQC is reasonable. This can be increased to two for larger test batches.

Acceptable limits for IQC

All analytic techniques are subject to variability. It is not possible to totally eliminate this but it is important to minimize variability by good laboratory practice. There are essentially two sources of variation in coagulation test analyses—random and systematic. Random error is described by the precision of the test. Systemic variation is a reflection of the accuracy of the test.

Since all tests suffer to a greater or lesser degree from variability, some authors prefer to use the term imprecision rather than precision. These describe the same effects in opposite ways, so low variability can be described either as high precision or as low imprecision. Precision can be defined as the closeness of agreement between independent results of measurements obtained under a particular set of conditions. For practical purposes this is measured by a number of replicate measurements on the sample. The degree of precision will normally depend on the analytical conditions. The precision of replicate measurements by one operator using a single set of reagents in a short time period of time (within run error) will normally be lower than a set of measurements made by different operators on different days using fresh reagent sets on each occasion (between run error). This means that setting acceptable limits for analysis of an IQC material must take account of day-to-day variability. The most commonly used measure of precision is the coefficient of variation (CV% = SD/mean × 100). Thus a high CV indicates poor reproducibility.

In the case of screening tests and occasionally assays, the results obtained will be dependent on the reagents and end-point detection system used to perform the tests. The target range must take account of these effects. For commercial IQC samples manufacturers often provide a target range of acceptable values; however, this should only be used as guide and the target range for any coagulation test should be established locally. The IQC material should be tested repeatedly (minimum 20 times) with testing spread over at least ten sessions. When collecting these data it is useful to have evidence that the method is under control and so any available IQC that has been used previously should be included and only if results on this previous material are within limits can the results on the material under evaluation be used. This may not always be possible, for example, when establishing a method for a new analyte. In this case any outliers amongst the data should be excluded from the calculation of target values. Identification of outliers can be done by statistical methods but visual inspection of the data may well be sufficient.

It is not recommended to use the observed range of results obtained to define the limits of the target range. Once the raw data are collected some form of data analysis is used to set the limits of the acceptable range. The mean and standard deviation (SD) of the results are calculated. The SD is a measure of the spread of results; the larger the SD, the greater is the spread of results. Random variation follows a Gaussian distribution, that is, the classical bell-shaped normal distribution. In this case the mean ±2SD encompasses 95.5% of the values. This is the most commonly used range so that intervention occurs if an IQC result is more than 2SD above or below the mean. The mean ±3SD encompasses 99.7% of the values and could be considered as overtolerant in respect of the target range that has to be exceeded before suspension of patient sample testing and subsequent method investigation. The acceptable limits of variation for an IQC material are therefore statistically based and reflect the causes of error. These limits reflect how reproducible the process is and do not describe the accuracy of the test, accuracy being how close the measured test result is to the true value.

Storage and processing of IQC results

The most convenient way to record and visualize IQC results is by using a chart. The most widely used system is the Levey–Jennings chart. First reported more than 50 years ago [9], its continued and widespread use in an essentially unchanged format is good evidence of its ease of use and fitness for purpose. A more recent perspective on this has been published [10] that reminds the reader that Levey and Jennings

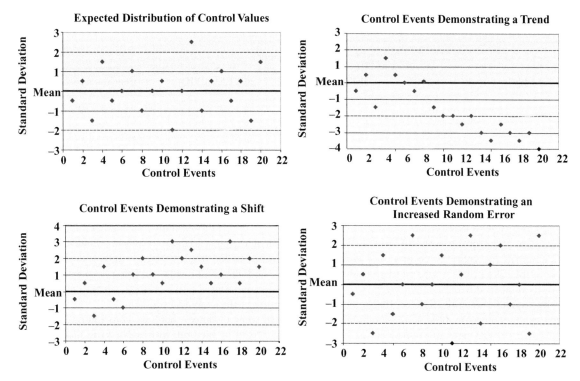

Figure 6.1 Examples of Levey–Jennings charts recording control values. This shows the expected distribution and examples where problems have occurred indicating that a method is moving out of control. In each case the dotted lines show the 2SD limits of acceptable results.

in their original publication comment that review of IQC results helps in the development of an appreciation of quality issues. This in turn helps improve patient care through increased pride amongst laboratory workers as a consequence of good IQC data and records.

Although originally designed for several biochemistry tests Levey–Jennings charts are suitable for a wide range of analytes including coagulation tests. Control charts are useful to judge what has happened to an analytical process in the past, and are useful for ongoing evaluation of the process over time. Ongoing evaluation can be used to help document the improvement over time as a consequence of any interventions, actions or efforts to reduce the causes of variation. The Levey–Jennings chart is constructed to show the mean value of initial testing performed to define the acceptable limits. The chart should also have lines showing the upper and lower limits of acceptable results—these being 2SD above and 2SD below the

mean. An example is shown in Figure 6.1 that illustrates the expected distribution of control values as well as examples where problems are occurring (see also out of limits section below).

There are a number of changes that can be made to a test system with the potential to alter the bias between a measured IQC result and the target or true value. These include a change in the calibration of the method, a change in lot number of reagents or consumables, or even a change in operator where there is potential for different operators to perform tasks differently. Many of these would be apparent as systematic shifts in the means of IQC results placed on a typical chart.

Out of limits IQC results

As soon as an out of limits IQC result is obtained all patient testing must be suspended pending identification and correction of the problem. When

Table 6.1 Troubleshooting IQC problems: how different patterns of IQC error for two levels of IQC material tested for PT and aPTT can direct the sequence of investigations required to correct the problem

IQC troubleshooting				
PT level 1 IQC	PT level 2 IQC	aPTT level 1 IQC	aPTT level 2 IQC	Conclusion/check
Out	In	In	In	PT level 1 IQC material
Out	Out	In	In	PT reagent
In	In	Out	In	aPTT level 1 IQC material
In	In	Out	Out	aPTT reagent
Out	Out	Out	Out	Instrument

an individual IQC test result falls outside limits then either there is a problem with the individual vial of IQC material, the entire batch of IQC has deteriorated, or there is a problem with the analytical system. It is important to differentiate among these possibilities by sequential investigations so that appropriate action can be taken. Analysis of a second vial of the same batch of IQC with the same reagents/method should be the first action. If this is within limits then it is highly likely that the test system is under control but the IQC sample analyzed earlier had deteriorated or been contaminated and should be discarded. This should be confirmed by performing a third IQC test. If this is within limits then patient testing can be safely resumed.

If on the other hand a second out of limits result is obtained on the replacement IQC vial of the same batch then the most likely explanation is that the test system is out of control. In this case analysis of a second lot or batch of IQC material would also give out of limits results.

If further vials of the first batch give out of limits results but the second batch of material gives within limits results, then the entire batch of the first IQC material may have deteriorated. This is normally a rare occurrence. Thus having more than one level of IQC available can be very useful when investigating the cause of out of limits IQC results.

The most common cause of an out of control test system in hemostasis laboratories is reagent deterioration or contamination. As mentioned above, all IQC results will be out of limits and in this case reagents should be discarded. Patient testing should only be safely resumed after the problem has been identified and rectified.

In many centers PT and aPTT methods are in operation on the same analyzer at the same time. In this case scrutiny of the whole pattern of IQC results for both methods may be informative. Table 6.1 illustrates how different patterns of IQC results can help identify the nature of the analytical problem.

In some instances there are compelling reasons to investigate a method with subsequent intervention even though recent IQC results are within the target range. For an IQC sample with appropriate target limits, analyzed with a well-controlled method, the results obtained should fluctuate around the mean (Figure 6.1). However, a series of seven to ten results on the same material showing a progressive trend in one direction, that is, gradually increasing or decreasing over time (Figure 6.1) may be an indication of drift in the analytical process. A gradual deterioration of a particular reagent over time or gradual change in an analyzer could be associated with such a pattern of IQC results. On other occasions there may be a series of individual IQC results all within limits but consistently lying above or consistently below the mean (Figure 6.1). This may indicate that there has been a change in the method since the target range was established. In this case a new target range should be established and investigation of recent changes in the method as well as an assessment of the accuracy of the test is merited (e.g., through external quality assessment or analysis of reference samples/materials). Where a batch or lot number of IQC is used for more than 3–4 months a recalculation of mean and SD is useful to confirm that the original range remains appropriate.

When the cause of out of limits IQC results has been identified it is necessary to assess which patient results need to be repeated. If the problem relates to the deterioration of IQC material no retesting is required. If the problem relates to reagents then all patient results obtained since the last within limits IQC result should be reviewed. One practical approach is to retest every tenth sample in reverse order to establish at which point the problem might have developed. Any patient samples from that point onward require retesting.

The comments above involve use of a single rule for intervention—if a single result exceeds a particular threshold then intervention follows. There are more complex procedures for assessing a series of IQC results based on multiple rules. These have come into use because IQC results may fall outside a target range by chance alone, without any problem being present in the analytical system. This is statistically inevitable from time to time and represents a false alarm. This is a limitation of using a single rule when assessing IQC results. The so-called Westgard rules [11] are an example that uses a combination of decision criteria from five different control rules. These have the advantage of fewer false rejections whilst maintaining a high rate of error detection. These were originally described for use with clinical chemistry testing with two to four control measurements per run. Some centers make use of multiple rules in coagulation testing but these have not been widely adopted in hemostasis laboratories.

Accreditation and regulatory bodies

The program of IQC employed within the laboratory should comply with any local legislation, regulations, guidelines, or standards issued by relevant bodies. In many countries there are local standards that are often constructed to be compatible with ISO 15189 (2003) Medical Laboratories—Particular requirements for quality and competence or ISO 17025: 2005; General requirements for the competence of testing and calibration laboratories. In the United Kingdom, for example, the accreditation process is undertaken by Clinical Pathology Accreditation ((CPA), www.cpa-uk.co.uk) who require written procedures to include records of the date, source and storage of IQC materials; the process used to validate IQC material prior to use; details of the statistical procedures employed; acceptance criteria for results obtained on IQC material in use. This body also requires that all IQC results

shall be recorded, regularly evaluated, and subsequent corrective and/or preventative actions taken recorded, and requires that laboratories shall determine the uncertainty of results, where relevant and possible. The CPA standards indicate that a laboratory shall have a program of calibration of measuring systems. This is of great importance in relation to pipette volumes and thermometer temperatures, where inaccuracies can have important implications for test results. We strongly recommend use of such an error log that can be extremely useful for informing the troubleshooting process. The above CPA standards further require that the period of retention for records should be defined. These recommendations and requirements should be followed in addition to any other local recommendations from relevant accreditation or professional bodies, or legislation.

Conclusion

Any out of limits IQC result should lead to an immediate investigation together with suspension of patient testing pending resolution of the problem. This whole process helps to establish well-controlled methods. Recognition of the causes of problems facilitates the process of minimizing errors in the future. All of this serves to improve the overall quality of the service but IQC testing and regular scrutiny of results obtained should be merely one component of the quality assurance and quality management program. Quality control is a continuous process and is the responsibility of all staff at all levels in the hemostasis laboratory. The wider issues around quality management are dealt with in Chapter 1 of this text.

References

1. Woodhams B, Girardot O, Blanco BJ, et al. Stability of coagulation proteins in frozen plasma. *Blood Coag Fibrinolysis.* 2001;12:229–236.
2. CLSI Document H47—A2. Marler KA, Cook J, Johnston M, et al. One stage prothrombin time and activated partial thromboplastin time test: approved guideline—second edition. 2007.
3. Mackie I, Cooer PC, Lawrie A, Kitchen S, Gray E, Laffan M, British Committee for Standards in Haematology. Guidelines on the laboratory aspects of assays used in haemostasis and thrombosis. *Int J Lab Hematol.* 2012. doi: 10.1111/ijlh.12004. [Epub ahead of print]

4. Parvin CA, Robbins S. Evaluation of the performance of randomised versus fixed time schedules for quality control procedures. *Clin Chem*. 2007;53:575–580.

5. NCCLS Document H30A. Day J; Arkin CF, Bovill EG, et al. Procedure for the determination of fibrinogen in plasma: approved guideline. 1994.

6. NCCLS, Arkin CF, Bowie EJW, Carroll JJ, et al. Determination of factor coagulant activator: approved guideline NCCLS/CLCI Document H48-A. 1997.

7. Bolton-Maggs P, Perry DJ, Chalmers EA, et al. The rare coagulation disorders—review with guidelines for management. *Haemophilia*. 2004;10:1–36.

8. Kitchen S, McCraw A, Echenagucia M. Diagnosis of haemophilia and other bleeding disorders. World Federation of Haemophilia. Second edition. 2010. (http://www.wfh.org/en/page.aspx?pid=1270).

9. Levey S, Jennings ER. The use of control charts in the clinical laboratory. *Am J Clin Path*. 1950;20:1059–1066.

10. Barger JD. Levey and Jennings revisited. *Arch Pathol Lab med*. 1992;116:799–803.

11. Westgard JO, Barry PL, Hunt MR, Groth T. A multi-rule Shewart chart for quality control in clinical chemistry. *Clin Chem*. 1981;27:493–501.

7

External quality assessment in hemostasis: its importance and significance

F. Eric Preston[1,2], Steve Kitchen[2,3,4], & Alok Srivastava[5]

[1]University of Sheffield, Sheffield, UK
[2]WHO and WFH International External Quality Assessment Programs for Blood Coagulation, Sheffield, UK
[3]Sheffield Hemophilia and Thrombosis Centre, Royal Hallamshire Hospital, Sheffield, UK
[4]UK National External Quality Assessment Scheme (NEQAS) for Blood Coagulation, Sheffield, UK
[5]Department of Hematology, Christian Medical School, Vellore, India

Overview

The coagulation laboratory plays a vital role in the diagnosis and management of patients with familial and acquired hemorrhagic and thrombotic disorders. Its involvement in oral anticoagulant control is of particular importance.

For all clinical laboratories, the results generated should be accurate, reliable, and reproducible. This applies to all laboratory investigations and particularly to those performed to diagnose, or to exclude, a possible familial disorder. The workload and scope of the coagulation laboratory has increased substantially over recent years and this has been accompanied by the introduction of increasingly sophisticated automated equipment employing a variety of technologies. The potential for error is therefore considerable. Consequently, it is essential to monitor a laboratory's performance through its participation in an external quality assessment (EQA) program [1].

EQA provides a comparison of results obtained on the same sample among different laboratories. Consequently, it provides information in respect of the accuracy of results produced by the participating laboratories. Of equal importance is that the larger programs also provide comparisons of results obtained with different reagents and different instrument–reagent combinations on a single sample.

In hemostasis EQA programs, plasma samples, usually lyophilized, are distributed to participating laboratories and these are instructed to perform specific tests using their standard methods. It is important that the EQA samples are tested in the same way and by the same personnel as for patient samples. In most programs the laboratory is requested to return its results to the program organizer for detailed analysis.

It is important to stress that, for obvious reasons, the samples that are distributed to participating laboratories are not identical to routine patient samples. The plasma samples are usually obtained by single donor plasmapheresis but occasionally it is necessary to pool donations, for example, for heparin dosage monitoring. In general genuine patient samples such as these are preferable to samples that have been created by manipulation of normal plasma, for example, by artificial depletion. Unless it is impossible to avoid, all distributed samples should be negative for HIV, HCV, and HBV. If this cannot be avoided then prior approval for the distribution of infected material should be obtained from the participant.

In most programs the distributed samples are lyophilized. Consequently, it is incumbent on the EQA providers to ensure that following reconstitution, the results obtained on their materials are similar to those obtained on the native plasma before lyophilization and also following reconstitution [2, 3]. Very rarely, a matrix effect is responsible for differences in EQA results. This has been noted by UK National External Quality Assessment Scheme (NEQAS) with respect to a particular thromboplastin for INR testing [4].

It is also important to establish the stability of the lyophilized samples over a range of different temperatures, especially where distributed materials may be exposed to higher temperatures for prolonged periods of time.

Target values

The most important component of any EQA program is the assignment of the target value, that is, the "correct" result since this is the yardstick by which all laboratories are assessed. Target value assignment is difficult. Possible candidates include results obtained using an approved reference method results obtained by "expert laboratories" and overall consensus results.

Although target values derived from results obtained through reference methods is acceptable for EQA programs in clinical chemistry, this approach is not feasible for EQA programs in hemostasis and thrombosis. Although common principles are employed for all tests of hemostasis, the number of variables operating within most, if not all, laboratory procedures is extremely large and there is no consensus for specific reference methods.

Another possible approach to target value assignment is to deploy the results obtained by laboratories recognized for their expertise in the area. Although this sounds reasonable there is no unanimous agreement as to what constitutes an expert laboratory. There is no guarantee that because a laboratory has a long-standing reputation in hemostasis and thrombosis it is able to produce accurate and reliable results across a broad spectrum of investigations. Indeed, when we explored this possibility in an EQA program, it was soon apparent that the results obtained by internationally accepted expert laboratories were as diverse as those derived from smaller institutions. When using expert laboratories it is vital that the participating centers in any EQA program accept the validity of target results derived from these laboratories. In respect of this, difficulties may arise and the efficiency of the EQA program compromised when professional rivalries exist between different high-profile centers.

The overall consensus value of the results obtained by all participants can also be adopted as the target value for EQA participants. This can be the mean, the median, or, after the removal of statistical outliers, the truncated mean value of the overall results.

However, even this approach is not without its problems. In any large EQA program the number of variables with respect to reagents, instruments, and calibrants is extremely large and major differences may be observed in the results obtained with different combinations. For example, in the UK NEQAS program for INR testing, participants used at least 27 different thromboplastins and 35 different coagulometers in at least 110 different combinations during 2006. Although the INR system is designed to give identical results with different thromboplastins this ideal situation is not always realized (Chapter 18) [5]. Consequently if different results are obtained with different reagent–calibrant–instrument combinations then the overall consensus result will be influenced by the numbers of participants employing any single combination of these variables.

An example of this is provided by the results obtained by UK NEQAS participants in an exercise of unfractionated heparin monitoring by aPTT (activated partial thromboplastin time). In this exercise participants received a lyophilized plasma sample derived from patients receiving unfractionated heparin. They were asked to perform an aPTT using their usual reagent. Results were expressed as a ratio of the sample aPTT divided by the midpoint of their reference range using the same reagent. Six reagents were used by ten or more participants. These results are presented in Table 7.1.

It can be seen from Table 7.1 that there were major differences in the results obtained by users of the different reagents, ranging from 1.30 to 1.93. This means that the median aPTT ratio of users of reagent "B" was 1.3 compared with a median aPTT ratio of 1.93 for users of reagents "IL" and "ML." The overall median aPTT for all participants was 1.7. Thus, if

Table 7.1 NEQAS results—pooled *ex vivo* heparinized plasmas

Reagent	N	Median aPTT ratio
IL	143	1.93
ML	10	1.93
MS	47	1.67
DB	37	1.55
DK	62	1.45
B	35	1.30

a user of reagent "B" obtained a ratio of 1.3 and this was assessed against the overall median of 1.7 then this would constitute "poor performance" since the result is 23.5% lower than the overall median. However, the median aPTT ratio for "B" reagent users was 1.3 and therefore if this result (1.3) is assessed against the group reagent median then it clearly represents a good performance.

Conversely, if the result of a reagent "B" user was 1.7 this would constitute a good performance if assessed against the overall median but a poor performance if assessed against the group median.

It is clear from this example that there are inherent flaws in assessing results against the overall median (or mean) result for tests such as the prothrombin time and aPTT. Whenever possible, therefore, it is more appropriate to assess results against the peer group median result. An assessment against the overall median, that is, all-methods analysis, is appropriate only where the number of laboratories deploying a specific method with the same reagents is too small, that is, less than ten, for an accurate statistical analysis or when all methods are known to give the same result for any given analyte. Separate peer group analyses is therefore appropriate for tests whenever there are ten or more users of any given combination.

The evaluation of laboratory performance

The methods by which individual EQA providers evaluate performance are very variable. Commonly used examples include a fixed percentage on either side of the overall or peer group mean or median and the application of the so-called z score. This is calculated from the formula $z = (R - T)/\sigma$ where R is the participants' result, T is the target value, and σ is the standard deviation for proficiency. Using the "z score" model, performance is evaluated as follows:

$$0 < z < 2 \quad \text{(acceptable)}$$
$$2 < z < 3 \quad \text{(questionable)}$$
$$3 < z \quad \text{(unacceptable)}$$

Some programs adopt a different approach in their assessment of performance analysis of simple tests such as the prothrombin time and the aPTT compared with that adopted for specific clotting factor assays

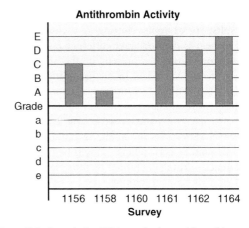

Antithrombin Activity

Figure 7.1 Cumulative EQA results for antithrombin activity. In the final three surveys (1161, 1162, and 1164) the laboratory has obtained grades E, D, and E for each of the test samples (see text for explanation of the grading system), indicating persistent poor performance over this period of time.

such as FVIII:C or FIX:C. The UK NEQAS program, for example, employs a grading system of A–E for clotting factor assays (Figure 7.1). This is based on the difference between the laboratory result and the overall median value. An "A" result covers all results that are either 25% above or below the overall median value. Conversely, an "E" grade is allocated to those laboratories that obtain the extreme 5% of results above and below the overall median result. The designation "persistently outwith consensus" is then based on the results of three consecutive surveys. For the simple tests such as the prothrombin time or aPTT, results are considered satisfactory if the fall within 15% above or below the peer group median result. Following statistical analysis the results are then forwarded to the participating laboratories. Most EQA providers also provide a corresponding performance analysis (see below).

For those laboratories that participate in more than one EQA program the different approaches adopted by the providers may result in some ambiguity in that a satisfactory performance may be achieved in one program and an unsatisfactory performance in another. In our experience this often relates to differences between results assessed against the overall median compared with results analyzed against a method-specific peer group median.

For some analytes different methods produce different results. For example, clotting- and chromogenic-based protein C methods give different results when other abnormalities are present in the sample, for example, factor V Leiden. In the case of Von Willebrand Factor Activity measurements we have shown that different results are produced by different methods, particularly in patients with type 2 VWD [6]. Where such differences occur, the assessment of individual laboratory performance should be determined by reference to results obtained by those laboratories that deploy the same technique.

In respect of the analysis of results and the evaluation of laboratory performance two quite distinct approaches are taken by EQA providers [7]. Some EQA providers set standards for satisfactory performance for individual analytes. The laboratory results are analyzed and the laboratory performance is graded according to the criteria established by the EQA program. The terms employed for performance analysis are extremely varied and include expressions such as "pass" or "fail," "desirable" or "undesirable," "within consensus" or "outwith consensus." Some of the programs do not perform a separate performance analysis for every analyte.

Other EQA providers adopt a different approach. These analyze the entire data set of results and report the statistics to the participating laboratory. The laboratory then assesses its own performance relative to the other results. Using this approach the laboratory thus assesses itself.

A questionnaire distributed by the recently formed EQATH (External Quality Assurance in Thrombosis and Hemostasis) has revealed that of the 11 EQA programs contacted, 6 were responsible for the analysis of performance of those participating whereas the remaining 5 reported the overall statistics to the participating laboratories for their own evaluation [7].

The criteria for the designation of poor performance by different EQA providers are extremely varied. In some programs, the method of performance analysis will always identify an apparent poor performer in each survey. For example, in the A–E system employed by UK NEQAS there will always be a number of laboratories that obtain results that are at the extreme 5% above and below the overall median result. However, contact is not made with participants until they are classified as being "persistently outwith consensus." As already indicated, the designation

"persistently outwith consensus" is based on the results of three consecutive surveys. The overall probability of a laboratory obtaining three consecutive very low gradings by chance alone is 0.014.

Following their identification of persistently poor performance a very small number of EQA providers make direct contact with the laboratory, drawing attention to the problem and offering repeat samples and technical advice.

Irrespective of the manner in which an EQA program evaluates performance, this activity is of vital importance since it enables laboratories to recognize unsuspected analytical problems. Separate evaluation should be made for each analyte. There is no ambiguity when EQA programs adopt a pass/fail approach but some consider this to be somewhat too rigid. Some parameters are not easily assessed. In particular, the assessment of lupus anticoagulant detection has proved to be particularly difficult for EQA providers [8, 9].

In those instances where the interpretation of EQA results and corresponding performance analysis is performed by the participating laboratory rather than by the EQA provider there appears to be an assumption that the laboratory will recognize its own unsatisfactory performance. In view of the many regulatory and fiscal pressures that are brought to bear on clinical laboratories we wonder whether absolute objectivity can always be maintained. This is clearly a controversial area.

In many countries the grading of laboratory performance is an essential prerequisite for accreditation or licensure requirements. This has largely occurred because it was noted by regulatory authorities that laboratories were not voluntarily including EQA in their quality programs [7]. This enforcement of EQA has consequently resulted in increasing regulation and a corresponding reduction in its educational component and, possibly, limiting the program's ability to actually improve quality in the participant laboratory. Participation in EQA programs that are essential for accreditation is therefore mandatory and the professional relationship that exists between participants in these programs and the EQA provider will be quite different from that which exists between those involved in those EQA programs where these requirements do not operate. Understandably, the former group will view EQA as potentially punitive whereas the latter will be stimulated by the educational support of the latter. Stated another way, the former program will attempt to "drive" the laboratory to better quality while the latter will "lead" the program to better quality. Which approach provides better success in actually improving laboratory quality is not known, one hopes that it would be the latter, less punitive one; however, that may be wishful thinking.

Monitoring results: the role of the laboratory

EQA programs enable laboratories to assess their results against those obtained by other laboratories using the same reagents and the same methodology. This allows them to adjust their procedures and/or change their reagents in order to improve their quality of service. Poor performance, however defined, demands some response from the laboratory. A single poor result should be noted and consideration given to possible causes.

It is particularly important for a laboratory's performance to be monitored over time. Results that are consistently above or below the peer group median may indicate either a systematic or a calibration error and therefore provide information that is not apparent from single assessments. The limitations of a single assessment are supported by reports that in approximately 25% of cases it was not possible to identify the cause of a single poor performance [10–12]. A center with consistently poor performance should examine its internal quality control records over the relevant time frame. This will help distinguish between imprecise and inaccurate results. Assay imprecision is likely when sequential EQA results fluctuate above and below the target values. In this case internal quality control (IQC) results will usually be variable with low precision. EQA results that are consistently higher or lower than those of the appropriate peer group indicate probable high precision in the assay. In this case consistent internal quality control results indicate that the method is precise, which contrasts with the EQA results that demonstrate their inaccuracy. In these circumstances all of the components of the assay system should be investigated and, where necessary, replaced.

If a center obtains EQA results for a particular test that fluctuate above and below the median by a considerable degree then the method is poorly controlled and it is likely that the corresponding internal quality results will also show a high degree of imprecision. In this case the center needs to consider whether a particular analyzer is variable in its performance or whether there is instability in the reagents used. It is also necessary to ensure that staff performing the investigations are properly trained and competent. Serial monitoring of EQA results also allows laboratories to assess the impact of any method or reagent change or modification.

In general terms an unsatisfactory laboratory performance may be caused by a clerical error, or else some problem in the laboratory or a problem with the EQA specimen. Unsatisfactory performance may reflect errors arising out of internal quality control, pipettes, instruments, and inadequately trained or inexperienced laboratory staff. Most EQA samples are lyophilized and therefore require reconstitution prior to analysis. Occasionally poor performance in EQA can be caused by inferior/contaminated distilled water, by incorrect diluent volume, or by failure to analyze the EQA sample within the stated period where sample stability is guaranteed. Some of these errors would not affect patient sample analysis because there is no requirement to reconstitute the plasma and in this case poor performance may not automatically confirm that patient results are unsafe.

In order to improve the quality of service it is clearly incumbent on the laboratory to reconcile the cause of its poor performance, particularly when this is recurrent. For some laboratories an additional and arguably more pressing imperative is the maintenance of its accreditation status. In some countries, clinical laboratories are required to provide documentary evidence of satisfactory participation in an EQA program operated by the regulatory agency or else in a program that is approved by a government agency such as CAP (College of American Pathology) in the United States. In the United States all laboratories must participate in proficiency testing and be inspected and accredited. This is undertaken by the government inspection program, run by the federal agency. The federal government does provide for EQA; this must come from an EQA provider that has been approved (i.e., has "deemed status"). There are 14 programs in the United States that have deemed status, one of which is the CAP. The CAP is, by far, the most comprehensive with about 6000 participants, mostly hospital or reference laboratories.

Of the 11 EQA programs participating in the EQATH initiative 7 have been granted "deemed" status by a governmental agency that allows participating laboratories to cite their results for continued EQA accreditation [7].

The educational role of EQA

EQA programs have an important educational role but this aspect may be minimal or even absent in those programs in which participation and success are essential for accreditation. Educational support is provided by printed or electronic commentaries and by regular participant meetings. A small number of EQA providers also offer technical support and repeat samples. Some of the EQA programs undertake supplementary exercises in which samples are distributed in order to address specific issues such as use of a common calibration plasma set for local calibration of INR, use of a common normal plasma for normalized ratios in detection of lupus anticoagulant or APC resistance testing, and so on.

Total confidentiality of results is usually maintained by those programs that are essentially educational in nature and the communication of EQA results and corresponding performance analysis is restricted to the individual nominated by the laboratory itself. The only exception to this approach is when a laboratory is financially sponsored by some agency such as WFH (World Federation of Hemophilia).

Additional advantages of EQA programs

In addition to their role in identifying poor laboratory performance, the larger EQA programs have the important and added advantage of being able to identify problems relating to instruments, reagents, and reference plasmas. This is achieved by comparing results obtained by peer group analysis. Persistent and significant differences of results between groups serves as an alert to the possibility of anomalies arising out of the method itself, rather than unsatisfactory laboratory performance. Some years ago in the UK NEQAS program the INR results obtained with a commonly used thromboplastin were significantly and consistently higher than those obtained by the users of a different thromboplastin [13]. In addition

to determining the INRs, participants were provided with a clinical history and were asked, on the basis of their results, to state whether the patient was over-, under-, or adequately anticoagulated. The differences in the INR results proved to be of considerable clinical importance since markedly differing conclusions were drawn by the two groups. For example, with one sample, 73% of the users of one of the thromboplastins concluded that the patient was over-anticoagulated whereas 71% of users of the other thromboplastin expressed the view that the patient was adequately anticoagulated. Following discussions with the Program Director, the matter was resolved by the manufacturers.

Discrepancies in clotting factor assays may also, on occasion, be attributed to anomalies relating to the use of commercial reference plasmas. In the UK NEQAS program this has been noted in respect of factors VIII:C and V:C assays. In a recent exercise the median factor VIII:C results obtained with six commonly used commercial reference plasmas varied from 72 to 86 u/dL. All the other assay components were similar. Similar observations have also been noted in respect of factor V:C assays in that the use of different commercial reference plasmas was associated with markedly differing results.

The discrepant FV:C results focused attention on the need for an international standard for FV:C [14]. This has now been implemented through the auspices of WHO [15].

It is clear that a comprehensive EQA program in hemostasis and thrombosis serves a number of important functions. By identifying, and assisting, those laboratories that fail to achieve satisfactory results it serves to improve laboratory performance and therefore patient care. Larger programs are able to identify unsatisfactory reagents, reference materials, and methods and therefore are able to assist laboratories in their choice of reagents and instrument–reagent combinations. EQA data also identifies poor methods and facilitates their elimination from laboratory practice.

Table 7.2 What does EQA not accomplish?

- EQA does not test the quality of the lab
- EQA does not test pre- and postanalytical steps
- Limitations in evaluation of analytical step (i.e., sample handled differently)
- EQA does not test staff competency

Table 7.3 What does EQA accomplish?

- Assess current state of the art in laboratory medicine
- Provides information on reagents, calibrants, and instruments
- Provides information to assist method selection
- Provides educational support
- Satisfies regulatory and accreditation requirements

It is important to appreciate the limitations of EQA programs (Tables 7.2 and 7.3) [16–18]. EQA does not test the efficiency of participating laboratories [7]. Nor does it test the important pre- and postanalytical steps of any analytical procedure [19]. There will always be some limitations in the actual analytical process since EQA samples are different from patient samples and are therefore handled differently. The concept of EQA is that the samples are tested alongside routine samples by the laboratory staff who routinely perform the tests. We are well aware that this does not always occur. Finally, EQA provides no information in respect of staff competency.

Recent developments

Within the last decade there has been a considerable increase in the number and complexity of tests performed by hemostasis laboratories [20]. These have included point-of-care (POC) testing for oral anticoagulant control, D-dimer assays for the exclusion of venous thrombovascular disease, lupus anticoagulant testing, familial thrombophilia testing, molecular genetic analysis, and thromboelastography. These have presented EQA providers with a number of difficult challenges to which they have responded with varying degrees of success.

In the developed world EQA programs in hemostasis and thrombosis are widely available but their coverage of tests of hemostasis and thrombosis is extremely variable [20–24]. Some attempt to cover virtually all routine tests of coagulation whereas others are more narrowly focused. One important area that does not receive EQA support is platelet function testing. We are unaware of any programs that distribute samples for this purpose. This undoubtedly reflects not only problems relating to sample collection, preparation, and transportation but also to the time-consuming tests of platelet function [25].

A recent initiative has been an evaluation of the performance characteristics of the Platelet Function Analyzer-100 (PFA-100; Dade Behring), introduced by the College of American Pathologists (CAP) program in 2006 [22].

POC testing for oral anticoagulant control represents a major growth area in hemostasis and thrombosis and worldwide there is an increase in the number of individuals who are using POC devices to monitor their oral anticoagulant control. Although most laboratory scientists recognized the necessity for an EQA program for these monitors, an important initial drawback was that most of the devices were calibrated for whole blood rather than anticoagulated lyophilized plasma, which is distributed in most EQA surveys. This means that participants were not testing "like for like" materials. However, different EQA programs have demonstrated that with these monitors INR results on whole blood are similar to results on the corresponding plasma [26, 27]. They have also demonstrated that EQA is achievable for POC/INR testing [26, 27]. Currently, UK NEQAS provides EQA support for the CoaguChek series (Roche Diagnostics) including the recent XS models and Hemochron Signature series (International Technodyne). In the United States, many tests have been classed as "waived" by the federal agency that oversees laboratory testing. These waived tests, including some POCT INR instruments, are not required to participate in EQA.

A wide variety of molecular genetic defects is now recognized in respect of both inherited hemorrhagic and thrombotic disorders. As a consequence of this, molecular genetic testing represents another important growth area in hemostasis and thrombosis. It is also clear that as a direct consequence of the improved technology and simplification of molecular genetic techniques more of these investigations are now being performed in the hemostasis laboratory.

The accuracy and reliability of molecular genetic testing is of particular importance since clinicians appear to place particular reliance on these investigations and, surprisingly, the result is rarely questioned. Also, the results of these tests have important clinical and social implications, not only for the index patient but also for other family members. With these considerations it is clear that those laboratories that provide a diagnostic service by genetic analysis have an even greater responsibility for accurate testing and reporting than "routine" coagulation laboratories.

A number of EQA providers now provide molecular genetic programs for the diagnosis of familial thrombophila [28, 29]. Although the majority of laboratories report accurate results there can be no sense of complacency. In respect of this, Preston et al. [28] reported that in the UK NEQAS program 3–6% of laboratories failed to correctly identify samples for DNA analysis for familial thrombophilia in three distributions to 47 laboratories. Two types of error were noted. Four laboratories failed to make the correct diagnosis through analytical errors and confirmed transcription errors occurred in four other laboratories. We do not share the view held by some that a transcription error is less serious than an analytical error. Similar concerns regarding the reliability of DNA testing have been expressed by Tripodi et al. [29].

An EQA program for the molecular genetics of hemophilia A was established by UK NEQAS in 2003. To date there have been 17 distributions involving whole blood or immortalized cell line DNA. The latter was satisfactorily introduced in 2005. The EQA exercises have focused on screening for intron 1 and intron 22 inversions and also sequence analysis [30]. In addition material has been distributed in respect of F9 and VWF gene analysis. Errors of both interpretation and analysis have been noted.

It is essential that participants in EQA programs should have total confidence in their efficiency and effectiveness. EQA surveys should be sufficiently frequent to make sequential performance analysis meaningful. Routine tests of hemostasis and thrombosis should be distributed at least quarterly and data processing must be as rapid as possible, with prompt returns to participants. Industry may provide a useful service by organizing a program for users of their equipment but it is our strongly held view that the financing of an independent EQA program should remain totally independent of industrial support.

Establishing EQA programs in developing countries

The need and the challenges

Hemostasis laboratories are generally less developed in many developing countries [31]. This is related to many factors such as low clinical demand for these tests due to lack of awareness about bleeding disorders among physicians or laboratories using inappropriate techniques or imprecise technology with inadequate understanding of quality requirements. This is further complicated by erratic supply of reagents and often poor technical support for maintenance from equipment manufacturers. It is important to appreciate therefore that while there is a great need to have a good EQA program in these circumstances, this needs to be created in an environment that may not be fully ready for it.

Initiating an EQA program in a developing country therefore has several challenges. The first of these is to convey the concept to the laboratories that should participate in it. This requires a local champion, a person, and a center that can conceptualize the need for EQAS and communicate it to colleagues in the country. It is important that this group also understands the technicalities of running such a program, even if they are not involved in the preparation of the samples. This person or center should have the trust and confidence of the participating laboratories and should have the logistics support to be able to coordinate such a program. It can greatly help the cause if such help comes from a government agency or a nongovernmental organization that has strong credibility in the scientific community. While over a period of time, the program can become self-sustaining, there is a need for funds to support the EQA program from the outset. This is necessary for staff salaries as well as for the preparation and transport of samples and other logistic requirements.

The second issue is with regard to recruitment of laboratories. As participation is not mandatory in most developing countries, significant effort is required to persuade individual laboratories to participate in EQAS programs. It is particularly important to educate people about EQA particularly with respect to its importance in improving and maintaining laboratory performance. One has to emphasize that the aim is educational and supportive and not regulatory and explain how confidentiality will be maintained. Support of the local professional societies can be very useful in achieving this.

The next important aspect is with regard to the service itself. Most importantly, the cost has to be maintained at a level that the community will be able to bear. If this is borne by governmental agencies, then it can be a great help but such examples are not common. Therefore, the service has to be designed in a way that the costs are kept low. The program therefore needs to start with the minimum number of technical and clerical staff, some of whom will only be part-time. The scientists and physicians involved with the program will initially often give "volunteer" time. Sample preparation is best outsourced, if possible, rather than invested in a high-end lyophilizer in the beginning. Systems are also needed to be established for these samples to be appropriately stored and transported in a way that they reach all participants in time and are stable through this process. Special attention needs to be given when ambient temperatures are over 40°C in some months of the year. Such periods are best avoided for sample transportation.

Another challenge is to ensure that reports are received consistently and punctually from all participants, especially for factor assays. Reported reasons for nonreturn of responses include the inability of some laboratories to obtain reportable results with the volume of sample provided even though other laboratories are able to with the same samples or lack of reagents needed for the tests or the samples just not reaching the laboratories. Technical support and advice is needed to help laboratories with these problems.

Finally reports of performance need to be provided on time and in a format that is easily understood by the participants. The service provider must appreciate that the knowledge of the theoretical aspects of the tests of hemostasis are not necessarily the same in all laboratories and that very basic issues may need emphasis and clarification for some participants.

The establishment of an EQA program in India: a successful model

When initiated in the year 2000, the program was limited to laboratories associated with the chapters of the Hemophilia Federation (India) (HFI). Samples were obtained from UK NEQAS in Sheffield, UK, and distributed to 27 such laboratories in different parts of the country. Results were then collected and sent to UK NEQAS for analysis, which then provided a report for each laboratory [32]. At the request of the Indian Society of Haematology and Transfusion Medicine, the program was converted into a national one in 2003 and called the ISHTM–CMC EQAS for Haemostasis [33]. The program aims to provide external

proficiency testing to all laboratories in India providing diagnostic services for hemostatic disorders.

Samples for EQAS

From 2000 until 2003, lyophilized samples for this EQA program were provided through UK NEQAS, a critical reason this program could sustain itself at that stage. The cost of distribution and data analysis was covered by a grant from a charitable trust. Local logistics were supported from the infrastructure available at the Christian Medical College, Vellore, with some support from the HFI. The EQA program ran without any cost to the participant laboratories that were supporting people with hemophilia in India. However, when the scheme expanded in 2003 into a national program for all laboratories performing tests of hemostasis, this model was modified. The program needed to sustain itself, in terms of both technology and finances. The team at the Christian Medical College, Vellore, was expanded to include technical and scientific personnel in addition to staff for data management and a statistician. Over the last 5 years the program has expanded to include over 300 laboratories in India. Only the technical staff work full-time in the program, which also has a transfusion medicine module with about 100 participants as well as a molecular genetics in hematology module with about 15 participants. The other members of the team (scientific, data management, and clerical) are part-time and supported for their employment by the hospital. It is for this reason that we are able to keep costs low but believe that it is our duty to support this program that provides an opportunity for developing countries to participate in it while they develop one of their own.

Local production of samples for the scheme started in India in 2004 since it was not financially viable to obtain samples from overseas. Appropriately derived plasma for lyophilization is now sent to a suitable facility in the industry. Following receipt of the lyophilized samples from this source, they are evaluated for their suitability for the EQAS. Apart from assessment of their physical characteristics and stability at different temperatures and interval variability, the coagulation parameters are also tested. These include PT, INR, aPTT, FVIIIC, FIXC after storage under a variety of conditions. Samples are distributed three times in a year. This is easily organized with an arrangement with local courier services. We avoid the hottest months for such distribution. Laboratories are asked to perform the tests listed above.

Assignment of target value

This is undertaken in a manner similar to the UK NEQAS program. However, given the wide heterogeneity of the participating laboratories we have considered taking the "expert lab" approach, as mentioned above, as well.

Profile of participants

The number of participating laboratories has increased from 35, in 2003, to more than 300 in 2011. The vast majority are active in responding to all surveys. The participants range in size and function, for example, very small laboratories (<20 samples/day); medium laboratories (20–200 samples/day); large laboratories (>200 samples/day) [34], with 48% of them serving as stand-alone laboratory services and 52% being associated with hospitals, both in the public and in the private healthcare systems.

Range of tests offered

Starting with PT, aPTT, and factor VIII and IX assays in 2003, we have gradually added fibrinogen, VWF:Ag and VWF:RCo to the tests that we provide. We offer these tests for EQA in two different modules. All laboratories perform the clotting times and correction studies but only about a sixth of the total registered laboratories participate in the factor assays and only about 5% of the laboratories perform the VWF assays.

The program and its impact

Participation in an EQA program is not currently mandatory in India. Awareness of its necessity and its significance in ensuring quality of results is also not widely understood. This is reflected in the small number of participants in a national EQA scheme for hemostasis. However, greater awareness of quality requirements and the demand within the community for it has led to a gradual increase in the number of registered participants over the years to over 300 in 2011. Information about this program needs to be further disseminated to increase participation. However, it is only with mandatory requirements for accreditation that participation is likely to become universal. The program is now self-sufficient in so much as it does need any external support but is subsidized by the hospital and is in fact helping, at similar subsidized costs, other developing countries start their own efforts.

The major impact of the program has been in raising awareness of the concept of EQAS among Indian laboratories performing hemostasis tests. It has also had an impact on the performance of many of the laboratories that have been participating for many years in that they have been able to make changes that have led to a more consistent performance from their laboratories. Table 7.4 shows the overall performance comparison for the entire group over the last 5 years from 2007 to 2011. This data shows that while there is improvement in the deviation of the results from the target value for PT, aPTT, and fibrinogen values, there is actually a much higher variation in the FVIII, FIX, and VWF assays. This suggests that while most laboratories are performing well for plasma clotting time tests and fibrinogen assays, the newer

Table 7.4 Comparison of performance of laboratories in India in over 5 years

	2011			2007		
	Median	CV (%)	n	Median	CV	n
PT ratio	1.2 (1.01–1.37)	7.6	303	1.8 (1.55–2.09)	13.2	99
INR	1.22 (1.04–1.4)	9.0	306	1.94 (1.65–2.23)	16.5	99
aPTT ratio	1.51 (1.29–1.75)	13.8	301	2.08 (1.56–2.6)	17.8	99
Fibrinogen	200.5	29.2	110	136.0	37.8	42
F VIII:C	42.0	64.2	50	29.0	35	24
F IX	70.3	41.2	37	33.0	35.7	24
vWF:Ag	54.2	28.8	16	55.7	17	6

laboratories have greater challenges in the factor assays. This issue need is being addressed.

Extension to other developing countries

Based on specific requests received from other developing countries this program also helps them develop their own local schemes. The aim is help them replicate our experience if possible. Through this mechanism we have supported the development of EQAS for hemostasis in the Philippines and Thailand. While the former program could not be sustained, the latter is now a regular program that is locally managed. We are currently supporting EQAS for tests of hemostasis for a limited number of laboratories in China and also assisting a national program in Sri Lanka. The overall aim is to help as many developing countries introduce EQA programs with samples and services that can be obtained at costs that they can afford and in a way that suits their requirements at the national level and helps them move on to a self-sustaining program when they are ready for it.

References

1. Woods TAL, Kitchen S, Preston FE. Quality assessment of haemostatic assays and external quality assessment schemes. In: Jespersen J, Bertina RM, Haverkate F, eds. *Laboratory Techniques in Thrombosis*. 2nd revised ed. Dordrecht, The Netherlands: Kluwer Academic Publishers; 1999:29–36.
2. Thienpont LM, Stöckl D, Fridecký B, et al. Trueness, verification in European external quality assessment schemes: time to care about the quality of the samples. *Scand J Clin Lab Invest*. 2003;63:195–201.
3. Middle JG, Libeer JC, Malakhov V, et al. Characterisation and evaluation of external quality assessment scheme serum. Discussion paper from the European external quality assessment (EQA) organisers working group C. *Clin Chem Lab Med*. 1998;36:119–130.
4. Preston FE, Kitchen S. Personal communication; 2006.
5. Kitchen S, Walker ID, Woods TA, Preston FE. Thromboplastin related differences in the determination of international normalised ratio: a cause for concern? *Thromb Haemost*. 1994;72:426–429.
6. Preston FE. Assays for von Willebrand factor functional activity: a UK NEQAS survey. *Thromb Haemost*. 1998;80:863.
7. Olson JD, Preston FE, Nichols WL. External quality assurance in thrombosis and hemostasis: an international perspective. *Semin Thromb Hemost*. 2007;33:220–225.
8. Tripodi A, Biasiolo A, Chantarangkul V, et al. Lupus anticoagulant (LA) testing: performance of clinical laboratories assessed by a national survey using lyophilised affinity-purified immunoglobulin with LA activity. *Clin Chem*. 2003;49:1608–1614.
9. Jennings I, Kitchen S, Woods TA, Preston FE, Greaves M. Potentially clinically important inaccuracies in testing for the lupus anticoagulant: an analysis of results from the three surveys of the UK National External Quality Assessment Scheme (NEQAS) for Blood Coagulation. *Thromb Haemost*. 1997;77:934–937.
10. Clinical and Laboratory Standards Institute. Using proficiency testing to improve the clinical laboratory: approved guideline. 2nd ed. GP27-A2; 2007.
11. Hoeltgee GA, Duckworth JK. Review of proficiency testing performance of laboratories accredited by the College of American Pathologists. *Arch Pathol Lab Med*. 1987;111:1011–1014.
12. Steindel SJ, Howanitz PJ, Renner SW. Reasons for proficiency testing failures in clinical chemistry and blood gas analysis. *Arch Pathol Lab Med*. 1996;120:1094–1101.
13. Kitchen S, Walker ID, Woods TA, Preston FE. Thromboplastin related differences in the determination of international normalised ratio: a cause for concern, steering committee of the UK national external quality assessment scheme in blood coagulation. *Thromb Haemost*. 2002;87:921–922.
14. Preston FE, Jennings I, Kitchen DP, Woods TA, Kitchen S. Variability for factor V:C assays in UK national external quality assessment scheme surveys: there is a need for an international standard. *Blood Coagul Fibrinolysis*. 2005;16:529–531.
15. Hubbard AT, Weller LJ, Johnes S. Calibration of the WHO 1st international standard for blood coagulation factor V. *J Thromb Haemost*. 2007;5:1318–1319.
16. Ehrmeyer SS, Laessig RH. Inter-laboratory proficiency-testing programs: a computer model to assess their capability to correctly characterise intra-laboratory performance. *Clin Chem*. 1987;33:784–787.
17. Gambino SR, O'Brien JE, Mallon P. More on proficiency testing. *Clin Chem*. 1987;33:2321.
18. Klee GG, Forsman RW. A user's classification of problems identified by proficiency testing surveys. *Arch Pathol Lab Med*. 1988;112:371–373.
19. Shahangian S. Proficiency testing in laboratory medicine. *Arch Pathol Lab Med*. 1998;122:15–30.
20. Favaloro EJ, Bonar R. Emerging technologies and quality assurance in haemostasis: a review of findings from the Royal College of Pathologists of Australasia Quality Assurance Program. *Semin Thromb Hemost*. 2007;33:235–242.

21. Jennings I, Kitchen DP, Woods TA, Kitchen S, Walker ID. Emerging technologies and quality assurance: the United Kingdom National External Quality Assessment Scheme perspective. *Semin Thromb Haemost.* 2007;33:243–249.

22. Cunningham MT, Brandt JT, Chandler WL, et al. Quality assurance in hemostasis: the perspective from the college of American Pathologist Proficiency Testing Program. *Semin Thromb Hemost.* 2007;33:250–258.

23. Spannagl M, Dick Andrea, Reinauer H. External quality assessment schemes in coagulation in Germany: between regulatory bodies and patient outcome. *Semin Thromb Hemost.* 2007;33:259–264.

24. Meijer P, Haverkate F. An external quality assessment program for von Willebrand factor laboratory analysis: an overview from the European Concerted Action on Thrombosis and Disabilities Foundation. *Semin Thromb Hemost.* 2006;32:485–491.

25. Hayward CPM, Eikelboom J. Platelet function testing: quality assurance. *Semin Thromb Hemost.* 2007;33:273–282.

26. Kitchen S, Kitchen DP, Jennings I, Woods TA, Walker ID, Preston FE. Point of care international normalised ratios: UK NEQAS experience demonstrates necessity for proficiency testing of three different monitors. *Thromb Haemost.* 2006;96:590–596.

27. Tripodi A, Bressi C, Carpenedo M, et al. Quality assurance program for whole blood prothrombin time—international normalised ratio point-of-care monitors used for patient self-testing to control oral anticoagulation. *Thromb Res.* 2004;113:35–40.

28. Preston FE, Kitchen S, Jennings I, Woods TAL, et al. A UK national external quality assessment scheme (UK NEQAS) for molecular genetic testing for the diagnosis of familial thrombophilia. *Thromb Haemost.* 1999;82:1556–1557.

29. Tripodi A, Peyvandi F, Chantaranqkul V, et al. Relatively poor performance of clinical laboratories for DNA analyses in the detection of two thrombophilic mutations—a cause for concern. *Thromb Haemost.* 2002;88:690–691.

30. Perry DJ, Goodeve A, Hill M, et al. The UK national external quality assessment scheme (UK NEQAS) for molecular genetic testing in haemophilia. *Thromb Haemost.* 2006;96:597–601.

31. Srivastava A. Delivery of haemophilia care in the developing world. *Haemophilia.* 1998;4(suppl 2):33–40.

32. Jennings I, Kitchen S, Woods AL, Preston FE. Laboratory performance of haemophilia centers in developing countries: 3 years' experience of the World Federation of Hemophilia External Quality Assessment Scheme. *Haemophilia.* 1998;4:739–746.

33. Hertzberg MS, Mammen, J, McCraw A, Nair SC, Srivastava A. Achieving and maintaining quality in the laboratory [laboratory aspects of haemophilia therapy]. *Haemophilia.* 2006;12(suppl 3):61–67.

34. Mammen J, Nair SC, Srivastava A. External quality assessment scheme for hemostasis in India. *Semin Thromb Hemost.* 2007;33(3):265–272.

8
The unique challenges of hemostatic testing in children

M. Patricia Massicotte[1], Mary E. Bauman[1], Vanessa Chan[2], & Anthony K.C. Chan[3]

[1] Stollery Children's Hospital, University of Alberta, Edmonton, AB, Canada
[2] Department of Pediatric Laboratory Medicine, The Hospital for Sick Children, Toronto, ON, Canada
[3] McMaster Children's Hospital/Hamilton Health Sciences Foundation, Chair in Pediatric Thrombosis and Hemostasis, Department of Pediatrics, McMaster University, Hamilton, ON, Canada

Introduction

The normal hemostatic system in infants and children has a number of differences compared to adults that impact on the investigation and management of children with hemorrhage and thrombosis. Diagnosis of acquired or congenital disorders of hemostasis relies on hemostatic testing carried out in the laboratory. Hemostatic testing in children may be requested for the management of patients in a number of clinical scenarios, including presurgery, in the event of a bleeding or thrombotic history, and during the management of either a bleeding child such as factor VIII or FIX in a hemophiliac, or a child with thrombosis such as a child with a deep venous thrombosis, and a family history of thrombophilia.

In addition, the interaction of the hemostatic system with anticoagulation in children with or at risk for thrombosis requires laboratory monitoring to ensure safety and efficacy of management. Consequently, the laboratory plays a major role in the care of children with hemostatic abnormalities. Therefore, it is necessary that the clinician and the hemostatic experts in the laboratory have ongoing communication about these children to provide the best care.

This chapter will discuss normal hemostasis; developmental differences in children; laboratory testing; and issues including blood sampling, thrombophilia testing, and anticoagulant (AC) monitoring.

Normal hemostasis

Hemostasis is a complex process providing a balance between bleeding and thrombosis with integral components including platelets, hemostatic proteins within the medium of plasma that have contact with vascular endothelium during circulation. The main component of plasma is water with additional minerals, salt, glucose, fats, amino acids, hormones, enzymes, dissolved gases, cellular waste by-products (i.e., urea), and other proteins. In addition, plasma is also composed of erythrocytes and leukocytes that influence hemostasis. Hemostasis can be described as the reparative process for damaged vasculature in the closed high-pressure circulatory system [1]. Regulatory mechanisms of thrombin and fibrin production exist to contain the reparative process and restore vascular integrity (Figure 8.1). However, if these mechanisms are overwhelmed, excessive amounts of thrombin are produced, resulting in thrombosis [1]. Hemostasis is maintained through a normal vessel wall, blood composition, and blood flow. If any of these were abnormal, the balance of hemostasis would be disrupted resulting in either bleeding or thrombosis.

The endothelium of the vessel wall secretes three thrombo-regulating substances playing a major role in ensuring patency of vasculature. Platelet adherence to the endothelium is inhibited by nitrous oxide

Quality in Laboratory Hemostasis and Thrombosis, Second Edition. Edited by Steve Kitchen, John D. Olson and F. Eric Preston.
© 2013 John Wiley & Sons, Ltd. Published 2013 by Blackwell Publishing Ltd.

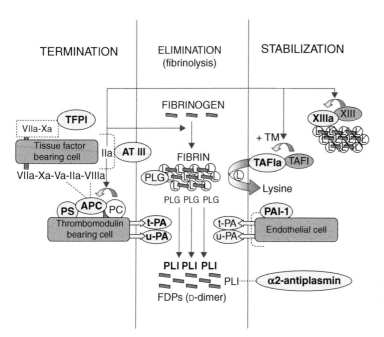

TERMINATION

ELIMINATION
(fibrinolysis)

STABILIZATION

FIBRINOGEN

TFPI

VIIa-Xa

Tissue factor
bearing cell

VIIa-Xa-Va-IIa-VIIIa

IIa

AT III

FIBRIN

PLG

PLG PLG PLG

XIIIa XIII

+ TM

TAFIa TAFI

Lysine

PS APC PC

Thrombomodulin
bearing cell

t-PA
u-PA

PAI-1

t-PA
u-PA

Endothelial cell

PLI PLI PLI

PLI

α2-antiplasmin

FDPs (D-dimer)

Figure 8.1 Regulation of thrombin and
fibrin production (From Reference 17,
with kind permission from Springer
Science + Business Media.).

[2, 3] and prostacyclin [4] while ectonucleotidase CD39 degrades adenosine triphosphate directly into adenosine monophosphate, thereby bypassing adenosine diphosphate production. This results in inhibition of adenosine diphosphate-induced aggregation by the platelet receptor P2Y1 [5].

Vessel wall damage may occur as a result of physical disruption such as injury or surgery. Furie et al. hypothesized that additional subtle endothelial cell alterations [1] also occur that cause activation of hemostasis. Damage to the vessel wall activates platelets activation through two distinct pathways. Collagen invokes the first pathway while the second pathway is invoked by tissue factor. The degree of vascular damage or the underlying disease entity will determine the main pathway for platelet activation [6, 7]. Platelets interact with exposed collagen in the subendothelial matrix resulting in adhesion through the following two mechanisms: binding to von Willebrand factor (VWF) followed by platelet glycoprotein 1b-IX-V, and through direct interaction with platelet glycoprotein VI [8]. Platelet tethering to the vessel wall is determined by shear force. Glycoprotein VI and glycoprotein 1_b are essential for platelet adhesion [6, 9, 10]. The integrin $\alpha_2\beta_1$ also plays a lesser role in platelet adhesion [11, 12].

Microparticles, remnants of cell membrane originating from white cells, endothelium, or platelets play a role in hemostasis. Tissue factor in microparticles requires activation [13, 14] from its circulating inactive form [15, 16], which has been hypothesized to occur through a protein disulfideisomerase released by activated endothelial cells and platelets [1, 14]. Activated tissue factor stimulates activation of factor VII and factor IX. The tenase complex then results from the combination of activated factor IX and factor VIII, which subsequently activates factor X. Activated factor X then combines with factor V to form the prothrombinase complex, which triggers a small amount of prothrombin conversion to thrombin. The trace amount of thrombin generated is a catalytic agent that activates factors V and VIII to their most active cofactor forms, factor VIIIa and factor Va as well as the activation of factor XI. Vast amounts of thrombin are then generated as a result of the ongoing action of the tenase and prothrombinase complexes (Figure 8.2) [17]. Fibrinogen is activated by thrombin to form non-polymerized thrombus, additionally activating platelets [18] through cleaving protease activating receptor 1 (PAR1), resulting in platelet granule release (adenosine diphosphate stored in the dense granules, and serotonin and thromboxane A_2 stored in

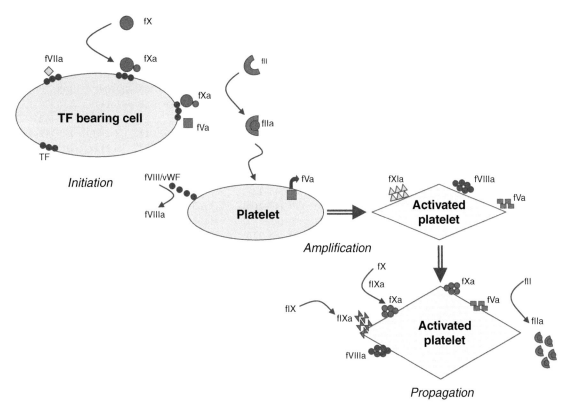

Figure 8.2 Coagulation phase of hemostasis. The coagulation phase of hemostasis occurs in three phases: initiation, amplification, and propagation. TF, tissue factor; VWF, von Willebrand factor. (Adapted from Reference 17, with kind permission from Springer Science + Business Media.).

the α granules) and further platelet activation. Adenosine diphosphate activates platelets through receptors P2Y1 and P2Y12. Serotonin activates platelets through 5 hydroxytryptamine 2A receptors. Thromboxane A_2 activates platelets through the thromboxane receptor.

Activated tissue factor then activates glycoprotein IIb/IIIa (integrin $\alpha_{IIb}\beta_3$) on platelets which then bind to ligands fibrinogen and VWF, thereby stimulating platelet recruitment to the thrombus and platelet–platelet interactions [19–21]. Platelets bound to the damaged vessel wall are activated and glycoprotein IIb/IIIa undergoes a transformational change increasing the affinity for the ligands [22]. Blood flow shear rates determine the binding ligand, with low and high shear rates binding with fibrinogen and VWF, respectively [8]. Tissue factor exposed on microparticles derived from monocytes stimulates further thrombin generation [13, 14].

Developmental hemostasis

Children have physiologic differences in hemostasis, compared with adults, which affect laboratory normal values of baseline tests (international normalized ratio (INR), activated partial thromboplastin time (aPTT)), hemostatic proteins, and response to anticoagulants. Specifically, there are decreased levels of factors XII, XI, X, IX, VII (Table 8.1), II (hemostatic proteins), plasminogen and tissue plasminogen activator (fibrinolytic proteins), antithrombin, and proteins C and S (hemostatic inhibitor proteins) (Table 8.2). As a result of these differences, known as developmental hemostasis [23], children generate less thrombin than adults when hemostasis is activated [24]. These differences result in different reference ranges for hemostatic tests (INR, aPTT; Table 8.3) and reference ranges for hemostatic protein levels (Tables 8.1 and 8.2).

79

Table 8.1 Coagulation factor reference values for neonates and children compared to results from Andrew et al.

Coagulation factors (%)	Day 1	1 mo to 1 yr	1–5 yr	6–10 yr	11–16 yr	Adults
II	54[a] (41–69)	90[a] (62–103)	89[a] (70–109)	89[a] (67–110)	90[a] (61–107)	110 (78–138)
II Andrew et al.	48[b] (37–59)	88[b] (60–116)	94[b] (71–116)	88 (67–107)	83 (61–104)	108 (70–146)
V	81[a] (64–103)	113 (94–141)	97[a] (67–127)	99[a] (56–141)	89[a] (67–141)	118 (78–152)
V Andrew et al.	72[b] (54–90)	91[b] (55–127)	103 (79–127)	90[b] (63–116)	77[b] (55–99)	106 (62–150)
VII	70[a] (52–88)	128 (83–160)	111[a] (72–150)	113[a] (70–156)	118 (69–200)	129 (61–199)
VII Andrew et al.	66[b] (47–85)	87[b] (47–127)	82[b] (55–116)	85 (52–120)	83[b] (58–115)	105 (67–143)
VIII	182 (105–329)	94[a] (54–145)	110[a] (36–185)	117[a] (52–182)	120[a] (59–200)	160 (52–290)
VIII Andrew et al.	100 (61–139)	73[b] (50–109)	90 (59–142)	95 (58–132)	92 (53–131)	99 (50–149)
IX	48[a] (35–56)	71[a] (43–121)	85[a] (44–127)	96[a] (48–145)	111[a] (64–216)	130 (59–254)
IX Andrew et al.	53[b] (34–72)	86[b] (36–136)	73[b] (47–104)	75[b] (63–89)	82[b] (59–122)	109 (55–163)
X	55[a] (46–67)	95[a] (77–122)	98[a] (72–125)	97[a] (68–125)	91[a] (53–122)	124 (96–171)
X Andrew et al.	40[b] (25–54)	78[b] (38–118)	88[b] (58–116)	75[b] (55–101)	79[b] (50–117)	106 (70–152)
XI	30[a] (7–41)	89[a] (62–125)	113 (65–162)	113 (65–162)	111 (65–139)	112 (67–196)
XI Andrew et al.	39[b] (24–52)	86[b] (49–134)	97 (56–150)	86 (52–120)	74 (50–97)	97 (67–127)
XII	58[a] (43–80)	79[a] (20–135)	85[a] (36–135)	81[a] (26–137)	75[a] (14–117)	115 (35–207)
XII Andrew et al.	53[b] (33–73)	77[b] (39–115)	93 (64–129)	92 (60–140)	81[b] (34–137)	108 (52–164)

For each assay the first row shows the mean and boundaries including 95% of the population.
[a]Denotes values that are significantly different from adult values ($p < 0.05$).
[b]Denotes values that are significantly different from adult values for Andrew et al. data.
Source: Modified from Monagle et al. (2006).

Pediatric reference ranges: challenges and deviations

There are a number of published studies determining the reference ranges for hemostatic tests and protein levels in infants and children [23, 25–29]. All studies confirm the above differences in children compared to adults. However, the absolute values for the proteins tested are not equivalent among studies due to varying test systems (reagents, techniques, and analyzers). As an example, this is demonstrated by the difference in published free protein S reference ranges

Table 8.2 Coagulation inhibitor reference values for neonates and children compared to results from Andrew et al.

Coagulation inhibitors (%)	Day 1	1 mo to 1 yr	1–5 yr	6–10 yr	11–16 yr	Adults
AT	76[a] (58–90)	109[a] (72–134)	116[a] (101–131)	114[a] (95–134)	111[a](96–126)	96 (66–124)
AT Andrew et al.	63[b] (51–75)	104 (82–124)	111 (82–139)	111 (90–131)	105 (77–132)	100 (74–126)
Protein C chromogenic	36[a] (24–44)	71[a] (31–112)	96[a] (65–127)	100 (71–129)	94[a] (66–118)	104 (74–164)
C chromogen, Andrew et al.	35[b] (26–44)	59[b] (37–81)	66[b] (40–92)	69[b] (45–93)	83[b] (55–111)	96 (64–128)
Protein C clotting	32[a] (24–40)	77[a] (28–124)	94[a] (50–134)	94[a] (64–125)	88[a] (59–112)	103 (54–166)
C clotting Andrew et al.	Not available	Not available	Not available	Not available	Not available	Not available
Protein S clotting	36[a] (28–47)	102[a] (29–162)	101[a] (67–136)	109[a] (64—154)	103[a] (65–140)	75 (54–103)
Protein S Andrew et al.	36[b] (24–48)	87 (55–119)	86 (54–118)	78 (41–114)	72 (52–92)	81 (60–113)

For each assay the first row shows the mean and boundaries including 95% of the population.
[a]Denotes values that are significantly different from adult values ($p < 0.05$).
[b]Denotes values that are significantly different from adult values for Andrew et al. data.
Source: Modified from Monagle et al. (2006).

Table 8.3 aPTT, PT, INR, and fibrinogen reference values for neonates and children compared to results from Andrew et al.

Coagulation tests	Day 1	1 mo to 1 yr	1–5 yr	6–10 yr	11–16 yr	Adults
aPTT (s)	38.7[a] (34.3–44.8)	39.3[a] (35.1–46.3)	37.7[a] (33.6–43.8)	37.3[a] (31.8–43.7)	39.5[a] (33.9–46.1)	33.2 (28.6–38.2)
aPTT Andrew et al.	42.9[b] (31.3–54.5)	35.5 (28.1–42.9)	30 (24–36)	31 (26–36)	32 (26–37)	33 (27–40)
PT (s)	15.6[a] (14.4–16.4)	13.1 (11.5–15.3)	13.3[a] (12.1–14.5)	13.4[a] (11.7–15.1)	13.8[a] (12.7–16.1)	13.0 (11.5–14.5)
PT Andrew et al.	13 (11.6–14.43)	12.3 (10.7–13.9)	11 (10.6–11.4)	11.1 (10.1–12.1)	11.2 (10.2–12.0)	12.0 (11.0–14.0)
INR	1.26[a] (1.15–1.35)	1.00 (0.86–1.22)	1.03[a] (0.92–1.14)	1.04[a] (0.87–1.20)	1.08[a] (0.97–1.30)	1.00 (0.80–1.20)
INR Andrew et al.	1[b] (0.53–1.62)	0.88[b] (0.61–1.17)	1 (0.96–1.04)	1.01 (0.91–1.11)	1.02 (0.93–1.10)	1.10 (10–1.3)
Fibrinogen (g/L)	2.80 (1.92–3.74)	2.42[a] (0.82–3.83)	2.82[a] (1.62–4.01)	3.04 (1.99–4.09)	3.15 (2.12–4.33)	3.1 (1.9–4.3)
Fibrinogen Andrew et al.	2.83 (2.25–3.41)	2.51 (1.5–3.87)	2.76 (1.70–4.05)	2.75 (1.57–4.0)	3 (1.54–4.48)	2.78 (1.56–4.0)

For each assay the first row shows the mean and boundaries including 95% of the population.
[a]Denotes values that are significantly different from adult values ($p < 0.05$).
[b]Denotes values that are significantly different from adult values for Andrew et al. data.
Source: Modified from Monagle et al. (2006).

between Andrew and Monagle (Table 8.2) [23, 27, 28, 30]. Although it is recommended that at least 40 normal people should be evaluated to establish a reference range (see Chapter 2), no studies in children have consistently evaluated this number of normal children within each age group [23, 27, 28, 30] due to challenges obtaining consent and blood samples from infants and children. Thus, the published ranges should be viewed in this context [31]. Furthermore, if published reference ranges are used, then patient test results should be interpreted with caution for reasons described in the following section.

Local pediatric reference range development

Published recommendations state that each laboratory should establish its own local pediatric reference ranges. The challenges with obtaining consent, samples, and associated amount of labor have resulted in the absence of local reference ranges in most pediatric centers. Without locally developed reference ranges, testing results should be cautiously interpreted (see Chapter 2). The health provider who interprets the

test result should ensure that the reference range accompanying the test result is a pediatric reference range as adult reference ranges differ. In addition, if a laboratory chooses to use a published pediatric reference range then a caution should accompany the report to inform the clinician that pediatric reference ranges are from the literature and not derived locally. Ideally each laboratory should develop an age-appropriate range for each baseline hemostatic screening test and protein level and report results for infants and children using these ranges. Furthermore, considering method differences that result in varying reference ranges, any test results at the high or low end of the published range may or may not indicate an abnormality (Table 8.2). For example, a protein S value of 54 U/mL for a 5-year-old child would be abnormal if referring to Monagle et al. but normal if referring to Andrew et al. [27, 29].

The effect of the assay method

If the laboratory elects to use a pediatric published reference range, the published range used as reference must have been developed using the same method or methodology as that used by the local laboratory. If the assay system of the laboratory is the same as the published age-appropriate reference range, the laboratory can be more comfortable using the published reference range as a comparator. If the same method/methodology is not used it is important to consider that the upper and lower limits of the reference range may be associated with some error and therefore caution should be used when interpreting the result. With markedly reduced test results (<20–30%) with repeated testing, a congenital defect may be considered. Then, with informed consent, the parents can be tested to determine if the patient's abnormality is inherited or acquired. If the test result is above the upper end of the reference range for hemostatic proteins, there are no data on children to suggest that the result is clinically relevant (i.e., antithrombin (AT) test result of 200%). However, if the INR or aPTT is prolonged in the absence of an antiphospholipid antibody or hemostatic protein inhibitor, the results may be abnormal but must be compared to pediatric reference ranges. Most commonly, local reference ranges posted by laboratories reflect adult and not pediatric normals. If a local age-appropriate range is not available, caution should be used to interpret the result when comparing to published reference ranges. Monagle et al. demonstrated that when comparing pediatric references ranges to Andrew et al., there were differences in the upper and lower range values. Differences in reagents and analyzers were felt to be the reason for these variations.

Test sampling

Quality of testing is influenced by preanalytical, analytical, and postanalytical variables. There are some variables unique to pediatric testing.

Preanalytical variables

Before the laboratory receives and processes samples, there are many preanalytical variables that can falsely elevate, decrease, or activate factor levels, hemostatic proteins, and/or platelets. With any laboratory test, the quality of the sample is crucial in providing accurate results. Small inconsistencies in coagulation sample collection can magnify inaccuracies in sample results. Proper coagulation sample collection has to be precise: the order of draw (refer to Chapter 5) and the ratio of blood to anticoagulant must be 9:1. After the sample is collected, prompt transportation at room temperature is also crucial to minimize cold activation of factor FVII, pre-activation of platelets, and loss of VWF (CLSI H21-A5) [32].

Sodium citrate, final concentration of 0.109 M (3.2%), is the recommended anticoagulant for hemostasis testing. Importantly, 3.8% sodium citrate should not be used since it produces differences in test results especially in the prothrombin time (PT)/INR and aPTT. Each institution should be using standardized 3.2%. Common tube sizes include 4.5, 2.7, or 1.8 mL. Neonates and infants have low blood volumes. Collecting large blood volumes can not only be unsafe for the patient, but also difficult because it takes longer for the blood to fill the tube leading to underfilled or clotted samples. If available, smaller volume collection tubes can alleviate these problems. Some tests require larger sample volumes (i.e., platelet aggregation testing) or extra sample volumes for lupus anticoagulant confirmatory testing. In these cases, samples are usually collected into syringes and then aliquoted into either commercial tubes or other in-house tubes or BD Vacutainers leading to more chances of improper filling and handling. Larger specimen tubes are more tolerant of variance of collection volume. Similar variance in collection may lead to specimen rejection when using smaller tubes.

Moreover, because children have much smaller veins than adults, smaller gauge needles are often recommended. For example, 19–21 gauge needles are recommended for adult blood collection to minimize hemolysis and sheer forces, but in pediatrics, 21–25 gauge, winged ("butterfly") needles are commonly used.

Collecting a proper coagulation sample from the pediatric population can be extremely challenging. Children may not understand why sample collection is necessary and they may be stressed, crying, restrained, or violent, resulting in activated, clotted, or improperly filled samples and/or falsely elevated acute phase reactant proteins. Falsely elevated VWF and FVIII levels can often result in a missed diagnosis of von Willebrand disease or hemophilia A due to falsely normal test results.

Neonates and infants have higher hematocrit levels compared to older children and adults. Patients with hematocrit >0.55 L/L require less anticoagulant in the collection tube and so special tubes need to be tailor-made for the patient's hematocrit level (see Chapter 4). The method of obtaining the blood sample from the child is extremely important in determining a representative test result. Many children have central venous or arterial catheters with a continuous infusion of low-dose unfractionated heparin (UFH) to maintain catheter patency. Studies in adults have demonstrated a failure to predict clearance of the UFH despite a discard blood sample prior to obtaining the test sample (see Chapter 4) resulting in an unreliable test result. If the central line from which the test sample was drawn contained UFH and was not adequately flushed to remove heparin, then the test affected by UFH becomes uninterpretable [33]. Even though manufacturers have sufficient heparin neutralizing agent in the reagent to inhibit up to 1 U/mL of heparin, caution is still necessary when performing PT/INR and antifactor Xa level in these specimens. Clotting factor assays are also problematic using specimens drawn from central catheters but may be reliable if two or more dilution points run parallel to the calibration line.

Due to the difficulty in obtaining blood samples in children, clinicians may attempt to persuade the laboratory to test samples that are improperly collected (blood sample insufficient, hematocrit slightly elevated, small clot in collection sample). However, the laboratory should not agree to this practice, because erroneous results would be reported in most cases.

Analytical variables

Samples should be tested promptly after collection and with minimal manipulation (see Chapter 5). Because the pediatric population comprises only a small percentage of global hemostasis testing, many companies do not tailor instruments for pediatric samples. If possible, samples should be tested in the original container (primary tube) without extra manipulation and to prevent possible contamination or mislabeling. Checking for clots before sample testing and aliquoting plasma can cause hemolysis and pre-activate the sample. Additionally, spinning the plasma off the cells is good practice and should not cause hemolysis unless some red cells are pipetted with the plasma. Also activation should not take place if all plastic surfaces are used. Small samples that are to be frozen for further analysis should be centrifuged twice to reduce platelets in the specimen.

Postanalytical variables

All test results are compared to a reference range and are dependent on effective quality control procedures that can be linked to each patient test. Whether the sample is classified as normal, slightly elevated, decreased, or critical is dependent on these reference ranges. If the ranges are not carefully calculated, it can lead to over- or underdiagnosis of certain conditions.

Global hemostasis parameters

Evaluation of hemostasis in the laboratory has been extrapolated from adult studies and, although similar, has not been well defined in the pediatric population. Global tests of hemostasis (e.g., thrombin generation or thromboelastography) have not been well characterized in children and are not currently used clinically. The activated clotting time (ACT) is a bedside test used primarily to monitor the UFH in adult and pediatric patients on extracorporeal devices. However, as in adults, the ACT correlates poorly with heparin concentration [34, 35].

The thromboelastogram uses activated whole blood to measure hemostasis (formation of a clot) as well as fibrinolysis (clot degradation). The most common devices used to measure thromboelastography are the ROTEM® (Pentafarm, Munich, Germany) and the TEG® (Hemonetics, Braintree, MA, USA). The application of thromboelastography in pediatric patients requires further evaluation.

Thrombophilia testing

Testing for thrombophilia is controversial in children. Highly thrombogenic yet rare abnormalities tested for include protein C, protein S, and antithrombin. As well, testing may be performed for the more common but less thrombogenic factor V Leiden and prothrombin gene 20210. Certain clinical scenarios, for example, aggressive thrombosis in an otherwise well child may lead to testing for antiphospholipid antibody (lupus anticoagulant and anticardiolipin antibody). Another abnormality that is tested for but for which less data regarding thrombogenicity exist is methylene tetrahydrofolate reductase (MTHFR).

When is thrombophilia testing indicated in children

Controversy exists in the pediatric literature and among experts as to when thrombophilia testing should be performed. Lack of longitudinal studies determining outcomes of children with thrombophilia has most certainly fostered this controversy. In addition, consequences of testing including financial cost, potential refusal of insurances (life, health, mortgage, etc.), and labeling patients as abnormal influence the decision to perform testing. Guidelines for determining when thrombophilic testing should be performed are individualized and have included the following. If the test results will have a direct impact on patient management then testing should be considered, such as antithrombin levels in a child who requires heparin therapy and is unable to achieve an anticoagulant effect as demonstrated by either aPTT or antifactor Xa level. In a child with purpura fulminans, testing for proteins C and S levels is appropriate as this clinical scenario is life threatening and treatable. In addition, a secondary thrombosis related to a particular disease entity such as nephrotic syndrome or low levels of protein C or S might influence patient management. In contrast, however, the utility of testing a child with thrombosis related to a central venous line is of no relevance to the immediate clinical management of the child. However, the central line thrombosis may be the result of thrombophilia that can be identified at a later date and/or discussed with the parents as to their preference of testing. Testing in a child who has a confirmed thrombosis is debatable and depends on the clinical setting. The family history of thrombosis in parents and siblings, if positive, can be very useful information to guide the clinician as to whether the child should be further investigated for thrombophilia.

Iatrogenic blood loss is a significant problem in children who are ill and testing for thrombophilia can require several specimens. In addition to using/designing assays that require minimal sample, the laboratory must also work with the clinicians and phlebotomists obtaining blood samples in children to test for thrombophilia to limit the amount of blood collected. In addition, the response time for the tests should not be excessive in order to provide clinical information important to the patient and clinician.

Monitoring currently administered anticoagulants

Currently, the most commonly administered anticoagulants in children are unfractionated heparin, low molecular weight heparin (LMWH), and vitamin K antagonists (VKAs). Laboratory monitoring of all of these agents is required to ensure optimal anticoagulation and minimize hemorrhagic or thrombotic complications. Each agent uses a specific laboratory test with a defined therapeutic range and minimizes bleeding and extension, recurrence, or development of thrombosis. The laboratory plays a unique important role in the management of children receiving anticoagulation by ensuring that the turnaround time for testing is rapid, whether the test is completed in the lab or sent to an outside lab for testing. Completion of the test and/or reporting of the result as quickly as possible will assist in providing optimal patient care.

Unfractionated heparin

The aPTT has been used in adults for a number of years to monitor UFH dosing and effect. In clinical scenarios where the aPTT may not be representative, for example, pregnancy, presence of antiphospholipid antibody, or high levels of FVIII, the heparin assay using the antifactor Xa method may be used. The more common measure of antifactor Xa uses a chromogenic test system with or without the addition of exogenous antithrombin with a therapeutic range of 0.3–0.7 U/mL corresponding to a therapeutic aPTT range (seconds). However, in children the age-appropriate aPTT baseline may be prolonged compared to adults and thus use of an adult therapeutic PTT range is not appropriate. Consequently, the use of heparin assay to monitor UFH has resulted in many centers. However, studies have demonstrated a poor correlation between aPTT and heparin concentration in children [36]. The actual therapeutic range of the aPTT in seconds depends on the responsiveness of the aPTT reagent.

Every hospital should determine their own aPTT therapeutic range for each lot of aPTT reagent using fresh or frozen samples from patients on unfractionated heparin therapy [37, 38] (see Chapter 22). In children, the heparin assay and the aPTT correlate even more poorly, possibly due to developmental differences, and the reference range used in adults for the aPTT (and the heparin assay) may not be appropriate for children. However, until properly designed clinical studies are completed determining the safety and efficacy of specific aPTT and heparin assay ranges for children receiving UFH, the adult ranges may be the only guide to managing UFH therapy. In the absence of evidence-based therapeutic aPTT and heparin assay ranges in children, the management of UFH using both the aPTT and heparin assay has resulted. The aPTT is impacted by many factors other than UFH (i.e., antiphospholipid antibody, elevated factor VIII levels) but may still be useful as part of a number of tests in managing children on UFH.

UFH potentiates antithrombin inhibition of all serine protease-activated coagulation factors but has the greatest inhibitory effect on factor Xa and thrombin. Monitoring antithrombin levels may be necessary when either larger doses than expected of UFH are required in a patient (1.5 × age-dependent doses) or there is an inability to achieve therapeutic heparin levels by either aPTT and/or heparin concentration.

The measured heparin concentration using the antifactor Xa-based assay depends upon the test system used. If the test system contains exogenous AT, the total amount of heparin that is available *in vivo* will be detected, which may not reflect the active amount of heparin *in vivo* that is complexing with the patient's antithrombin. This may occur if the antithrombin level is low *in vivo* and the antifactor Xa test system contains exogenous antithrombin; the measured antifactor Xa levels will appear to be within the therapeutic range, when in reality the patient may be sub-therapeutic. As a result, it is recommended that the antifactor Xa assay should be performed without the addition of exogenous antithrombin.

The consensus of the authors concerning the use of aPTT and/or heparin assay in managing children receiving UFH is as follows. If the aPTT and the heparin assay correspond, determined by performing both tests simultaneously in a child receiving UFH, then the health provider could continue titrating UFH using either test. The target heparin concentration using the antifactor Xa-based assay in children is suggested to be 0.35–0.7 U/mL which is slightly different than that for adults [39].

Low molecular weight heparin

The chemical or enzymatic alteration of unfractionated heparin (molecular weight 3–30 kDa; average 15 kDa) results in LMWH (molecular weight 2–9 kDa). LMWHs are most commonly used in infants and young children [40–47]. The use of LMWH compared with UFH has a number of advantages including subcutaneous administration, decreased immunogenicity, good bioavailability, and production of a more predictable anticoagulant response thus the requirement for less monitoring [48, 49]. Similar to UFH, the major anticoagulant action of LMWH results from the interaction of a unique pentasaccharide sequence with antithrombin causing antithrombin activation. A chain length of 18 saccharide units is necessary to bridge AT to thrombin as the first step in thrombin inactivation. In contrast, heparin chains of any length that contain the high-affinity pentasaccharide can catalyze activated factor X (FXa) inhibition by antithrombin. Two-thirds of LMWH fragments are smaller than 18 saccharide units. Consequently, LMWHs are unlike UFH in that they have reduced ability to inactivate thrombin as they bind simultaneously to antithrombin and thrombin much less efficiently [48]. As a result of this difference in composition, LMWH more specifically inactivates FXa resulting in variable prolongation of aPTT and necessitating measurement of the heparin concentration using antifactor Xa assay [48, 49]. Although the antifactor Xa-based heparin assay is recommended to monitor LMWH therapy in children, there are no properly designed clinical studies that correlate the levels with safety or efficacy. Current efficacy and safety data from case series or cohort studies using an antifactor Xa-based assay recommend a therapeutic range of 0.5–1.0 U/mL measured 4 hours after the second dose of LMWH which is administered every 12 hours [39] or at various age-appropriate time points for the LMWH, tinzaparin [39].

The mode of action of LMWH is similar to UFH and thus if large doses are required or the inability to achieve therapeutic heparin level occurs, the AT should be measured to ensure an adequate level.

Many children who require LMWH also require central venous catheters (CVCs) for their supportive care. Consequently, out of necessity, LMWH samples are often drawn from the CVC, resulting in more measurement challenges. Studies suggest a continuous infusion of low-dose UFH (1–3 U/mL infused at a rate of 1 mL/h) results in improved CVC patency and increased catheter indwell time [50–56]. As a result, many institutions infuse low-dose UFH through CVCs as standard of care. Since UFH influences the aPTT and the heparin level and LMWH has a minimal effect on the aPTT and influences the antifactor Xa-based heparin assay, blood samples to measure LMWH heparin levels drawn from CVCs may be artificially elevated by UFH contamination [57]. Consequently, LMWH dose changes based on UFH-contaminated CVC blood samples may result in inappropriate LMWH dose changes and adverse events. Measuring an aPTT in combination with a blood sample to measure LMWH level drawn from a CVC may identify UFH contamination and artificially elevated heparin levels.

Vitamin K antagonists

Warfarin, the most common VKA used in children for thromboprophylaxis, must be regularly monitored to avoid both thrombotic and bleeding complications and ensure safety and efficacy [29, 58–61]. Challenges with VKA therapy in children exist due to the presence of complex underlying health problems, receipt of multiple medications, having inconsistent nutritional intake, adherence, and the difficulties with phlebotomy [29, 62] that affect the level of anticoagulation and necessitate frequent monitoring. The gold standard method for monitoring VKA therapy is the PT testing of plasma collected via venipuncture and is expressed as the INR.

The INR was developed to help standardize the monitoring of VKA therapy among different PT methods. The calculation of the INR involves the International Sensitivity Index (ISI) of the reagent being used, the mean normal PT (MNPT), and the patient's PT:

$$INR = [(patient's\ PT)/(mean\ normal\ PT)]^{ISI}.$$

The ISI of reagents vary depending on how responsive the reagents are; the more responsive the reagent, the shorter the clotting time and the closer the ISI is to 1.0. Chest guidelines recommend using thromboplastins with an ISI range of 0.9–1.5 [63]. ISI validation and calibration should be performed if validation fails after a change in the lot of PT reagent and after all situations in which the PT, MNPT, and/or ISI can be affected [32]. For many labs in the United States, validation and calibration is still a challenge, because most manufacturers have not developed FDA-approved kits for this purpose. The possibility of using a direct INR curve with universal calibrants (calibrants that can be used for all/most instruments and reagents) would be ideal but are not currently on the horizon.

Laboratory monitoring of VKA requires a venipuncture sample from a child that may be impossible to obtain due to needle phobia and/or poor venous access. The use of point of care (POC) INR monitors has revolutionized VKA management in children with a capillary blood sample the only requirement to obtain an INR (see Chapter 14).

POC INR monitoring

POC INR monitors require a minimal blood sample volume, produce an INR result within 2–3 minutes, enable timely drug dosage adjustment, and prompt attention to critical values [64–68]. The POC INR monitor test can be performed at the patients' convenience and eliminates the need for the patient to visit the laboratory. This convenience facilitates more frequent INR testing, a requirement for children when illness is present or when there is a change in diet or medication [29, 58, 69]. For these reasons the use of POC INR monitors for INR measurement in children can be used as an option for improving oral VKA monitoring [29, 70–76].

The CoaguChek® POC INR system has generated the most published data in children. The INR is measured using 10 μL of whole blood obtained by finger prick that is easily applied to a test strip. The monitor has an embedded quality control (on board single-channel strip control) that tests the integrity of each single test strip while the test strip is being used for patient blood testing. Two levels of performance are evaluated. First, the amount of resazurin (resorufin), an oxidation/reduction inhibitor in the test area of each individual test strip, is quantified which corresponds with the quantity of all components in the formulation used for clot detection. Second, the strips integrated quality control function quantifies the amount of by-product resorufin it utilized to assess for incorrectly handled/stored test strips. The calibration concept of the new CoaguChek XS® system is in agreement with the "WHO guidelines for thromboplastins and plasmas used to control anticoagulant therapy" [77]. The manufacturer uses a master lot of test strips that is directly calibrated by comparison with international reference preparations (IRP) and represents the manufacturer's working standard. Further calibration in routine manufacturing of test strips is performed versus this master lot using whole blood samples from patients on oral anticoagulation and from normal donors. The mean ISI for the CoaguChek XS® PT test is 1.01 [78]. The monitor uses an amperometric (electrochemical) method to monitor blood clotting induced by thromboplastin within the test strip to determine the PT. The PT is then converted to an INR using the ISI previously determined and encoded on the chip for each lot of test strips. This meter has been evaluated in adults with favorable results [79, 80].

The average the CoaguChek XS® INR compared with a laboratory INR, if drawn at the same time, was on average 0.1 INR units lower than the laboratory INR. Ninety five percent of differences between the two methods fell within the range of −0.2 to 0.4 INR units [67]. Within meter calibration 91% of INR pairs fell within 0.3 units of each other, demonstrating good precision—further evidence of strong agreement between the two methods.

How often differences between the POC and laboratory INR will result in differing warfarin management decision is important clinically. Standard definitions for clinical agreement of INR tests exist and include expanded and narrow agreements [67].

Ensuring POC users have learned and demonstrated accurate testing technique may positively influence CoaguChek XS®–laboratory INR result concordance. User proficiency in testing technique improves the level of agreement between POC INR results generated at home compared with the laboratory INR [66, 67]. Documentation of competency in the laboratory and the POC is equally important. Performing and documenting competency is more frequently overlooked or done poorly with the POC and can result in erroneous test results exposing patients to serious adverse events, for example, hemorrhage or thrombosis.

New anticoagulants in children

There are new anticoagulant agents, parenteral and oral, that have been approved in adults and are being administered/or being considered for use in children. These agents can be classified according to their mechanism of action, that is, antifactor Xa (e.g., fondaparinux, rivaroxaban) or anti-IIa (e.g., dabigatran) agents. Testing these agents in proper clinical trials in children will be important as drug metabolism may be different and thus impact on efficacy and safety. Currently, there are a number of international investigational programs underway in children to determine pharmacokinetics, pharmacodynamics, and safety and efficacy of these agents. Laboratory monitoring of these agents in adults has demonstrated challenges in determining laboratory testing that results in accurate levels (see Chapter 24).

Agents that may currently be administered in children include the following. Fondaparinux is a pentasaccharide that functions like heparin. It inhibits factor Xa and relies on antithrombin levels. Monitoring blood levels using an antifactor Xa-based assay must be performed using a test system that includes a fondaparinux calibrator. In addition, rivaroxaban, apixaban, and edoxaban are oral factor Xa inhibitors [81] which do not require a cofactor. Monitoring of these agents is, at present, rarely performed in adults as testing methods have not yet been developed. However, test methods are being developed in order to monitor patients with complications such as bleeding and determine drug effect and concentration. Bivalirudin and dabigatran are inhibitors of factor IIa (direct thrombin inhibitor) that do not require a cofactor. Optimal monitoring of these agents is currently controversial with some centers using the aPTT, while the literature recommends an ecarin clotting time, an assay that is not available in most clinical laboratories.

Conclusion

Normal hemostasis in children is age related and differs from adults. Reference intervals for the premature infant and the different age groups of children are vital to correctly diagnose and manage thrombosis and hemostasis in newborns and children. These differences often lead to increased sample handling and time to lab test evaluation. The laboratory plays an extremely important role in hemostatic testing in children. Their knowledge about the challenges in pediatrics and liaison with the health provider will ensure the best care for children requiring hemostatic testing or management of anticoagulation.

References

1. Sacco RL, Adams R, Albers G, et al. Guidelines for prevention of stroke in patients with ischemic stroke or transient ischemic attack: a statement for healthcare professionals from the American Heart Association/American Stroke Association Council on Stroke: co-sponsored by the Council on Cardiovascular Radiology and Intervention: the American Academy of Neurology affirms the value of this guideline. *Circulation*. 2006;113(10):e409–e449.

2. Ignarro LJ, Buga GM, Wood KS, Byrns RE, Chaudhuri G. Endothelium-derived relaxing factor produced and released from artery and vein is nitric oxide. *Proc Natl Acad Sci U S A*. 1987;84(24):9265–9269.

3. Palmer RMJ, Ferrige AG, Moncada S. Nitric oxide release accounts for the biological activity of endothelium-derived relaxing factor. *Nature*. 1987;327(6122):524–526.

4. Marcus AJ, Broekman MJ, Pinsky DJ. COX inhibitors and thromboregulation. *New Engl J Med*. 2002;347(13):1025–1026.

5. Marcus AJ, Broekman MJ, Drosopoulos JHF, et al. Role of CD39 (NTPDase-1) in thromboregulation, cerebroprotection, and cardioprotection. *Semin Thromb Hemost*. 2005;31(2):234–246.

6. Dubois C, Panicot-Dubois L, Gainor JF, Furie BC, Furie B. Thrombin-initiated platelet activation in vivo is vWF independent during thrombus formation in a laser injury model. *J Clin Investig*. 2007;117(4):953–960.

7. Mangin P, Yap CL, Nonne C, et al. Thrombin overcomes the thrombosis defect associated with platelet GPVI/FcRγ deficiency. *Blood*. 2006;107(11):4346–4353.

8. Ruggeri ZM. Old concepts and new developments in the study of platelet aggregation. *J Clin Investig*. 2000;105(6):699–701.

9. Bergmeier W, Piffath CL, Goerge T, et al. The role of platelet adhesion receptor GPIbα far exceeds that of its main ligand, von Willebrand factor, in arterial thrombosis. *Proc Natl Acad Sci U S A*. 2006;103(45):16900–16905.

10. Massberg S, Gawaz M, Grüner S, et al. A crucial role of glycoprotein VI for platelet recruitment to the injured arterial wall in vivo. *J Exp Med*. 2003;197(1):41–49.

11. Holtkötter O, Nieswandt B, Smyth N, et al. Integrin α2-deficient mice develop normally, are fertile, but display partially defective platelet interaction with collagen. *J Biol Chem*. 2002;277(13):10789–10794.

12. Nieswandt B, Brakebusch C, Bergmeier W, et al. Glycoprotein VI but not α2β1 integrin is essential for platelet interaction with collagen. *EMBO J*. 2001;20(9):2120–2130.

13. Falati S, Liu Q, Gross P, et al. Accumulation of tissue factor into developing thrombi in vivo is dependent upon microparticle P-selectin glycoprotein ligand 1 and platelet P-selectin. *J Exp Med*. 2003;197(11):1585–1598.

14. Giesen PLA, Rauch U, Bohrmann B, et al. Blood-borne tissue factor: another view of thrombosis. *Proc Natl Acad Sci U S A*. 1999;96(5):2311–2315.

15. Bach R, Rifkin DB. Expression of tissue factor procoagulant activity: regulation by cytosolic calcium. *Proc Natl Acad Sci U S A*. 1990;87(18):6995–6999.

16. Maynard JR, Heckman CA, Pitlick FA, Nemerson Y. Association of tissue factor activity with the surface of cultured cells. *J Clin Investig*. 1975;55(4):814–824.

17. Becker RC. Cell-based models of coagulation: a paradigm in evolution. *J Thromb Thrombolysis*. 2005;20(1):65–68.

18. Stegner D, Nieswandt B. Platelet receptor signaling in thrombus formation. *J Mol Med*. 89(2):109–121.

19. Burgess JK, Hotchkiss KA, Suter C, et al. Physical proximity and functional association of glycoprotein 1bα and protein-disulfide isomerase on the platelet plasma membrane. *J Biol Chem*. 2000;275(13):9758–9766.

20. Chen VM, Hogg PJ. Allosteric disulfide bonds in thrombosis and thrombolysis. *J Thromb Haemost*. 2006;4(12):2533–2541.

21. Essex DW, Li M, Miller A, Feinman RD. Protein disulfide isomerase and sulfhydryl-dependent pathways in platelet activation. *Biochemistry*. 2001;40(20):6070–6075.

22. Du X, Gu M, Weisel JW, et al. Long range propagation of conformational changes in integrin αIIbβ. *J Biol Chem*. 1993;268(31):23087–23092.

23. Andrew M, Vegh P, Johnston M, Bowker J, Ofosu F, Mitchell L. Maturation of the hemostatic system during childhood. *Blood*. 1992;80(8):1998–2005.

24. Massicotte P, Leaker M, Marzinotto V, et al. Enhanced thrombin regulation during warfarin therapy in children compared to adults. *Thromb Haemost*. 1998;80(4):570–574.

25. Abstracts of the XXII Congress of the International Society of Thrombosis and Haemostasis. Boston, Massachusetts, USA. July 11–16, 2009. *J Thromb Haemost*. 2009;7:1261–1268.

26. Andrew M, Massicotte-Nolan PM, Karpatkin M. Plasma protease inhibitors in premature infants: influence of gestational age, postnatal age, and health status. *Proc Soc Exp Biol Med*. 1983;173(4):495–500.

27. Andrew M, Paes B, Milner R. Development of the human coagulation system in the full-term infant. *Blood*. 1987;70(1):165–172.

28. Andrew M, Paes B, Milner R, et al. Development of the human coagulation system in the healthy premature infant. *Blood*. 1988;72(5):1651–1657.

29. Monagle P, Barnes C, Ignjatovic V, et al. Developmental haemostasis. Impact for clinical haemostasis laboratories. *Thromb Haemost*. 2006;95(2):362–372.

30. Monagle P, Ignjatovic V, Savoia H. Hemostasis in neonates and children: pitfalls and dilemmas. *Blood Rev*. 2011;24(2):63–68.

31. Massicotte MP, Sofronas M, deVeber G. Difficulties in performing clinical trials of antithrombotic therapy in neonates and children. *Thromb Res*. 2006;118(1):153–163.

32. Adcock DM, Hoefner DM, Kottke-Marchant K, Marlar RA, Szamosi DI, Waruanek DJ. *Collection, Transport and Processing of Blood Specimens for Testing Plasma-Based Coagulation Assays and Molecular Hemostasis Assays: Approved Guideline*. 5th ed. Wayne, PA: Clinical and Laboratory Standards Institute; CLSI document H21-A5; 2008.

33. Bauman ME, Belletrutti M, Bauman ML, Massicotte MP. Central venous catheter sampling of low molecular heparin levels: an approach to increasing result reliability. *Pediatr Crit Care Med*. 2012;13(1):1–5.

34. Green TP, Isham-Schopf B, Steinhorn RH, Smith C, Irmiter RJ. Whole blood activated clotting time in infants during extracorporeal membrane oxygenation. *Crit Care Med*. 1990;18(5):494–498.

35. Nankervis CA, Preston TJ, Dysart KC, et al. Assessing heparin dosing in neonates on venoarterial extracorporeal membrane oxygenation. *ASAIO J*. 2007;53(1):111–114.

36. Newall F, Johnston L, Ignjatovic V, Monagle P. Unfractionated heparin therapy in infants and children. *Pediatrics*. 2009;123(3):e510–e518.

37. Brill-Edwards P, Ginsberg JS, Johnston M, Hirsh J. Establishing a therapeutic range for heparin therapy. *Ann Intern Med*. 1993;119(2):104–109.

38. Gausman JN, Marlar RA. Inaccuracy of a "spiked curve" for monitoring unfractionated heparin therapy. *Am J Clin Pathol*. 2011;135(6):870–876.

39. Monagle P, Chan AKC, Goldenberg NA, et al. Antithrombotic therapy in neonates and children: antithrombotic therapy and prevention of thrombosis, 9th ed: American College of Chest Physicians Evidence-Based Clinical Practice Guidelines. *Chest*. 2012;141(2 suppl):e737S–e801S.

40. Dix D, Andrew M, Marzinotto V, et al. The use of low molecular weight heparin in pediatric patients: a prospective cohort study. *J Pediatr*. 2000;136(4):439–445.

41. Massicotte P, Julian JA, Gent M, et al. An open-label randomized controlled trial of low molecular weight heparin compared to heparin and coumadin for the treatment of venous thromboembolic events in children: the REVIVE trial. *Thromb Res*. 2003;109(2-3):85–92.

42. Verso M, Agnelli G, Bertoglio S, et al. Enoxaparin for the prevention of venous thromboembolism associated with central vein catheter: a double-blind, placebo-controlled, randomized study in cancer patients [see comment]. *J Clin Oncol*. 2005;23(18):4057–4062.

43. Albisetti M, Andrew M. Low molecular weight heparin in children. *Eur J Pediatr*. 2002;161(2):71–77.

44. Michaels LA, Gurian M, Hegyi T, Drachtman RA. Low molecular weight heparin in the treatment of venous and arterial thromboses in the premature infant. *Pediatrics*. 2004;114(3):703–707.

45. Kuhle S, Massicotte P, Dinyari M, et al. Dose-finding and pharmacokinetics of therapeutic doses of tinzaparin in pediatric patients with thromboembolic events. *Thromb Haemost*. 2005;94(6):1164–1171.

46. Bauman M, Belletrutti M, Bajzar L, et al. Evaluation of enoxaparin dosing requirements in infants and children. Better dosing to achieve therapeutic levels. *Thromb Haemost*. 2009;101(1):86–92.

47. Bauman ME, Black KL, Bauman ML, Belletrutti M, Bajzar L, Massicotte MP. Novel uses of insulin syringes to reduce dosing errors: a retrospective chart review of enoxaparin whole milligram dosing. *Thromb Res*. 2009;123(6):845–847.

48. Hirsh J, Warkentin TE, Shaughnessy SG, et al. Heparin and low-molecular-weight heparin: mechanisms of action, pharmacokinetics, dosing, monitoring, efficacy, and safety. *Chest*. 2001;119(1 suppl):64S–94S.

49. Hirsh J, Bauer KA, Donati MB, Gould M, Samama MM, Weitz JI. Parenteral anticoagulants: American College of Chest Physicians Evidence-Based Clinical Practice Guidelines (8th edition). *Chest*. 2008;133(6 suppl):141S–159S.

50. Martinon-Torres F, Rodriguez Nunez A, Pekorikova J, Martinon-Sanchez JM. Is heparin daily flushing useful

to decrease the incidence of catheter-related infections? *Chest.* 1998;114(5):1498–1499.

51. Timsit JF, Farkas JC, Boyer JM, et al. Central vein catheter-related thrombosis in intensive care patients: incidence, risks factors, and relationship with catheter-related sepsis. *Chest.* 1998;114(1):207–213.

52. Delva R, Gamelin E, Lortholary A, et al. Suppression of heparinization of central venous catheters between cycles of chemotherapy: results of a phase I study. *Support Care Cancer.* 1998;6(4):384–388.

53. Randolph AG, Cook DJ, Gonzales CA, Andrew M. Review: Heparin reduces central venous and pulmonary artery catheter clots. *Evid Based Med.* 1998;3(4): 111.

54. Mudge B, Forcier D, Slattery MJ. Patency of 24-gauge peripheral intermittent infusion devices: a comparison of heparin and saline flush solutions. *Pediatr Nurs.* 1998;24(2):142–145, 149.

55. Randolph AG, Cook DJ, Gonzalez CA, Andrew M. Benefit of heparin in central venous and pulmonary artery catheters: a meta-analysis of randomized controlled trials. *Chest.* 1998;113(1):165–171.

56. Keller EG, DeFazio J, Jencks F, Steiner M, Rogers J, Ritchey AK. The use of heparinase to neutralize residual heparin in blood samples drawn through pediatric indwelling central venous catheters. *J Pediatr.* 1998;132(1):165–167.

57. Hirsh J, Guyatt G, Albers GW, Harrington R, Schünemann HJ. Executive summary: American College of Chest Physicians Evidence-Based Clinical Practice Guidelines (8th edition). *Chest.* 2008;133(6 suppl):71S–109S.

58. Streif W, Andrew M, Marzinotto V, et al. Analysis of warfarin therapy in pediatric patients: a prospective cohort study of 319 patients. *Blood.* 1999;94(9):3007–3014.

59. Andrew M, Marzinotto V, Brooker LA, et al. Oral anticoagulation therapy in pediatric patients: a prospective study. *Thromb Haemost.* 1994;71(3):265–269.

60. Errichetti AM, Holden A, Ansell J. Management of oral anticoagulant therapy. Experience with an anticoagulation clinic. *Arch Intern Med.* 1984;144(10):1966–1968.

61. Michelson AD, Bovill E, Monagle P, Andrew M. Antithrombotic therapy in children. *Chest.* 1998;114 (5 suppl):748S–769S.

62. Hamilton JG. Needle phobia: a neglected diagnosis. [see comment]. *J Fam Pract.* 1995;41(2):169–175.

63. Monagle P, Chan A, Massicotte P, Chalmers E, Michelson AD. Antithrombotic therapy in neonates and children: the Eighth ACCP Conference on Antithrombotic and Thrombolytic Therapy. *Chest.* 2008;133(6 suppl):645S–687S.

64. Bauman M, Conroy S, Massicotte M. Point of care INR measurement in children: what has been evaluated and future directions. *Ped Health.* 2008;2(5):651–659.

65. Bauman ME, Black K, Bauman ML, et al. EMPoWarMENT: Edmonton pediatric warfarin self-management pilot study in children with primarily cardiac disease. *Thromb Res.* 2010;126(2):e110–e115.

66. Bauman ME, Black K, Kuhle S, et al. Kidclot©: the importance of validated educational intervention for optimal long term warfarin management in children. *Thromb Res.* 2009;123(5):707–709.

67. Bauman ME, Black KL, Massicotte MP, et al. Accuracy of the CoaguChek XS for point-of-care international normalized ratio (INR) measurement in children requiring warfarin. *Thromb Haemost.* 2008;99(6):1097–1103.

68. Bauman ME, Conroy S, Massicotte MP. Point-of-care INR measurement in children requiring warfarin: what has been evaluated and future directions. *Ped Health.* 2008;2(5):651–659.

69. Newall F M.B. Point-of-care monitoring of anticoagulant therapy in paediatric patients. *Progr Pediatr Cardiol.* 2005;21(1):53–61.

70. Reiss N, Blanz U, Breymann T, Kind K, Bairaktaris A, Korfer R. Mechanical valve replacement of the systemic atrioventricular valve in children. *ASAIO J.* 2006;52(5):559–561.

71. Christensen TD. Self-management of oral anticoagulant therapy: a review. *J Thromb Thrombolysis.* 2004;18(2):127–143.

72. Christensen TD, Attermann J, Hjortdal VE, Maegaard M, Hasenkam JM. Self-management of oral anticoagulation in children with congenital heart disease. *Cardiol Young.* 2001;11(3):269–276.

73. Mahonen S, Riikonen P, Vaatainen RL, Tikanoja T. Oral anticoagulant treatment in children based on monitoring at home. *Acta Paediatr.* 2004;93(5):687–691.

74. Massicotte P, Marzinotto V, Vegh P, Adams M, Andrew M. Home monitoring of warfarin therapy in children with a whole blood prothrombin time monitor. *J Pediatr.* 1995;127(3):389–394.

75. Nowatzke W, Landt M, Smith C, Wilhite T, Canter C, Luchtman-Jones L. Whole blood international normalization ratio measurements in children using near-patient monitors. *J Pediatr Hematol/Oncol.* 2003;25(1):33–37.

76. Gunther T, Mazzitelli D, Schreiber C, et al. Mitral-valve replacement in children under 6 years of age. *Eur J Cardiothorac Surg.* 2000;17(4):426–430.

77. WHO. Guidelines for thromboplastins and plasmas used to control anticoagulant therapy. Technical Report Series. 1999.

78. Kitchen S, Unkrig V. Evaluation of the CoaguChek XS System. International Evaluation Workshop. Heidelberg, Germany; 2005.

79. Braun S, Watzke H, Hasenkam JM, et al. Performance evaluation of the new CoaguChek XS system compared with the established CoaguChek system by patients experienced in INR-self management. *Thromb Haemost.* 2007;97(2):310–314.

80. Leichsenring I, Plesch W, Unkrig V, et al. Multicentre ISI assignment and calibration of the INR measuring range of a new point-of-care system designed for home monitoring of oral anticoagulation therapy. *Thromb Haemost.* 2007;97(5):856–861.

81. Young G. New anticoagulants in children: a review of recent studies and a look to the future. *Thromb Res.* 2011;127(2):70–74.

PART 2

Quality in Coagulation Testing

Initial evaluation of hemostasis: reagent and method selection

Wayne L. Chandler

Coagulation Laboratory, Department of Pathology and Genomic Medicine, The Methodist Hospital Physician Organization, Houston, TX, USA

Introduction

The initial evaluation of hemostasis occurs in several situations including evaluation of patients that are bleeding, prior to invasive procedures and before starting antithrombotic medications. In these situations the initial assays used to assess hemostasis are selected to determine whether the patient has any evidence of a clinically significant acquired or hereditary deficiency of coagulation factors or platelets. The initial evaluation often includes measurement of the prothrombin time (PT), activated partial thromboplastin time (aPTT), fibrinogen, thrombin time, and platelet count. Whole blood viscoelastic assays have been developed for the rapid evaluation of hemostasis during surgery. This chapter focuses on the selection and evaluation of instruments and reagents for the PT, aPTT, fibrinogen, thrombin time, and viscoelastic assays.

In general there are two classes of instruments for determining PT and aPTT, manual analyzers for point of care or small laboratory use and automated or semi-automated analyzers for larger laboratories. Several different point-of-care analyzers are available for determining the PT, typically for oral anticoagulant monitoring. This chapter discusses the selection of assays based on citrate anticoagulated plasma or whole blood (viscoelastic assays) using clot-endpoint methods; other types of methods will not be discussed further.

Instrument selection

The first step in selecting a test methodology is determining what clinical questions the test will help answer and how the test will be utilized. Table 9.1 summarizes a number of questions related to hemostasis instrument selection. A test that is only run on day shift without the option for stat requests might use a batch analyzer methodology while a test that will run 24 hours per day with stat testing would be handled better on a sequential analyzer with stat interrupt capability. If more than one type of test is typically ordered at the same time, an analyzer that can do all the testing on a single platform may be best. Some analyzers are designed primarily to perform routine tests like the PT, aPTT, and fibrinogen, while others can be used for routine and more specialized assays like factor activity. Another important consideration is the assay types that will be needed including clot-based assays, chromogenic assays, and antigenic assays. Some instruments are capable of performing all three types simultaneously. The types of panels offered and the desired turnaround times will help determine the type of instrument required. For clot-based assays like the PT and aPTT, it is important to understand the mechanism of clot detection on the instrument (optical, mechanical, other) and potential sample interference problems that may affect the results such as sample hemolysis, icterus, or lipemia.

Quality in Laboratory Hemostasis and Thrombosis, Second Edition. Edited by Steve Kitchen, John D. Olson and F. Eric Preston.
© 2013 John Wiley & Sons, Ltd. Published 2013 by Blackwell Publishing Ltd.

Table 9.1 Considerations for new instrument selection

- Will the test be offered 24 hours per day?
- What is the anticipated test volume?
- Will the test be offered stat? If so what is the anticipated stat volume?
- What is the minimum sample volume anticipated for pediatric or other patients?
- What is the most common panel of tests that will be ordered? Can they all be done on the same instrument?
- What types of hemostasis testing are anticipated: clot-based, chromogenic, antigenic?
- How many samples and reagents will the instrument hold?
- Does the instrument utilize barcoded reagents?
- What sample preparation is required?
- How many samples are processed per hour, how many reaction cuvettes does the instrument hold, how many tests can be run prior to operator intervention?

There are other parameters to consider before selecting an instrument. Most modern instruments should be able to read barcoded samples and be interfaced to the laboratory information system reducing the chance for specimen identification and result reporting errors. After centrifugation, some instruments directly sample through the cap into the tube, other instruments require the cap be removed, while still others require the plasma be removed from the cells and put in another aliquot container that is put on the instrument. It is useful to know how many different tests the instrument can be set up to run and whether it can run tests from other manufacturers. Display, storage, and recall of calibration curves and quality control data should be reviewed. The rate of sample processing may be important in high-volume situations. Speed may vary with the assay type depending on the number of reagents needed for each assay. This in turn may depend on the number of sampling probes the instrument uses. Instruments with only a single probe used to pipette plasma and all reagents may be slower than instruments with multiple probes. Throughput on an analyzer may also depend on other factors including the number of reaction cuvettes the instrument can store on board, waste capacity, and so on. This may determine the number of assays the instrument can perform prior to operator intervention. Other sample parameters include the number of

samples that can be stored on the instrument, storage temperature and stability, minimum sample volume needed, and sample dead volume that cannot be utilized. Reagent parameters may be an important consideration including the number of different reagents and controls that can be stored on the instrument as well as the storage temperature and stability of the reagents. This is particularly important for reagents used for the PT and aPTT that may stay on the instrument 24 hours per day. When evaluating reagent usage it may be important to know the minimum reagent volume the instrument can use and dead volume the instrument cannot utilize. Most instruments can now read bar codes on the reagent vials with details of reagent type, lot number, expiration date, and other parameters to help reduce errors when placing new reagents on the instrument. This may only be available for reagents made by the same vendor as the instrument.

Evaluation of the method

For PT, aPTT, fibrinogen, and thrombin time assays, most instruments are sold in combination with coagulation reagents intended for use on that instrument. When selecting a methodology, a specific instrument–reagent combination is typically evaluated. Some companies offer several different versions of PT and aPTT reagents for their instruments. Some may choose to use only reagents from the same vendor as the instrument while others may choose to use a reagent from one company on an instrument from another company. Some instrument–reagent combinations may have disadvantages including lack of support if there are problems, inability to read bar codes between companies, and so on. Another consideration for laboratories that must meet regulatory and/or accreditation standards that require external proficiency testing is the lack of a peer group if the method is not used by many other laboratories, necessitating the development of an alternative assessment for the method.

A number of different organizations, including the Clinical and Laboratory Standards Institute (CLSI), provide protocols for evaluation of clinical laboratory tests [1]. The goal of the following sections is to provide overviews of method selection for initial assessment of hemostasis applicable to all clinical laboratories, but they are not intended to cover all the specific details found in evaluation or regulatory protocols from different countries. Each section is designed to provide a detailed review of method (instrument–reagent) selection for a given test followed at the end of the section by a summary of the minimum evaluation steps that are recommended.

Prothrombin time method selection

The principal uses for the PT assay include monitoring of vitamin K antagonist (VKA) therapy, evaluation of liver function, and the initial evaluation of hemostasis prior to surgery in patients with active bleeding or a prior history of bleeding. Typically the same PT reagent is used for all of these purposes. For VKA monitoring the PT result is typically converted to an international normalized ratio (INR). Details regarding monitoring of VKA can be found later in this book (Chapter 23).

The PT assay consists of combining citrated plasma with tissue factor, phospholipids, and calcium followed by detection of the clotting time using turbidometric (optical), nephelometric (optical), mechanical clot detection, or other methods. The two most common sources of tissue factor are rabbit brain and human recombinant preparations. To reduce interference from heparin, PT reagents often contain a heparin-neutralizing agent such as polybrene. The major differences among PT reagents are their analytic sensitivity to deficiencies of coagulation factors II, V, VII, X, and fibrinogen. Highly sensitive PT reagents prolong more for the same level of factor deficiency than low-sensitivity reagents. This is quantified to some extent for PT reagents used to calculate the INR by the International Sensitivity Index (ISI). A low ISI near 1 indicates a PT reagent with high sensitivity to factor deficiency. In general, PT reagents with a high ISI value (2 and greater) show higher levels of imprecision for the INR. It is recommended to use a lower ISI reagent to improve INR reproducibility. The current recommendation is to use an ISI of 0.9–1.7 [2]. An ISI of 1 or less can result in poor precision at INRs of 5 or above. Thus, the optimal ISI may be in the range of 1.3–1.6.

The initial evaluation of any new PT instrument–reagent combination should include the assessment of within-run and between-run imprecisions at normal and prolonged values, stability of the reagent on the instrument, and stability of the sample at room temperature and 4°C with respect to the PT. Imprecision for the PT assay should meet or exceed the manufacturer's specifications for the instrument–reagent combination. Modern automated instruments should show a between-run coefficient of variation less than 5% for the PT assay. It is useful to determine the shortest and longest PT values the instrument can produce and what the reportable range of the assay will be. Depending on the clinical setting it is also important to determine whether a critical value or cutoff will be used to alert clinicians to dangerously prolonged PT results.

If a new PT assay is being selected or a new lot of reagent evaluated it should be compared to the current assay across a wide range of possible values and patient types including patients on VKA. Both the PT and INR values should be compared among methods. Due to differences in the sensitivity of reagents (different ISI), it is possible that PT values may show a substantial bias between methods, but should still be highly correlated. In contrast, the INR between methods should show high correlation and little or no bias.

In some laboratories the INR is calculated by the instrument, which passes the INR value on to the laboratory information system. Another option commonly used is for the instrument to pass the PT result to the laboratory information system, which then calculates the INR. Whenever the PT reagent or method is changed it is important to verify that the INR is being correctly calculated and displayed in the instrument, the laboratory information system, and downstream electronic medical record systems. Sources of error include the equation used to calculate the INR and the values for the geometric mean normal PT and the ISI used in the calculation. It is critical to good patient care to trace an initial PT and INR result produced in the laboratory and see that it is faithfully reproduced in all downstream systems.

When evaluating possible coagulation factor deficiencies there are three common clinical situations: single factor deficiency (either acquired or hereditary), vitamin K-dependent factor deficiency (loss of factors II, VII, and X in the PT reaction), and all factor deficiency seen in bleeding patients. The more factors that are deficient, the greater the prolongation of the PT. For example, a PT reagent with an ISI of 1.3 gave a clotting time of 16 seconds when only factor VII was reduced to 0.3 U/mL of normal while all other factors were normal, compared to 21 seconds when factors

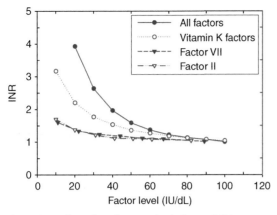

Figure 9.1 Effect of single- or multiple-factor deficiency on the PT/INR. The PT reagent used had an ISI of 1.3. Plasma samples with varying degrees of factor II, factor VII, vitamin K-dependent factor, or all factor deficiency were prepared by mixing pooled normal plasma with plasma deficient in the appropriate factor or factors.

Table 9.2 Factors potentially affecting the prothrombin time (PT) assay

- Coagulation factors II, V, VII, X, and fibrinogen deficiency
- Direct thrombin inhibitors, unfractionated heparin, low molecular weight heparin, heparinoids, pentasaccharides, and other anti-thrombotic medications
- Clotted sample
- Hemolyzed sample
- Over- or underfilled sample tube
- Lupus anticoagulants
- Recombinant human factor VIIa
- Daptomycin therapy

II, VII, and X were at 0.3 U/mL, versus 29 seconds when all factors were reduced to 0.3 U/mL of normal (Figure 9.1). How the PT assay will be used in a particular institution may determine how important it is to know the sensitivity of the assay to different types of factor deficiency. If the PT is only being used for VKA monitoring then knowledge of sensitivity to individual factors may not be needed. If the test is being used as an initial assay for unknown factor deficiency, or to assess factor deficiency in massively bleeding patients, knowledge of sensitivity to different forms of factor deficiency may be useful.

Strictly speaking the INR calculation is only calibrated for patients on stable VKA therapy and was only intended for VKA monitoring. Some groups have suggested that the INR should only be used for VKA monitoring, unless an alternate calibration is used, for example, in patients with chronic liver disease [3]. The reality of everyday laboratory practice is that it is difficult, if not impossible, to determine which PT orders are from patients on stable VKA therapy. The INR is calculated on every PT in most institutions and in many laboratories only the INR is reported on all PT samples. The INR is currently used in many different ways in the literature including as a cutoff for factor deficiency and fresh frozen plasma transfusion. How the INR is used clinically is still under discussion.

Table 9.2 shows a list of conditions that may potentially affect the PT result. Most PT reagents are relatively insensitive to unfractionated heparin due to the nature of the PT assay and inclusion of heparin-neutralizing agents in many PT formulations. The PT assay is typically even less sensitive to low molecular weight heparin, heparinoids, and pentasaccharides. While this is true, it is useful to know what heparin concentration prolongs the PT assay as this can occur if the assay is contaminated with concentrated heparin [2]. Likewise most PT reagents are relatively insensitive to lupus anticoagulants, but this varies with reagent. It is important to know how sensitive the PT reagent is to clotted or hemolyzed samples. Some instrument–reagent PT combinations are relatively insensitive to hemolysis [4, 5] while others may be more sensitive [6].

In samples that are preactivated before testing, often due to inadequate mixing of blood and citrate anticoagulant during blood draw, the PT may show slightly shorter results than in a properly collected sample [5]. Clotting in the tube may be identified from fibrin strands or visible clots. Modest underfilling of the 3.2% citrate sample tubes may have little effect on some PT reagents, but this needs to be carefully evaluated before any over- or underfilled tube is accepted [7]. A number of other medications may affect the PT including prolongations due to direct thrombin inhibitors like lepirudin, argatroban, bivalirudin, and oral agents like dabigatran [8]. Different PT reagents show highly variable results in response to new oral direct anti-Xa inhibitors like apixaban and rivaroxiban [9, 10]. PT results may be shortened due to recombinant human factor VIIa therapy.

Minimum evaluation, prothrombin time

Assuming an INR will be calculated with the PT result, the minimum assessment of a new PT instrument–reagent combination includes the determination of the geometric mean normal PT for INR calculations; PT and INR comparison with the current method; determination or validation of the reference interval; within-run and between-run imprecisions at normal and prolonged values; analytical measurement range (particularly the upper limit); and sample and reagent stability.

Activated partial thromboplastin time method selection

Whereas the PT assay is primarily used to assess coagulation factor levels, the aPTT has many uses including assessing coagulation factor levels, monitoring antithrombotic agents like heparin and direct thrombin inhibitors, and detecting lupus inhibitors. No standardization comparable to the INR is available for the aPTT, so each aPTT instrument–reagent combination potentially has different abilities related to these different uses. The aPTT is a two-stage assay using two reagents. The first reagent is an activator composed of phospholipids (partial thromboplastin) and a negatively charged substance like ground glass or kaolin to activate the contact system and form factor XIIa. The first reagent is added to citrate anticoagulated plasma and incubated for several minutes at 37°C, followed by the addition of a calcium solution that allows coagulation system activation by factor XIIa to proceed.

The initial evaluation of any new aPTT instrument–reagent combination should include the assessment of within-run and between-run imprecisions at normal and prolonged values, stability of the reagent on the instrument, and stability of the aPTT in the sample at room temperature and 4°C. An important separate consideration for the aPTT is the stability of heparinized aPTT samples. Activated platelets can release platelet factor 4 that reacts with and neutralizes heparin. If citrate anticoagulated plasma is not removed from the platelets, the heparin level in the sample can fall over time giving falsely reduced aPTT results. Imprecision for the aPTT assay should meet or exceed the manufacturer's specifications for the instrument–reagent combination. Modern automated instruments should show a between-run coefficient of variation

less than 5% for the aPTT assay. If a new aPTT assay is being selected or a new lot of reagent evaluated it should be compared to the current assay across a wide range of possible values and patient types, including patients with lupus inhibitors and patients on warfarin, heparin, and other antithrombotic agents.

The composition of the aPTT reagent may show different analytic sensitivity to deficiencies of coagulation factors II, V, VIII, IX, X, XI, and fibrinogen. In particular, different reagents can show substantial differences in sensitivity to factors VIII and IX [11–13]. Like PT reagents, the more factors that are deficient, the greater the prolongation of the aPTT will be. For example, an aPTT reagent with a mean normal value of 30 seconds gave a clotting time of 37 seconds when only factor VIII was reduced to 0.3 U/mL of normal while all other factors were normal, compared to 48 seconds when factors II, IX, and X were all at 0.3 U/mL, versus 75 seconds when all factors were reduced to 0.3 U/mL of normal (Figure 9.2). How the aPTT assay will be used in a particular institution may determine how important it is to know the sensitivity of the assay to different types of factor deficiency. If the aPTT is only being used for heparin monitoring then knowledge of sensitivity to individual factors may not be needed. If the test is being used as an initial assay for unknown factor deficiency, or to assess factor deficiency in massively bleeding patients, knowledge of sensitivity to different forms of factor deficiency may

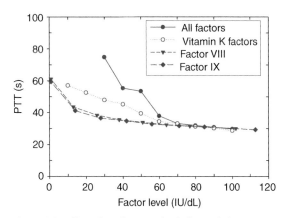

Figure 9.2 Effect of single- or multiple factor deficiency on the aPTT. Plasma samples with varying degrees of factor VIII, factor IX, vitamin K-dependent factor, or all factor deficiency were prepared by mixing pooled normal plasma with plasma deficient in the appropriate factor or factors.

99

Table 9.3 Factors potentially affecting the activated partial thromboplastin time (aPTT) assay

---

- Coagulation factors VIII, IX, and XI deficiency. Also useful to know the sensitivity to factors II, V, X, XII, prekallikrein, and high molecular weight kininogen and fibrinogen deficiency
- Lupus anticoagulants
- Direct thrombin inhibitors, unfractionated heparin, low molecular weight heparin, heparinoids, pentasaccharides, and other anti-thrombotic medications
- Clotted sample
- Hemolyzed sample
- Over- or underfilled sample tube
- Elevated factor VIII levels

---

be useful. In particular, aPTT reagents should produce abnormal prolonged results in plasmas that have less than 0.3 U/mL factors VIII, IX, or XI. The reagent used in Figure 9.2 shows similar factors VIII and IX sensitivity. Some aPTT reagents are less sensitive to factor IX. While factor deficiencies can prolong the aPTT, increases in factor VIII due to an acute phase response can shorten the aPTT, complicating the interpretation. Patients with deficiencies of factor XII, prekallikrein, and high molecular weight kininogen do not have increased bleeding, but the aPTT will be variably prolonged depending on the degree of deficiency and the sensitivity of the particular reagent.

Table 9.3 shows a list of conditions that may potentially affect the aPTT result. Different aPTT reagents show wide variations in their sensitivity to heparin [14–16]. When the aPTT is used to monitor unfractionated heparin therapy, care must be taken to accurately determine the heparin therapeutic range using one of several different methods as discussed later in this book (Chapter 22). Determination of aPTT heparin therapeutic ranges should always be performed using *ex vivo* samples from patients on stable heparin therapy, and not by spiking heparin into individual or pool samples [17].

aPTT reagents show different sensitivities to direct thrombin inhibitors including argatroban, lepirudin, bivalirudin, and new oral forms like dabigatran [8]. If direct thrombin inhibitors will be monitored using the aPTT, then the sensitivity of aPTT to these medications will need to be determined. Other assays like plasma-diluted thrombin times may be needed for monitoring these drugs [18].

If the aPTT will be used as an initial step in a lupus anticoagulant assay, then its sensitivity to lupus anticoagulants should be determined and compared to current reagents (Chapter 21) [19]. It is important to know how sensitive the aPTT reagent is to clotted or hemolyzed samples. In samples that are preactivated before testing, often due to inadequate mixing of blood and citrate anticoagulant during blood draw, the aPTT may show substantially shorter results than in a properly collected sample. Clotting in the tube may be identified from fibrin strands or visible clots. Samples with short aPTT results, often less than 25 seconds, should be checked for preactivation or clotting. Some instrument–reagent aPTT combinations are relatively insensitive to hemolysis while others may be more sensitive [4, 6]. Modest underfilling of the citrate sample tubes may have little effect on some aPTT reagents [7], but this needs to be evaluated before any over- or underfilled tube is accepted.

Minimum evaluation, activated partial thromboplastin time assay

Assuming the aPTT is used to monitor unfractionated heparin therapy, the minimum assessment of a new aPTT instrument–reagent combination includes the determination of the heparin therapeutic range using *ex vivo* samples from patients on stable heparin therapy; comparison with current method; determination or validation of the reference interval; within-run and between-run imprecision at normal and prolonged values; analytic measurement range (particularly at the upper end of the assay); and sample and reagent stability.

Fibrinogen method selection

Fibrinogen assays are most often used during the evaluation of hemostasis in patients with active bleeding or a prior history of bleeding. Low fibrinogen levels may occur due to blood loss, excessive intravascular coagulation activation, and consumption or reduced production of fibrinogen as a result of hereditary fibrinogen abnormalities or liver disease (cirrhosis or others). Fibrinogen may appear low using kinetic or activity assays in some patients with fibrinogen abnormalities that slow cleavage by thrombin. Fibrinogen is an acute phase reactant; its concentration rises during a variety of clinical syndromes including inflammation, infection, and cancer.

Fibrinogen concentration in plasma can be measured in several ways including immunoassays for antigenic concentration, total clottable assays, and activity or functional assays. Antigenic and total clottable fibrinogen assays are typically used only for research or the evaluation of dysfibrinogens. They are too slow and expensive for routine clinical use. Most clinical laboratories measure fibrinogen using a functional assay, either a kinetic method or a turbidity method derived from the PT assay. For the kinetic fibrinogen method, citrated plasma is diluted in buffer then clotted using a relatively high concentration of thrombin. The time required for the clot to form is inversely proportional to the fibrinogen concentration. For the PT-derived fibrinogen, a standard PT is run on the sample. The change in total light scattering or turbidity in the sample is proportional to the fibrinogen concentration [20].

The initial evaluation of any new fibrinogen instrument–reagent combination should include calibration of the fibrinogen assay using a reference plasma calibrated against a standard plasma of known fibrinogen concentration. At least five points should be used to determine the fibrinogen calibration curve and the upper and lower limits of the reportable range determined for the standard dilution of plasma. If the fibrinogen falls outside this range, lower or higher dilutions of plasma can be used. It is possible to extend the kinetic fibrinogen calibration curve on some instruments from about 50 to 1000 mg/dL, reducing the number of dilutions, repeat assays, and prolonged turnaround times on samples with low fibrinogens, but this needs careful evaluation on each instrument–reagent combination [5]. New reference curves should be prepared with each change of reagent lot, any change in instrument, or with any deviation from quality control or proficiency testing limits. Next the assay should be evaluated for within-run and between-run imprecisions at normal and reduced fibrinogen values, stability of the reagent on the instrument, and stability of fibrinogen in the sample at room temperature and 4°C. In most clinical settings the fibrinogen assay is used to assess low fibrinogen as a cause of bleeding. The ability to accurately and precisely measure fibrinogen levels below 1 g/L is important. At least one control for the fibrinogen assay should be a low control near or below 1 g/L in concentration.

If a new fibrinogen assay is being selected or a new lot of reagent evaluated it should be compared to the current assay across a wide range of possible values and patient types, including patients on heparin and other antithrombotic agents [21].

Underfilled tubes can result in falsely low fibrinogen due to dilution of the plasma by citrate. In samples that are preactivated before testing, often due to inadequate mixing of blood and citrate anticoagulant during blood draw, the fibrinogen may show falsely low fibrinogen due to consumption of fibrinogen in the *in vitro* clot [5]. Clotting in the tube may be identified from fibrin strands or visible clots. The effect of hemolysis, icterus, and lipemia should be evaluated. Some fibrinogen assays based on optical clot detection or total light scattering may be affected by plasma interference more than methods using mechanical clot detection. Due to the dilution of the plasma and relatively high concentrations of thrombin used, kinetic fibrinogen assays are relatively insensitive to heparin contamination. It is important to know the level of heparin that interferes in the fibrinogen assay. High levels of direct thrombin inhibitors may interfere in fibrinogen assays including the new oral inhibitors like dabigatran [8].

Several studies have reported problems with PT-derived fibrinogen assays. Variable results have been reported depending on the type of thromboplastin used for the PT assay and the patient group studied producing clinically unreliable results in some situations [22, 23]. How the fibrinogen assay will be used clinically and in which patient populations should be considered before selecting an assay.

Minimum evaluation, fibrinogen assay

The minimum assessment of a new fibrinogen assay includes the calibration of the standard curve; comparison with the current method; determination or validation of the reference range; within-run and between-run imprecisions at normal and reduced values; determination of the analytic measurement range; and sample and reagent stability. If a PT-derived fibrinogen is selected, it should be evaluated in different patient groups to assure accuracy.

Thrombin time method selection

The principal uses of the thrombin time in the initial evaluation of hemostasis include detection of

101

anticoagulants in the sample including antithrombin antibodies, heparin, and direct thrombin inhibitors; acquired and hereditary abnormalities of fibrin formation; or polymerization including higher levels of fibrin degradation products, paraproteinemias, and dysfibrinogens. The thrombin time assay consists of adding a dilute solution of thrombin to undiluted citrate anticoagulated plasma. The thrombin used in the assay may come from human or animal sources (often bovine thrombin). The thrombin time assay is not sensitive to deficiency of any coagulation factor except fibrinogen, but may also be prolonged in some cases when fibrinogen levels are more elevated. The initial evaluation of any new thrombin time instrument–reagent combination should include assessment of within-run and between-run imprecisions at normal and prolonged values, stability of the reagent on the instrument, stability of the sample at room temperature and 4°C and, if applicable, comparison of the new instrument–reagent combination with the existing method across a wide range of possible values and patient types, including both high and low fibrinogen levels. Most thrombin time assays are sensitive to heparin in the sample, including many low molecular weight heparins. The sensitivity of the thrombin time depends on the amount of thrombin used in the assay. Higher thrombin concentrations are less sensitive to heparin and other anticoagulants but may be used to monitor heparin therapy. Lower concentrations of thrombin make the assay more sensitive to heparin to improve the assay's performance in detecting low-level heparin contamination, but make it too sensitive for heparin monitoring. It is important to know how sensitive the thrombin time reagent is to clotted or hemolyzed samples. Some thrombin time assays are relatively insensitive to modest overfilling or underfilling of the sample tube, as citrate and calcium concentration are not important in the thrombin time assay, but this needs to be carefully evaluated before any over- or underfilled tube is accepted.

Minimum evaluation, thrombin time

The minimum assessment of a new thrombin time instrument–reagent combination includes comparison with the existing method; determination or validation of the reference range; within-run and between-run imprecisions at normal and prolonged values; and sample and reagent stability.

Whole blood viscoelastic assays

Several different manual whole blood viscoelastic assays have been developed, primarily for monitoring of coagulation during cardiac, liver transplantation, and trauma surgery. These include the TEG® Hemostasis Analyzer (Haemonetics Corp, Braintree, MA, USA), the ROTEM® (Pentapharm GmbH, Munich, Germany), and the Sonoclot (Sienco Inc., Arvada, CO, USA) [24–29]. Several different reagent combinations are available including native whole blood clotting, recalcification of citrated blood with no activator, contact activators like kaolin (similar to an aPTT), and tissue factor activators (similar to a PT).

These instruments measure viscoelastic properties of clotting whole blood producing estimates of time to initial clot formation, rate of clot formation, maximum clot viscoelasticity, and degree of clot lysis. Time to initial clot formation correlates best with coagulation factor levels. Maximum amplitude is related to fibrinogen concentration, platelet count, and hematocrit [24, 30]. Some methods include reagents that block platelet function or only activate fibrinogen resulting in a maximum amplitude that is correlated with fibrinogen concentration. In whole blood assays, including viscoelastic measurements, measured fibrinogen concentration is inversely related to hematocrit which in effect dilutes the plasma-lowering viscoelastic amplitude (Figure 9.3) [29]. Factors that may affect viscoelastic assays are shown in Table 9.4. Hematocrit must be taken into account if fibrinogen estimates are made from whole blood measurements [31]. Viscoelastic assays can detect clinically significant, severe fibrinolysis not easily detectable by other routinely available assays, but they only detect severe lysis [27, 32].

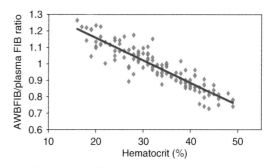

Figure 9.3 Relationship between hematocrit and measured fibrinogen level in whole blood assays (from Reference 31).

Table 9.4 Factors potentially affecting viscoelastic assays

- Coagulation factor deficiency
- Lupus anticoagulants
- Direct thrombin inhibitors, unfractionated heparin, low molecular weight heparin, heparinoids, pentasaccharides, and other anti-thrombotic medications
- Clotted sample
- Hemolyzed sample
- Over- or underfilled sample tube
- Hematocrit
- Platelet count
- Fibrinogen concentration
- Anti-GPIIbIIIa inhibitors

The different viscoelastic methodologies are not well standardized [25], report different parameters, and thus results from one method show only limited correlation with other viscoelastic methods and standard assays like PT, aPTT, and fibrinogen. In proficiency testing results, there is substantial variation even within one manufacturer's system. This indicates that imprecision is so great for these methods that variability in patient specimens could result even when one repeats the testing of a single sample [25, 29, 33, 34]. Normal parameters from these assays vary with age and sex [29]. High levels of assay imprecision combined with limited reference range studies have led to a high proportion of normal subjects being diagnosed as abnormal in some studies [29]. Standard viscoelastic measurements are insensitive to von Willebrand factor levels, aspirin, and clopidogrel [26]. Highly modified assays are required to detect antiplatelet effects from these drugs.

Minimum evaluation, viscoelastic assays

The minimum assessment should include within- and between-run imprecisions at normal and abnormal values for each parameter, whole blood sample and reagent stability, determination or validation of reference ranges, and comparison with an existing method. Sensitivity of the parameters to heparin, direct thrombin inhibitors, and other anticoagulants should be evaluated. If the method will be used to estimate fibrinogen concentration, it should be compared to a standard fibrinogen assay and the sensitivity of the method to heparin, direct thrombin inhibitors, and sample hematocrit should be determined.

References

1. Krouwer JS. EP10-A3, Preliminary Evaluation of Quantitative Clinical Laboratory Measurement Procedures: Approved Guideline. Wayne, PA: Clinical and Laboratory Standards Institute; 2006.
2. Shahangian S, Labeau KM, Howerton DA. Prothrombin time testing practices: adherence to guidelines and standards. Clin Chem. 2006;52:793–794.
3. Tripodi A, Baglin T, Robert A, et al. Reporting prothrombin time results as international normalized ratios for patients with chronic liver disease. J Thromb Haemost. 2010;8:1410–1412.
4. Laga AC, Cheves TA, Sweeney JD. The effect of specimen hemolysis on coagulation test results. Am J Clin Pathol. 2006;126:748–755.
5. Chandler WL, Ferrell C, Trimble S, et al. Development of a rapid emergency hemorrhage panel. Transfusion. 2010;50:2547–2552.
6. Lippi G, Montagnana M, Salvagno GL, et al. Interference of blood cell lysis on routine coagulation testing. Arch Pathol Lab Med. 2006;130:181–184.
7. Adcock DM, Kressin DC, Marlar RA. Minimum specimen volume requirements for routine coagulation testing: dependence on citrate concentration. Am J Clin Pathol. 1998;109:595–599.
8. Lindahl TL, Baghaei F, Blixter IF, et al. Effects of the oral, direct thrombin inhibitor dabigatran on five common coagulation assays. Thromb Haemost. 2010;105:371–378.
9. Barrett YC, Wang Z, Frost C, et al. Clinical laboratory measurement of direct factor Xa inhibitors: anti-Xa assay is preferable to prothrombin time assay. Thromb Haemost. 2010;104:1263–1271.
10. Hillarp A, Baghaei F, Fagerberg Blixter I, et al. Effects of the oral, direct factor Xa inhibitor rivaroxaban on commonly used coagulation assays. J Thromb Haemost. 2010;9:133–139.
11. Sibley C, Singer JW, Wood RJ. Comparison of activated partial thromboplastin reagents. Am J Clin Pathol. 1973;59:581–586.
12. Hathaway WE, Assmus SL, Montgomery RR, et al. Activated partial thromboplastin time and minor coagulopathies. Am J Clin Pathol. 1979;71:22–25.
13. Barrowcliffe TW, Gray E. Studies of phospholipid reagents used in coagulation I: some general properties and their sensitivity to factor VIII. Thromb Haemost. 1981;46:629–633.
14. Triplett DA, Harms CS, Koepke JA. The effect of heparin on the activated partial thromboplastin time. Am J Clin Pathol. 1978;70:556–559.

15. Barrowcliffe TW, Gray E. Studies of phospholipid reagents used in coagulation II: factors influencing their sensitivity to heparin. *Thromb Haemost*. 1981;46:634–637.

16. Brandt JT, Triplett DA. Laboratory monitoring of heparin. Effect of reagents and instruments on the activated partial thromboplastin time. *Am J Clin Pathol*. 1981;76:530–537.

17. Gausman JN, Marlar RA. Inaccuracy of a "spiked curve" for monitoring unfractionated heparin therapy. *Am J Clin Pathol*. 2011;135:870–876.

18. Love JE, Ferrell C, Chandler WL. Monitoring direct thrombin inhibitors with a plasma diluted thrombin time. *Thromb Haemost*. 2007;98:234–242.

19. Mannucci PM, Canciani MT, Mari D, et al. The varied sensitivity of partial thromboplastin and prothrombin time reagents in the demonstration of the lupus-like anticoagulant. *Scand J Haematol*. 1979;22:423–432.

20. De Cristofaro R, Landolfi R. Measurement of plasma fibrinogen concentration by the prothrombin-time-derived method: applicability and limitations. *Blood Coagul Fibrinolysis*. 1998;9:251–259.

21. Arkin CF, Adcock DM, Day HJ, et al. *H30-A2, Procedure for the determination of fibrinogen in plasma*; Approved Guideline–2nd Edition. *NCCLS*, 2001.

22. Mackie J, Lawrie AS, Kitchen S, et al. A performance evaluation of commercial fibrinogen reference preparations and assays for Clauss and PT-derived fibrinogen. *Thromb Haemost*. 2002;87:997–1005.

23. Lawrie AS, McDonald SJ, Purdy G, et al. Prothrombin time derived fibrinogen determination on Sysmex CA-6000. *J Clin Pathol*. 1998;51:462–466.

24. Chandler WL. The thromboelastograph and the thromboelastographic technique. *Semin Thromb Hemost*. 1995;21(suppl 4):1–6.

25. Chitlur M, Lusher J. Standardization of thromboelastography: values and challenges. *Semin Thromb Hemost*. 2010;36:707–711.

26. Wegner J, Popovsky MA. Clinical utility of thromboelastography: one size does not fit all. *Semin Thromb Hemost*. 2010;36:699–706.

27. Adams M, Ward C, Thom J, et al. Emerging technologies in hemostasis diagnostics: a report from the Australasian Society of Thrombosis and Haemostasis Emerging Technologies Group. *Semin Thromb Hemost*. 2007;33:226–234.

28. Nair SC, Dargaud Y, Chitlur M, et al. Tests of global haemostasis and their applications in bleeding disorders. *Haemophilia*. 2010;16(suppl 5):85–92.

29. MacDonald SG, Luddington RJ. Critical factors contributing to the thromboelastography trace. *Semin Thromb Hemost*. 2010;36:712–722.

30. Chandler WL, Patel MA, Gravelle L, et al. Factor XIIIA and clot strength after cardiopulmonary bypass. *Blood Coagul Fibrinolysis*. 2001;12:101–108.

31. Amukele TK, Ferrell C, Chandler WL. Comparison of plasma with whole blood prothrombin time and fibrinogen on the same instrument. *Am J Clin Pathol*. 2010;133:550–556.

32. Spiess BD, Wall MH, Gillies BS, et al. A comparison of thromboelastography with heparinase or protamine sulfate added in-vitro during heparinized cardiopulmonary bypass. *Thromb Haemost*. 1997;78:820–826.

33. Kitchen DP, Kitchen S, Jennings I, et al. Quality assurance and quality control of thrombelastography and rotational thromboelastometry: the UK NEQAS for blood coagulation experience. *Semin Thromb Hemost*. 2010;36:757–763.

34. Chen A, Teruya J. Global hemostasis testing thromboelastography: old technology, new applications. *Clin Lab Med*. 2009;29:391–407.

10 Assay of factor VIII and other clotting factors

Steve Kitchen[1,2] & F. Eric Preston[3,4]

[1] Sheffield Hemophilia and Thrombosis Centre, Royal Hallamshire Hospital, Sheffield, UK
[2] UK National External Quality Assessment Scheme (NEQAS) for Blood Coagulation, WHO and WFH International External Quality Assessment Programs for Blood Coagulation, Sheffield, UK
[3] University of Sheffield, Sheffield, UK
[4] WHO and WFH International External Quality Assessment Programs for Blood Coagulation, Sheffield, UK

This chapter will deal with issues relating to the assay of clotting factors in plasma with particular emphasis on FVIII:C. This will include assays of plasma from patients treated with concentrates but will not address the assignment of potencies to concentrates which is addressed elsewhere in this book (Chapter 4).

Pretest variables

The recommended anticoagulant for collection of blood samples for assays of clotting factors, including factor VIII:C and factor IX:C, is normally tri-sodium citrate [1] at a concentration of 0.105–0.109 M (3.2%) [2, 3]. It is likely that the use of 3.8% citrate has less impact on factor assay results than on the aPTT (see Chapter 5) since the test plasma is diluted in buffer before testing. For the same reason, factor assays may be more tolerant of tube underfilling or extremely low hematocrits, although there are few data to confirm this.

For factor assays it is essential that blood is collected as rapidly as possible by clean venipuncture. Any delay in mixing blood with the anticoagulant may affect the results. Before assaying, the blood samples should be inspected for the presence of clots by gentle inversion or by sweeping the tube with a wooden stick. Samples containing clots or exhibiting marked hemolysis should be discarded. Tests performed on partially clotted or activated samples can lead to overestimation of the activity present and activated clotting factors may be associated with nonparallelism in the assay graphs.

Samples should be stored at room temperature (20–25°C) before testing. Storage of blood at 2–8°C leads to significant loss of both factor VIII and VWF and should be avoided [4] (see also Chapter 5). If assays are not performed within 2–3 hours of collection plasma can be stored deep frozen for longer periods at −70°C, since clotting factors including VIII:C and IX:C have been shown to be stable for at least 18 months [5]. Frozen plasma should be transferred immediately to a 37°C waterbath, thawed for 4–5 minutes at 37°C and mixed by gentle inversion prior to analysis. A slow thaw at lower temperature must be avoided to prevent the formation of cryoprecipitate that reduces the FVIII concentration in the supernatant plasma.

Factor VIII is an acute phase reactant [6] and is increased in pregnancy and by exercise. Caution is therefore required when interpreting factor VIII assays when investigating for possible hemophilia A or von Willebrand disease and these diagnoses should not be confirmed or excluded on the basis of a single result.

For a general discussion of preanalytical variables in relation to coagulation tests see Chapter 5.

One-stage assay of factor VIII:C or factor IX:C

The most commonly performed assay for factor VIII:C worldwide for many years has been the one-stage

Quality in Laboratory Hemostasis and Thrombosis, Second Edition. Edited by Steve Kitchen, John D. Olson and F. Eric Preston.
© 2013 John Wiley & Sons, Ltd. Published 2013 by Blackwell Publishing Ltd.

assay [7, 8]. The following observations, relating to FVIII:C assays, can also be applied to one-stage assays of FIX:C or FXI:C. The one-stage assay is based on the aPTT and depends on the ability of a sample containing factor VIII to correct or shorten the delayed clotting of a plasma which has a complete lack of factor VIII (FVIII-deficient plasma). It is important that the concentration of FVIII in this mixture is rate-limiting in its influence on the clotting time, as measured by the aPTT.

The assay requires a reference or standard plasma of known factor VIII concentration. The preparation of several different dilutions of the reference plasma allows the construction of a calibration curve in which the clotting time response depends on the concentration (dose) of factor VIII:C. If plasma is not sufficiently diluted then the other clotting factors in the test plasma will influence the clotting time and the assay is no longer specific for factor VIII and is therefore invalid. For this reason most assays operate with a minimum dilution of 1 in 5. At very low concentrations of factor VIII the clotting time may not be influenced by factor VIII and the aPTT is similar to the aPTT of the factor VIII-deficient plasma. If doubling dilutions of 1/5, 1/10, 1/20, 1/40, 1/80, 1/160, and 1/320 are selected then this may occur when dilutions of 1 in 160 or 1 in 320 are analyzed (depending on the reagent). The use of stored calibration curves on analyzers is widespread and under carefully controlled evaluation conditions it may be possible to obtain acceptable FVIII assay precision by using a stored calibration curve [9]. However, there are insufficient published data for different measurement systems and assays to extrapolate these findings to all test systems and some authors recommend that stored calibration curves generated in a different assay batch should not be used [3]. The safest approach is making a calibration using the same vials of reagent used for test samples and to perform these analyses at essentially the same time.

In order to obtain a linear relationship the data normally require transformation. Linearity of the reference or calibration curve is required for a valid assay. The most appropriate data transformation is that which gives the closest fit to a straight-line relationship as indicated by an r value (relating clotting times to concentration) that is close to 1.0. This is most commonly achieved using log transformation so that the log of concentration is plotted against the log of the clotting times. For some assay systems the use of non-transformed data (linear scale) for the clotting times with log-transformed concentrations may be suitable. Correlation coefficients of $r > 0.99$ are easily achievable and calibration curves with r values of <0.98 should be rejected. Some systems calculate a slope ratio (calibrator slope/test sample slope) from the regression calculations as an estimate of parallelism. This should normally be in the range 0.9–1.1 [3].

Guidelines recommend that test plasmas be analyzed using at least three dilutions [3, 10–12]. This is essential to confirm that two critical criteria for a valid assay have been met, namely, that there is a straight-line relationship through clotting times at different dilutions and second that the line through patient times is parallel to the calibration line. An example is shown in Figure 10.1. If a test and standard line are parallel this indicates that the two materials have behaved in a similar way under the test conditions. Comparing unlike materials such as concentrate against a plasma standard or comparing plasmas containing animal clotting factors against a human plasma standard often leads to nonparallel lines, indicating that the criteria for a valid assay have not been met. Identifying parallelism is only possible if several test dilutions are analyzed. Nonparallel one-stage

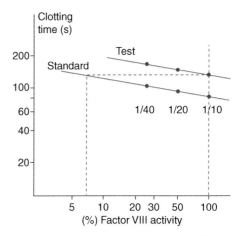

Figure 10.1 Factor assay dose–response curve. Three dilutions of standard and test plasma are plotted with concentration (dose) on the horizontal axis and clotting time (response) on the vertical. In the example above the concentration of FVIII:C in the test sample is 7% of the activity in the standard plasma.

assays can also occur in the presence of heparin or thrombin inhibitors such as lepirudin [13].

A second important reason to include multiple test dilutions is to improve the precision of the assay. In a UK NEQAS exercise a test sample with FIX:C of 6 IU/dL was assayed in approximately 90 hemophilia centers. The CV of the FIX:C results in the 22 centers performing a single test dilution was 54%, compared with a CV of 22% for the 42 centers that performed the analysis using three test dilutions. The difference was statistically significant ($p < 0.05$). This indicates that the precision of assays is much improved by testing multiple dilutions. Similar advantages of better precision were noted in relation to FVIII:C assays in a second exercise.

If only one dilution is analyzed there can also be important errors in the accuracy of the assay, particularly if lupus inhibitors are present (see below).

Assays in the presence of strong lupus anticoagulant

Since lupus anticoagulant (LAC) can prolong phospholipid-dependent tests, and in particular the aPTT, it is not surprising that in some cases these antibodies can compromise the quality of assay results by interfering in aPTT-based one-stage assays. In extreme cases such antibodies can completely block the reactions even when the test plasma has been diluted for analysis in a one-stage assay and in this case assay results of <1 IU/dL are obtained in both FVIII and FIX assays [14]. More typically, some clotting factor activity is detectable but the estimate of potency depends on the dilution of test plasma, with different results being obtained at different plasma dilutions [15]. The measured activity increases at higher dilutions. An example of LAC effect on a one-stage FVIII assay is shown in Figure 10.2. LAC typically interferes to a similar extent in all one-stage PTT assays, so the nonparallel effects in Figure 10.2 occur in assays of FIX:C, FXI:C, and FXII:C in addition to FVIII:C. An accurate assay result can be obtained only if two different plasma dilutions give the same activity.

There are three possible solutions to this problem. One is to employ a chromogenic assay where the initial plasma dilution is high and the inhibitory effect of LAC is diluted out [13]. In a report of ten cases where LAC led to interference and underestimation of the FVIII:C, reliable estimates could be obtained in a chromogenic assay, including a

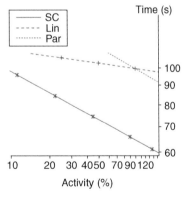

Factor VIII MDA		
ID No 7004	[0004–04]	
29/9/27	16:03	37.1°C

MDA ratio	Clot time	Activity (%)
1/1	99.0 (s)	9.5
1/2	103.0 (s)	15.3
1/4	106.0 (s)	26.1
		Mean 17.0
SCr = −1.000	Test r = −0.996	

Figure 10.2 This shows a printout from an auto analyzer for a FVIII:C assay using a lupus-sensitive aPTT reagent. On the plot SC = standard curve; Lin is the line of best fit through the three test dilutions; Par is a line drawn parallel to the SC through the first test dilution clotting time. In this example the Lin through patient dilution clotting times is not parallel to the SC. In the table 1/1 represents the 1 in 10 dilution which in this case is the first test dilution and which suggests a FVIII test result of 9.5% of the standard. 1/2 and 1/4 are the next two dilutions (1 in 20 and 1 in 40, respectively) that suggest test results of 15% and 26%, respectively. Two further test dilutions of 1/80 and 1/160 gave test results of 43% and 106% of standard (not shown in the figure above). This patient has a normal level of FVIII:C and a strong LAC which is causing the nonparallel assay effect and underestimation of activity in lower dilutions.

case where the one-stage assay suggested that FVIII was completely absent even at a plasma dilution of 1/80 [15].

In respect of factor VIII:C a second way to obtain accurate assay results in the presence of LAC is to employ a two-stage clotting assay that is rarely affected by LAC despite the fact that phospholipid is required in the assay. The absence of LAC interference is related to the high initial test dilution (typically 1 in 50 or 1 in 100) used in two-stage clotting assays. Chromogenic assays are not widely used for FIX:C or FXI:C determination.

The final option, which may be the favored choice for all one-stage aPTT-based assays, is to perform the assay in the presence of a high concentration of phospholipid so that there is an excess of PL beyond the concentration that can be blocked by LAC. This can be done by the addition of platelet-derived phospholipid [16] or more simply by using an aPTT reagent known to be insensitive to LAC as a consequence of higher PL concentration. We have reported that Actin FS has approximately 20-fold more PL than a number of other aPTT reagents [17] and one-stage assays performed with this reagent are only very rarely affected by the presence of LAC. A recent UK guideline has recommended that aPTT reagents with LAC sensitivity should be used in one-stage assays to improve specificity unless the presence of LAC has been excluded [3].

One-stage assay components

The quality of assay results is very much influenced by laboratory reagents currently in use. One-stage aPTT-based assays can be performed with any of the available aPTT reagents although it should be noted that they contain different types of activator including kaolin, celite, silica particle, and ellagic acid. Reagents employing ellagic acid as activator are unsuitable for assay of prekallikrein since activation by ellagic acid is largely independent of PK.

There is considerable variation in the concentration and composition of phospholipids [17] in widely used reagents. Since the phospholipids support the clotting reactions through bound clotting factors, different phospholipid preparations have the potential to give different assay results depending on the aPTT reagent used. One example we have reported is that

in subjects with VWD Normandy higher one-stage FVIII:C results were obtained with the DAPTTIN aPTT reagent compared to the results obtained with other aPTT reagents [18].

In general, differences between one-stage results of factor VIII:C assays performed using different types of aPTT reagent are not sufficient to influence patient management [19].

In the case of factor IX:C assays differences between results obtained using different aPTT reagents are also minor [20]. The selection of aPTT reagent can influence the precision of both FVIII:C and FIX:C assays [7, 20, 21]. In both cases precision is better for reagents where there is a greater increase in clotting time for a given change in concentration. Calibration curves of assays performed with such reagents have steeper slopes. While many different aPTT reagents are suitable for use in assays of factor VIII:C and IX:C it remains important to select a reagent for which there is evidence (e.g., through proficiency testing surveys) that results are in agreement with those obtained with an alternative reagent.

For PT-based assays the results may be influenced, albeit rarely, by the nature of the tissue factor present in the thromboplastin reagent. Some patients have normal levels of FVII:C (and normal PT) when the test is performed with a reagent containing human tissue factor, whereas reduced activity in both factor VII:C assay and the PT is obtained with a thromboplastin of rabbit origin. Interestingly, in cases such as these bleeding symptoms normally correlate with the results obtained with reagents of human origin [12].

One-stage assays require an appropriately deficient plasma. This should have a total lack of the factor being assayed, normal levels of other relevant clotting factors, and no evidence of coagulation factor inhibitor. Even 1–2 IU/dL residual activity of the factor being assayed makes this unsuitable for use, leading to nonparallel assays and possible overestimation of the factor under analysis. In one UK NEQAS proficiency testing survey center using FVIII-deficient plasma from one particular manufacturer, obtained results spread around 30 U/dL whereas results obtained with five other widely used deficient plasmas were close to 15 U/dL. When this was investigated it was noted that the level of FV in the FVIII-deficient plasma was not normal (as required) but was unexpectedly low (around 3 U/dL). This caused FV from the test sample to influence the clotting time during the assay and led to overestimation of apparent FVIII activity in the test sample.

Most commercially available factor-deficient plasmas are now prepared by immunodepletion of one factor from normal plasma. In general this works well and in a study reported by Barrowcliffe et al. [22] no differences were observed between FVIII:C assay results obtained with a deficient plasma from severe hemophilia A patients and five different immunodepleted FVIII-deficient plasmas.

Some FVIII:C-deficient plasmas are prepared using an anti-VWF antibody. Such plasmas are deficient in both FVIII:C and VWF. This might influence the results of FVIII:C assays in some hemophilia patients. A normal level of VWF in the FVIII:C-deficient plasma may be of particular importance when performing FVIII:C assays on concentrates.

It has been reported that the antibody against FVIII:C used to produce deficient plasma can leach off the column used for the depletion and then be present in the FVIII:C-deficient plasma. This can cause problems in FVIII:C inhibitor assays [23, see also Chapter 20] and would therefore be unsuitable for use in one-stage FVIII:C assays of any kind.

The accuracy of all factor assays is dependent on the use of reference or calibration plasma that has an accurately assigned potency, which should be traceable to the relevant WHO international standard. For commercial materials this is the responsibility of the manufacturer. Most often results in proficiency testing exercise confirm that results obtained by centers using different sources of reference plasma are in good agreement but this is not always the case. On rare occasions results obtained using one reference plasma are consistently different from results obtained against all others [8]. This is normally caused by inaccurate assignment by the manufacturer, and in the U K, at least, some manufacturers have issued revised potencies after correcting errors in the original assignment process. In an assessment by the Scientific and Standardization Committee (SSC) of International Society for Thrombosis and Haemostasis (ISTH) of six commercial reference plasmas the observed potency as determined in nine expert centers differed from the labeled potency by as much as 17% for FVIII:C and 16% for FIX [24], indicating that the problems above are not restricted to the U K.

Factor assays in the presence of severe deficiency

The SSC has defined severe hemophilia A and B as being less than 0.01 IU/mL (<1% or <1 IU/dL), with levels of FVIII:C/FIX:C being 0.01–0.05 IU/mL (1–5%) defined as moderate and >0.05–0.40 IU/mL (5–40%) as mild [25]. The same publication points out that classification based on clinical symptoms has sometimes been used because some patients with reported levels of <0.01 IU/mL exhibit little or no spontaneous bleeding whereas some patients with reportedly moderate, or even mild disease, have frequent spontaneous bleeds and appear to be clinically severe. It may be that this discrepancy between laboratory assay and clinical phenotype arises out of the difficulties in accurately assaying FVIII and FIX at very low levels. Following a proficiency testing survey we reported that approximately one-third of expert hemophilia centers wrongly classified two severe hemophilia A patients as mild or moderate [26]. There are particular difficulties in performing assays at levels below 0.03 IU/mL (3%). One way to improve the accuracy of results in such samples is to extend the calibration curve and include reference plasma dilutions with activities of 1% or 2% as recommended by NCCLS [10]. If the patient results are more prolonged than the clotting time of the lowest dilution then the patient result can be reported as less than that activity [10]. It is also useful to perform a test using all the same reagents but with dilution buffer in place of the test plasma dilution. This is sometimes referred to as the blank time of the assay. Only patient dilutions with clotting times shorter than this blank can be properly interpreted. When the level of FVIII:C and FIX:C is genuinely <0.01 IU/mL then it is not usually possible to obtain clotting times on test plasma dilutions which are clearly shorter than this blank time. The comments in relation to FVIII:C assays above also apply to other factor assays.

For FVIII:C assays in the presence of severe deficiency there is also the option to use a modified chromogenic assay as described by Yatau and colleagues [27] who used the Coamatic chromogenic assay with a lower dilution of 1 in 30 (rather than the recommended 1 in 80) and prolonged the incubation time with chromogenic substrate to 30 minutes (rather than the recommended 10 min). The modified assay allowed precise and accurate determinations in the range 0.001–0.02 IU/mL (0.1–2%).

Assay of elevated factor VIII:C

The recognition that elevated levels of FVIII:C are risk factors for thrombovascular disease has resulted in an increased demand, by clinicians, for FVIII:C determinations in individuals with both venous and arterial vascular disease. The same assay design used for investigation of bleeding disorders is generally suitable for assay of elevated levels of FVIII:C (and other factors) although the dilution of test plasma should be increased accordingly so that the clotting times of at least two of the three patient dilutions lie within the range covered by the calibration curve. The calibration curve should not be extended by testing dilutions lower than 1 in 5 since clotting factors in the test sample other than the one under assay may begin to influence the clotting time obtained and assay specificity is lost. For FVIII:C activities of 150 IU/dL or more chromogenic assays may be more precise than one-stage clotting methods [13].

Two-stage clotting assay for FVIII:C

Mild hemophilia A is not excluded by the finding of a normal FVIII:C level by one-stage assay. Several groups have reported that a subgroup of mild hemophilia A patients have discrepant FVIII:C results, as determined using different types of assay [28–30]. More than 20% of mild hemophilia A patients are associated with assay discrepancy if a twofold difference between results obtained with different assay systems is used to define this [28]. In some cases the one-stage assay result may be five times higher than the two-stage clotting or chromogenic assay [28]. The most common manifestation of assay discrepancy is one-stage assay results that are more than twofold higher than those of two-stage clotting or chromogenic assays. In more than 75% of such patients all assay results are reduced below the lower limit of the reference range so that a diagnosis can be reliably made irrespective of which method is employed for analysis. However, a small proportion of patients have results by the one-stage assay which are well within the

Table 10.1 Comparison of factor VIIIC assays using three methods

Case	One-stage assay (IU/dL)	Two-stage clotting assay (IU/dL)	Chromogenic assay (IU/dL)[a]
A	101	34	13
B	88	15	28
C	63	30	40
D	55	24	40
E	58	21	33
F	72	21	36
G	84	19	45

[a]Chromogenic assay (Dade–Behring Ltd).

normal range with reduced levels by a two-stage clotting or chromogenic assays [29, 31]. These patients usually have bleeding histories compatible with the lower levels obtained in two-stage clotting or chromogenic assay. In many cases the genetic defect has been identified so there is no doubt that these subjects do indeed have hemophilia [31, 32]. About 5–10% of mild hemophilia A patients have a normal one-stage assay result [33, 34]. We screened 60 patients with mild hemophilia A and found 7 patients from 6 families in whom the result by one-stage assay was within the normal range and was at least twice the level obtained by two-stage clotting assay. Results are shown in Table 10.1.

Since FVIII:C activity is normal in the one-stage aPTT-based assay it is not surprising that the aPTT is also normal in such patients. This means that patients with a clinical history compatible with hemophilia A should have a two-stage clotting or chromogenic assay even if the aPTT and one-stage assay are normal.

There are a small number of mild hemophilia A patients with the reverse pattern, that is, reduced activity by one-stage but normal results by the two-stage assay [35–38]. In these cases the clinical phenotype once again correlates with the two-stage result in that there is no personal or family history of bleeding with no requirement for FVIII:C replacement therapy [39], although other such cases with different genetic defects may have bleeding consistent with mild hemophilia A.

The two-stage clotting assay was developed as a modification of the now rarely used thromboplastin generation test by Rosemary Biggs and co-workers in Oxford and reported in the very first issue of the *British Journal of Haematology* [40]. It is a testament to the usefulness of this assay that after more than 50 years it continues to be used in some hemophilia reference centers largely unchanged except for a minor modification proposed by Ken Denson [41] to facilitate automation of the test. Chromogenic FVIII assays were later developed from two-stage clotting assays using similar principles.

As the name implies there are two distinct stages to the assay. The first stage involves creation of a reaction mixture that contains an excess of the components required for the generation of the prothrombinase complex with the exception of FVIII:C. The initial reagent therefore needs to contain activated factor IX (FIXa), factor X (FX), phospholipid (PL), calcium ions, and factor V. The FIXa and FX are provided by diluted activated human serum which has been fully clotted to remove all the FII, fibrinogen, and FVIII, followed by incubation to allow antithrombin to neutralize thrombin and activated FX formed during the clotting process, and to allow activation of FIX to IXa via contact activation. This manipulated serum contains FX but not Xa and most of the FIX in the active form. For a full description of the reagent see Barrowcliffe [42].

In the first stage of the assay the rate at which FIXa activates FX depends on the amount of FVIII which has been added. The Xa generated is bound through FV and calcium to PL. This first stage must not contain factor II and fibrinogen or else the mixture will clot. Test and reference plasma are therefore mixed with alumina hydroxide to remove prothrombin, with other vitamin K clotting factors being removed as a side effect of this. Such adsorption also removes any trace quantities of thrombin or FXa. Barrowcliffe [42] provides a full description of the assay details.

Chromogenic assay for factor VIII:C in plasma

The chromogenic assay method is based on the ability of FVIII to act as a cofactor in promoting the activation of FX:C by FIXa. The FXa generated in the assay is detected by the cleavage of a chromogenic substrate and the generation of color. The assay method ensures that the color development is dependent only on the concentration of FVIII:C in the test sample. The chromogenic method has some similarities to the two-stage clotting assay. In the first stage the test sample containing FVIII:C is incubated in the presence of phospholipid, calcium, and purified coagulation factors IXa and X. This mixture leads to the generation of FXa in amounts proportional to the concentration of FVIII:C in the test sample. The second stage of the assay involves the estimation of FXa by the cleavage of a chromogenic substrate and the generation of color by the release of *p*-nitroaniline (pNa) which is measured photometrically at 405 nm.

There are several different chromogenic assays available and there are important differences in the composition of the reagents so that results obtained using different chromogenic assays are not always interchangeable. Some chromogenic assays include added thrombin to fully activate FVIII:C whereas in the original Chromogenix system thrombin is not added and must be generated in the first stage for FVIII:C activation.

For most (but not all) chromogenic assays the second stage includes a thrombin inhibitor in order to prevent cleavage of the chromogenic substrate by any thrombin that might be present. The generation of color may either be measured continuously or as an end point perhaps with an acid-stopped reaction. The generation of color in the second stage is directly proportional to the concentration of FVIII in the test sample. The data from calibration curves do not normally require transformation and can be plotted on a simple linear scale to give a straight-line relationship.

The chromogenic method differs from the one-stage clotting method in that it is not sensitive to the presence of activated FVIII:C in the test plasma sample. A gross discrepancy between results of a one-stage and chromogenic assay may be caused by the activation of FVIII:C during sample collection, although this can be a genuine finding in certain hemophilia A patients (see section on two-stage clotting assays).

The chromogenic assay is currently recommended by the European Pharmacopoeia [43] and by SSC of ISTH for assignment of potency to FVIII:C concentrates [44], though SSC are reviewing guidance on this area at the time of writing with a new published guidance possible (earliest 2013).

In addition to the lack of interference by LAC (see above) chromogenic FVIII:C assays may also be unaffected by the presence of heparin or lepirudin [13], making them the method of choice if assay is required in the presence of these kinds of anticoagulants.

Factor VIII:C and FIX:C assays following clotting factor infusions

In most cases the same factor assay design and reagents should be used for measuring samples from treated hemophiliacs as for other test samples. Issues related to the assay of such samples have been extensively reviewed [45, 46]. There are particular issues related to the assay of samples containing recombinant FVIII:C. When measuring full-length recombinant FVIII:C in plasma, results of some chromogenic assays may be 40–50% higher than by one-stage clotting assays [47].

A further issue relates to B-domain-depleted recombinant FVIII:C where results of one-stage assays were approximately 30% greater than results by chromogenic assay in plasma samples containing this material in an SSC/ISTH field study [48]. This discrepancy could be substantially reduced by calibrating the assay using B-domain-depleted material as calibrator. There is evidence that the higher result by one-stage assay (with the usual plasma standard) is a consequence of the artificial phospholipids present in the reagent [49]. The more appropriate result is considered to be the lower activity obtained by either chromogenic assay or one-stage clotting assay when calibrated against the B-domain-depleted standard. We have noted that there are differences between results of different chromogenic assays in samples from patients treated with this product. The SSC field study [48] concluded that the one-stage assay, when calibrated with the B-domain-depleted standard, provides an accurate and precise assessment of FVIII:C in plasma samples containing this material. Following reformulation of this B-domain-depleted FVIII in an albumin-free material (ReFacto AF), it has been established that a product-specific standard continues to be required for one-stage assays to deliver agreement with chromogenic assay results [50].

It is highly likely that a number of other product-specific laboratory standards will be required in future for successful monitoring of at least some of the newer long-acting products which are in clinical trials at the time of writing. The UK guideline recommends that concentrate-specific standards should be used when

recommended by the manufacturer for FVIII assays in patients treated for hemophilia A [3]. In future this may need to be extended to include FIX products containing modified forms of the protein.

References

1. World Health Organisation Report Use of anti-coagulants in diagnostic laboratory investigations. WHO/DIL/LAB/99, 1 Perl. 1999.
2. CLSI. *H21-A5, Collection, Transport and Processing of Blood Specimens for Testing Plasma-Based Coagulation Assays and Molecular Haemostasis Assays: Approved Guideline.* 5th ed. Wayne, PA: Clinical and Laboratory Standards Institute; 2008.
3. Mackie I, Cooper PC, Lawrie A, Kitchen S, Gray E, Laffan M. On behalf of British Committee for Standards in Haematology. Guidelines on the laboratory aspects of assays used in haemostasis and thrombosis. *Int J Lab Hematol.* 2012. doi: 10.1111/ijlh.12004. [Epub ahead of print].
4. Bohm M, Teaschner S, Kretzschmar E, Gerlach R, Favaloro EJ, Scharrer I. Cold storage of citrated whole blood induces drastic time-dependent losses of factor VIII and von Willebrand factor: potential for misdiagnosis of haemophilia and von Willebrand disease. *Blood Coagul Fibrinolysis.* 2006;17:39–45.
5. Woodhams B, Giradot O, Blanco MJ, Colesse G, Gourmelin Y. Stability of coagulation proteins in frozen plasma. *Blood Coagul Fibrinolysis.* 2001;12:229–236.
6. Gallus AS, Hirsh J, Cade J. Relevance of pre-operative and post-operative blood tests in post-operative leg vein thrombosis. *Lancet.* 1973;2:805–809.
7. Brandt JT, Triplett DA, Musgrave K, et al. Factor VIII assays. Assessment of variables. *Arch Pathol Lab Med.* 1988;112:7–12.
8. Preston FE, Kitchen S. Quality control and factor VIII assays. *Haemophilia.* 1998;4:651–653.
9. Lattes S, Appert-Flory A, Fischer F, Jambou D, Toulon P. Measurement of factor VIII activity using one-stage assay: a calibration curve has not to systematically included in each run. *Haemophilia.* 2011;17:139–142.
10. National Committee for Clinical Laboratory Standards (USA). *Determination of Factor Coagulant Activities: Approved Guidelines,* NCCLS document H48–A; 1997.
11. Kitchen S, McCraw A, Echenagucia M. *Diagnosis of Haemophilia and Other Bleeding Disorders: A Laboratory Manual.* 2nd ed. Montreal, Canada: World Federation of Haemophilia; 2010.
12. Bolton-Maggs PH, Perry DJ, Chalmers EA, et al. The rare coagulation disorders–review with guidelines for management. *Haemophilia.* 2004;10:1–36.

13. Chandler WL, Ferrell C, Lee J, Tun T, Kha H. Comparison of three methods for measuring FVIII levels in plasma. *Am J Clin Pathol.* 2003;120:34–39.

14. Kazmi MA, Pickering W, Smith MP, Holland LJ, Savidge GF. Acquired haemophilia A: errors in the diagnosis. *Blood Coagul Fibrinolysis.* 1998;9:623–628.

15. De Maistre E, Wahl D, Perret-Guillaume C, et al. A chromogenic assay allows reliable measurement of FVIII levels in the presence of strong lupus anticoagulant. *Thromb Haemost.* 1998;79:237–238.

16. Armitage J, Ashcraft J, Kim A, Kaplan HS. An approach to factor assays in patients with strong lupus anticoagulant. *Clin Appl Thromb Hemost.* 1995;1:125–130.

17. Kitchen S, Cartwright I. Wood TAL, Jennings I, Preston FE. Lipid composition of seven aPTT reagents in relation to heparin sensitivity. *Br J Haematol.* 1999;106:801–808.

18. Bowyer AE, Cartwright I, Kitchen S, Makris M. FVIII:C assay discrepancy in type 2N VWD is reagent dependant. *J Thromb Haemost.* 2007;5(suppl 2).

19. Arkin CF, Bovill EG, Brandt JT, Rock WA, Triplett DA. Factors affecting the performance of factor VIII coagulant activity assays. Results of proficiency surveys of the College of American Pathologists. *Arch Pathol Lab Med.* 1992;116:908–915.

20. Brandt JT, Atkin CF, Bovill EG, Rock WA, Triplett DA. Evaluation of aPTT reagent sensitivity to factor IX and factor IX assay performance. *Arch Pathol Lab Med.* 1990;114:135–141.

21. Brandt J.T. Measurement of factor VIII: a potential risk factor for vascular disease. *Arch Pathol Lab Med.* 1992;117:48–51.

22. Barrowcliffe TW, Tubbs JE, Wong MY. Evaluation of FVIII deficient plasmas. *Thromb Haemost.* 1993;70:433–437.

23. Verbruggen B, Giles A, Samis J, Verbeek K, Menisink E, Novakova I. The type of factor VIII deficient plasma used influences the performance of the Nijmegen modification of the Bethesda assay for factor VIII inhibitors. *Thromb Haemost.* 2001;86:1435–1439.

24. Kasper C, Aronson DL, Davignon G, et al. Comparison of six commercial reference plasma for FVII, factor IX and von Willebrand factor, on behalf of the Subcommittee for FVIII and IX of the SSC of the ISTH. *Thromb Haemost.* 1995;74:987–989.

25. White GC, Rosendaal F, Aledort LM, Lusher JM, Rothschild C, Ingerslev J. Definitions in hemophilia. Recommendations of the Scientific Subcommittee on FVIII and FIX of the SSC of ISTH. *Thromb Haemost.* 2001;85:560.

26. Preston FE, Kitchen S, Jennings I, Woods TAL, Makris M. SSC/ISTH classification of hemophilia A: can hemophilia center laboratories achieve the new criteria? *J Thromb Hameost.* 2004;2:271–274.

27. Yatau R, Dayan I, Baru M. A modified chromogenic assay for the measurement of very low levels of factor VIII activity (FVIII:C). *Haemophilia.* 2006;12:253–257.

28. Parquet-Gernez A, Mazurier C, Goudemand M. Functional and immunological assays of FVIII in 133 haemophiliacs–characterisation of a subgroup of patients with mild haemophilia A and discrepancy in 1-stage and 2-stage assays. *Thromb Haemost.* 1988;59:202–206.

29. Duncan EM, Duncan BM, Tunbridge LJ, Lloyd JV. Familial discrepancy between one-stage and two-stage factor VIII assay methods in a subgroup of patients with haemophilia A. *Br J Haematol.* 1994;87:846–848.

30. Keeling DM, Sukhu K, Kemball-Cook G, Waseem N, Bagnall R, Lloyd JV. Diagnostic importance of the two-stage FVIII:C assay demonstrated by a case of mild haemophilia associated with His[1954]–Leu substitution in the FVIII A3 domain. *Br J Haematol.* 1999;105:1123–1126.

31. Mazurier C, Gaucher C, Jorieux S, Parquet-Gernez A. Mutations in the FVIII gene in seven families with mild haemophilia A. *Br J Haematol.* 1997;96:426–427.

32. Rudzi Z, Duncan EM, Casey GJ, Neuman M, Favaloro RJ, Lloyd JV. Mutations in a subgroup of patients with mild haemophilia A and familial discrepancy between one-stage and two-satge factor VIII:C methods. *Br J Haematol.* 1996;94:400–406.

33. Rodgers SE, Duncan EM, Sobieraj-Teague M, Lloyd JV. Evaluation of three automated chromogenic FVIII kits for the diagnosis of mild discrepant haemophilia A. *Int J Lab Hematol.* 2009;31:180–188.

34. Kitchen S., Hayward C., Negrier C, Dargaud Y. New developments in laboratory diagnosis and monitoring. *Haemophilia.* 2010;16(suppl 5):61–66.

35. Goodeve AC, Hinks JL, Nesbitt IM, et al. Unusual discrepant factor VIII:C assays in haemophilia A patients with Tyr346Cys and Glu321Lys FVIII gene mutations. *Thromb Haemost.* 2001;86(suppl 1).

36. Mumford AD, Kemball-Cook G, O'Donnell J, et al. A novel factor VIII variant Tyr346Cys in the acidic a1 domain is associated with an unusual one-stage/two-stage assay discrepancy and delayed thrombin activation. *Thromb Haemost.* 2001;86(suppl 1):1370

37. Mumford AD, Laffan M, O'Donnell J, et al. A Tyr346Cys in the interdomain acidic region a1 of FVIII in an individual with FVIII:C assay discrepancy. *Br J Haematol.* 2002;118:589–594.

38. Bowyer AE, Goodeve A, Liesner R, Mumford AD, Kitchen S, Makris M. Tyr365Cys change in factor VIII:

haemophilia A, but not as we know it. *Br J Haematol.* 2011;154:618–625.

39. Lyall H, Hill M, Westby J, Grimley C, Dolan G. Tyr346–Cys mutation results in factor VIII:C assay discrepancy and a normal bleeding phenotype – is this mild haemophilia A? *Hemophilia.* 2008;14:78–80.

40. Biggs R, Eveling J, Richards G. The assay of antihaemophilic globulin activity. *Br J Haematol.* 1955; 1:20–34.

41. Denson KWE. Human blood coagulation. In: Biggs R, ed. *Haemostasis and Thrombosis.* Oxford: Blackwells; 1976:682–692.

42. Barrowcliffe TW. Methodology of the two-stage assay of FVIII (FVIII:C). *Scand J Haematol Suppl.* 1984;41:25–38.

43. Assay of blood coagulation factor VIII. In: *European Pharmacopoeia.* 3rd ed. Strasbourg: Council of Europe; 1997:111–114.

44. Barrowcliffe TW On behalf of the factor VIII and IX subcommittee of SSC of ISTH. Recommendations for the assay of high-purity FVIII concentrates. *Thromb Haemost.* 1993;70:876–877.

45. Lundblad RL, Kingdom HS, Mann KG, White GC. Issues with the assay of FVIII activity in plasma and FVIII concentrates. *Thromb Haemost.* 2000;84:942–948.

46. Barrowcliffe TW, Raut S, Sands D, Hubbard AR. Coagulation and chromogenic assays of FVIII activity: general aspects standardisation and recommendations. *Semin Thromb Haemost.* 2002;28:247–256.

47. Hubbard AR, Bevan SA, Weller LJ. Potency estimation of recombinant FVIII: effect of assay method and standard. *Br J Haematol.* 2001;113:533–536.

48. Ingerslev J, Jankowski MA, Weston SB, Charles LA. Collaborative field study on the utility of a BDD factor VIII concentrate standard in the estimation of BDDr factor VIII:C activity in hemophilic plasma using the one-stage clotting assay. *J Thromb Haemost.* 2004;2:623–628.

49. Mikaelsson M, Oswaldson U, Sanderg H. Influence of phospholipids on the assessment of factor VIII activity. *Haemophilia.* 1998;4:646–650.

50. Pouplard C, Caron C, Aillaud MF, et al. The use of the new ReFacto AF laboratory standard allows reliable measurement of FVIII:C levels in ReFacto AF mock plasma samples by a one-stage assay. *Haemophilia.* 2011;17:e958–e962.

11 Application of molecular genetics to the investigation of inherited bleeding disorders

Stefan Lethagen[1], Morten Dunø[2] & Lars Bo Nielsen[3]

[1]Copenhagen University, Copenhagen, Denmark; Medical and Science, Haemophilia R&D, Novo Nordisk A/S, Denmark

[2]Department of Clinical Genetics, Copenhagen University Hospital (Rigshospitalet), Copenhagen, Denmark

[3]Department of Clinical Biochemistry, Rigshospitalet and Department of Biomedical Sciences, University of Copenhagen, Copenhagen University Hospital (Rigshospitalet), Copenhagen, Denmark

Hemophilia A and B

Hemophilia is an X-linked inherited bleeding disorder, with female carriers and affected males. There are two clinically indistinguishable forms. Hemophilia A is characterized by a deficiency of coagulation factor VIII (FVIII) and hemophilia B by a deficiency of FIX. The incidence of the diseases is about 1:5000–1:10 000 and 1:30 000–1:50 000 boys, respectively.

FVIII is synthesized as a single-chain precursor glycoprotein with 2351 amino acids ($\approx$330,000 Da). It has a domain structure with three A domains, one B domain, and two C domains and circulates as a dimer composed of one heavy chain (A1-A2-B domains) and one light chain (A3-C1-C2 domains) in a concentration of 150 ng/mL. In plasma (Figure 11.1), FVIII is noncovalently bound to von Willebrand factor (VWF), which protects FVIII from inactivation and clearance. VWF is required for normal release of FVIII and also targets FVIII to the site of vascular damage. FVIII is activated to FVIIIa initially by thrombin, which releases FVIII from VWF. FVIIIa is an unstable heterotrimer consisting of the A1, A2, and A3-C1-C2 chains. Inactivation is caused by either spontaneous dissociation of the A2 domain or cleavage of FVIIIa by activated protein C (APC) [1] (Figure 11.2).

FIX, a single-chain glycoprotein with 461 amino acids ($\approx$55,000 Da), is one of the vitamin K-dependent coagulation factors and contains 12 gamma-carboxyglutamate (gla) residues. The gla-domain, which requires vitamin K for normal synthesis, is essential for normal protein conformation and for binding to phospholipid membrane surfaces via calcium. Other important functional regions are the catalytic and activation domains. FIX circulates as an inactive zymogen in a concentration of about 3–5 μg/mL. FXa or FVIIa in complex with tissue factor activates the zymogen FIX to FIXa by cleavage of two peptide bonds and release of an activation peptide [2].

In the coagulation process, FVIIIa associates with FIXa on a phospholipid surface (physiologically the surface of the activated platelets) and forms the tenase complex that activates FX to FXa.

Depending on the factor activity in plasma, hemophilia is divided into severe (factor levels <1 IU/dL), moderate (factor levels of 1–4 IU/dL), and mild (factor levels of 5–40 IU/dL). The range of FVIII and FIX in plasma of normal healthy individuals is usually about 50–150 IU/dL (0.50–1.50 IU/ml). One (1) international unit (IU) is defined as the activity of the respective factor in 1 mL of normal plasma and calibrated to an international standard.

Inhibitors to FVIII develop in about 20–30% of patients with severe hemophilia A [3] and in about 9–23% of those with severe hemophilia B [4]. Inhibitors are antibodies against FVIII or FIX that neutralize the coagulant activity of the respective factor and develop in response to exogenous administration of

Quality in Laboratory Hemostasis and Thrombosis, Second Edition. Edited by Steve Kitchen, John D. Olson and F. Eric Preston.
© 2013 John Wiley & Sons, Ltd. Published 2013 by Blackwell Publishing Ltd.

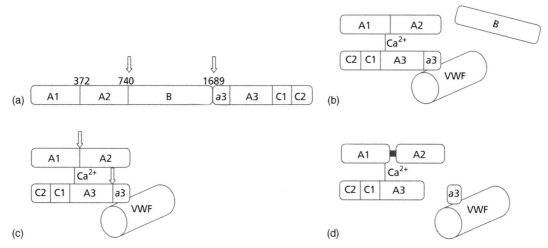

(a) (b) (c) (d)

Figure 11.1 Schematic cartoon of the activation steps of FVIII. (a) After cleavage of a 19-residue signal peptide the mature FVIII protein contains 2332 amino acids arranged in the main domains A1, A2, A3, B, C1, and C2.
It is activated mainly by thrombin and FXa cleavage at positions 372, 740, and 1689. (b) FVIII circulates as a heterodimer consisting of a heavy chain (A1, A2, and B domains) and a light chain (A3, C1, and C2 domains) in complex with the von Willebrand factor (VWF). The *a3* region within the A3 domain contains the VWF binding site. During activation, the B domain is cleaved off. (c and d) The A2 domain is cleaved off at position 372 and stays loosely bound to the relatively stable A1/A3-C1-C3 dimer via weak electrostatic interaction. Activation of FVIII involves release from the VWF.

the factor. Exogenous FIX may even cause anaphylactic reactions. About one-third to half of patients with inhibitors have low titers that may resolve spontaneously. High-titer inhibitors (>5 Bethesda Units, BU) preclude the effect of factor VIII or IX concentrates. Instead, bypassing agents, that is, activated prothrombin complex concentrates (APCC), or recombinant FVIIa (rFVIIa), are used to treat bleeding episodes. Different immune tolerance induction regimes are in use to eliminate the inhibitor, but are not always successful. Several risk factors for inhibitor development have been identified, including both genetic risk factors and non-inherited risk factors. The genetic factors include certain high-risk mutations in the *F8* or *F9* genes, inhibitors amongst first-degree relatives,

variation in some immune response genes (IL-10, TNF-α), and Native American or African ethnicity [3]. Non-inherited risk factors are less well documented. Proposed risk factors are age at first exposure, immunological challenge at the time of early factor substitution (e.g., infections or recent vaccinations), continuous infusion in mild hemophilia, and type of factor concentrate.

Factor concentrates as a cause of inhibitor development has only been documented for two intermediate plasma-derived FVIII concentrates that had undergone a combined solvent/detergent and pasteurization process. This altered the antigenic presentation of the C2 domains in the FVIII molecule [5]. Apart from that, any proposed difference in risk of inhibitor

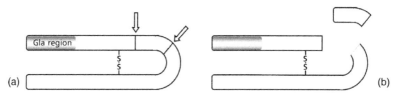

(a) (b)

Figure 11.2 Schematic cartoon of the activation steps of FIX. FIX is a single-chain glycoprotein with 415 amino acids (≈55,000 Da). It is activated by cleavage of two peptide bonds and release of an activation peptide.

development between plasma-derived and recombinant factor concentrates has not been proven in sufficiently powered controlled prospective trials [6, 7].

The genes and their mutations

Both the *F8* and *F9* genes are located on the long arm of the X chromosome at Xq28 and Xq27, respectively. *F8* (NM_000132) spans 186 kb and is comprised of 26 exons, ranging in size from exon 5 with 69 bp to the large exon 14 of 3106 bp [8]. The *F9* (NM_000133) gene is much smaller with 8 exons spanning 33.5 kb [8, 9].

Most common mutations

Hemophilia A
Today more than 2100 different mutations have been described and compiled in the HAMSTeRS (http://hadb.org.uk) and in the Human Gene Mutation databases (http://www.hgmd.org). The latter is commercially administrated and requires subscription. The most common mutation is a 500 kb inversion involving exon 1–22 and is found in 30–45% of patients with severe hemophilia A [9, 10]. The second most common mutation is likewise an inversion involving intron 1 and found in 1–3% of patients with severe disease [11, 12]. Except for these two inversions the remaining mutations are primarily point mutations and small insertions or deletions (Table 11.1). The most common insertion/deletion is a frame shift mutation in the tract of nine adenosine bases

Table 11.1 Number of unique mutations in *F8* as of June 2011

Type	Number
Mis-sense/nonsense	1324
Splicing errors	144
Regulatory	4
Small deletions	348
Small insertions	105
Small insertion/deletions	25
Gross deletions	199
Gross insertions	22
Complex rearrangements	12

Table 11.2 Number of unique mutations in *F9* as of June 2011

Type	Number
Mis-sense/nonsense	701
Splicing errors	98
Regulatory	26
Small deletions	139
Small insertions	39
Small insertion/deletions	15
Gross deletions	63
Gross insertions	7
Complex rearrangements	13

(codons 1210–1213) in exon 14 (c.3637_3638insA/c.3637delA, p.I1213fs).

Hemophilia B
Presently more than 1100 unique mutations have been described (Table 11.2). The mutations are scattered throughout the entire *F9* gene. There are no common mutations as for HA, although some of the mutations have been identified several times in different families. A subset of these relatively abundant mutations might be founder mutations, particularly those associated with a mild clinical course. The vast majority of mutations are minor sequence changes whereas only 2–4% are large structural rearrangements. A list of the mutations can be found in the Haemophilia B Mutation database (http://www.kcl.ac.uk/ip/petergreen/haemBdatabase.html) and in the Human Gene Mutation Database (http://www.hgmd.org).

Molecular diagnosis
Knowing the causative mutation in a patient suffering from hemophilia A or B is now considered part of good practice in larger clinics. However, a molecular genetic test is not absolutely necessary for establishing the diagnosis or further treatment. In a few rare cases with mild symptoms a molecular genetic analysis can be used for establishing, and thus confirming, the diagnosis. For carrier analysis, genetic counseling and prenatal and preimplantation genetic diagnoses, it is, however, important to know the disease-causing mutation.

Traditionally, a molecular diagnosis of HA has been hampered by the relatively large size of the gene, and several presequencing screening methods have been employed over the years [13–16], but with the development of high-throughput sequencing techniques, direct sequencing of the coding and exon-flanking sequences is now considered the gold standard for mutation detection. The introduction of multiplex ligation-dependent probe amplification (MLPA) has likewise simplified the detection of large deletions and duplications, and especially provided a quick and robust assay for carrier analysis of these structural mutations [17].

A diagnostic approach for mutation detection in a new HA patient (or obligate carrier) should start with a long-range PCR for detection of the common intron 22 inversion [18, 19] followed by an investigation of the intron 1 inversion [11, 12]. If negative, all coding and flanking intron regions should be investigated by PCR and direct sequencing. Due to the relatively large size of exon 14 and the presence of the commonly mutated polyA tract (c.3626–c.3637) this exon is typically sequenced initially. The overall mutation detection rate using this approach reaches >98% but is obviously dependent on a correct clinical assessment.

Similarly, the molecular analysis of *F9* is performed by conventional PCR and direct sequencing. If no mutation is identified an investigation of large structural abnormalities should be performed by MLPA. If the patient is suspected of hemophilia B Leyden type, the *F9* promoter should be included in the mutation screening. Overall, the mutation detection rate is very high, >99%.

Genotypic–phenotypic relationship

The two common inversions in HA are always associated with a severe disease. This is also, with a few exceptions, the case for nonsense mutations, frame shift mutations, and splice-site mutations in both *F8* and *F9*, since these are invariably predicted to result in the absence of a protein product or, at best, a truncated enzyme.

Depending on the type of the missense mutation these are associated with severe, moderate, and mild forms of the diseases, but the structure–function relationship of most missense mutations remains unknown. The role of novel mutations, especially missense mutations, may therefore be difficult to interpret as disease causing and great care has to be taken before using this knowledge in genetic counseling and carrier diagnosis. When a novel missense mutation

is found, the type of amino acid change (conservative/nonconservative) and the position in the protein should be taken into consideration. Furthermore, the conservation of the involved amino acid across several species should be assessed. Several software tools have been developed aimed at predicting a possible pathogenic effect of novel changes. However, great care must be taken as these in silico analyses are merely predictions. If possible, the pathogenic effect of a novel sequence change could be assessed by extended familial analysis. This should only be undertaken after sufficient genetic counseling.

The individual patient's *F8* or *F9* gene defect is probably the single most important risk factor for inhibitor development. In hemophilia A, mutations that completely preclude the synthesis of FVIII, that is, large deletions/duplications/inversions and nonsense and splice-site mutations, are associated with a higher incidence of inhibitor formation. In such patients, infused FVIII will appear as a foreign protein.

With respect to hemophilia B, the causative mutation can be identified by direct sequencing in about 97% patients, whereas only 2–4% harbor large structural mutations. In severe hemophilia B, a much larger proportion of patients have detectable FIX antigen and, therefore, exhibit immunological tolerance to infused factor IX, as compared to FVIII antigen in hemophilia A. This may, at least partly explain the much lower inhibitor incidence in hemophilia B.

Genetic counseling and prenatal and preimplantation diagnoses

Hemophilia A and B are both X-linked recessive diseases. It is generally assumed that one-third of all isolated cases would arise by a *de novo* mutation. One-third of the remaining cases are due to a new mutation in the grandparental generation. The mothers of severe hemophiliacs with the intron 22 inversion mutation are nearly all carriers.

If the mutation in the family is known, carrier diagnosis is straightforward. However, this is not always the case. In larger families with several known patients or obligate carriers linkage analysis is still a rather powerful method especially to exclude a possible female carrier status. Although such studies have been superseded by direct mutation analysis, linkage analysis protocols using intragenic linked markers should be considered when the causative mutation has not been identified. Linkage analysis always requires the involvement of other family members, which is not always possible, and is only useful where a *de novo* mutation has been ruled out.

Linkage analysis is highly reliable when intragenic polymorphisms are used and is a cheap and easy approach for countries (clinics) with a low budget and without access to more expensive methods as direct sequencing [20].

Linkage analysis is highly dependent on informative intragenic markers. The mother of the index case must be heterozygous for the polymorphism and often several markers have to be tested in order to find an informative marker. Although several very useful polymorphisms are known for both *F8* and *F9*, the frequency of heterozygous individuals varies considerably among different ethnic groups, which has to be considered [21].

Prenatal diagnosis is possible either as a direct mutation test if the disease-causing mutation is known or by marker analysis if informative linked markers have been identified.

Chorionic villus biopsy is performed in weeks 11–13 of pregnancy. Mutation analysis as well as sex determination is usually done within 2–3 days. Due to the greatly improved treatment of the diseases during the last 10–20 years, a fetal diagnosis of hemophilia does not always lead to termination of pregnancy. Prenatal diagnosis is, however, indicated for necessary precautions during delivery.

Preimplantation genetic diagnosis (PGD) has become attractive for female carriers [22, 23]. This method implies *in vitro* fertilization followed by an embryo biopsy at the 6–12 cell stage. There are two approaches in PGD: (1) a single blastomere is analyzed by FISH analysis to determine the sex of the embryo, where only female embryos are transferred to the uterus and (2) direct mutation detection using single-cell PCR and transfer of unaffected male/female embryos.

Other rare bleeding disorders

Hemophilia A and B and von Willebrand disease (VWD) are the most prevalent inherited bleeding disorders, together covering about 95–97% of all inherited deficiencies of coagulation factors. The remaining defects are generally recessively inherited by both sexes. They are rare, with prevalence ranging from approximately 1 in 2 million for factor II (prothrombin) and FXIII deficiency to 1 in 500,000 for FVII deficiency. Prevalence may be higher in areas with a high frequency of consanguineous marriages, for example, FXI deficiency in some Jewish communities, and also other deficiencies in the Middle East or Southern India. Being so rare, most centers have limited experience of their management. Some large, international registries have enhanced our knowledge about these rare bleeding disorders [24–26].

In contrast to hemophilia A where 30–45% of the patients have the same inversion of exon 1 to exon 22, the rare inherited bleeding disorders are often caused by mutations that are specific for each family, and mutations are scattered throughout the genes. The mutations can be missense, nonsense, or insertion/deletion types or mutations in noncoding regions affecting mRNA splicing. Gross deletions or large inversions have rarely been described, but this may to some extent reflect that such gene rearrangements will often escape detection with the conventional DNA sequencing strategies used in molecular diagnostics. Indeed, conventional DNA sequencing fails to identify specific mutations in ~10–20% of patients with rare coagulation factor deficiencies. The Institute of Medical Genetics in Cardiff maintains a large database of mutations in coagulation factors and a comprehensive summary of mutations described up to 2002 has been provided by Peyvandi and coworkers [27]. Table 11.3 shows the occurrence of different mutation types in various types of rare bleeding disorders adapted from Reference 25.

Severe deficiency of coagulation factors is mostly caused by large deletions. Null mutations may result in the production of truncated proteins and very low or undetectable plasma factors and may cause severe bleeding symptoms. Missense mutations are less predictable and may lead to both mild and severe deficiencies.

Fibrinogen deficiency can present as afibrinogenemia, hypofibrinogenemia, or dysfibrinogenemia, depending on the causing mutation. In contrast to other rare bleeding disorders, fibrinogen disorders are often inherited as autosomal dominant traits. Some patients have a bleeding tendency, others have thrombotic tendency, and some may have both [28].

Prothrombin deficiency is either characterized by a parallel decrease of activity and antigen levels or a dysfunctional protein with normal antigen levels. There

Table 11.3 Mutations in genes causing rare bleeding disorders (adapted from the Human Gene Mutation Database at the Institute of Medical Genetics in Cardiff, January 2008)

Coagulation factor	Frequency of homozygous deficiency[a]	Gene	Type of mutation					
			Missense/ nonsense	Small insertion/ deletion	Splicing	Gross insertion/ deletion/ rearrangement	Regulatory	Total
Fibrinogen	1:1,000,000	FGA	29	20	3	4	1	57[b]
		FGB	27	0	4	1	2	42[b]
		FGG	50	2	5	0	0	57
Prothrombin	1:2,000,000	F2	36	5	3	0	3	47[b]
V	1:1,000,000	F5	28	17	6	1	0	52[b]
VII	1:500,000	F7	104	18	21	2	10	156[c,b]
X	1:1,000,000	F10	64	6	3	3	0	76
XI	1:1,000,000	F11	69	10	10	1	0	90[b]
XIII	1:2,000,000	F13A1	39	18	8	1	0	66
		F13B	2	3	0	0	0	5
V + VIII	1:2,000,000	LMAN1	5	10	4	0	0	19
		MCFD2	2	3	2	0	0	7
Vitamin K dependent	1:2,000,000	GGCX	3	1	1	0	0	5[c,d]
		VKORC1	6	0	1	0	1	8[d]

[a]Adapted from Reference 28.
[b]Rarely mutations have been detected in individuals with increased plasma concentrations or a history of thrombosis.
[c]Includes one repeat variation.
[d]Mutations have also been described in individuals with altered sensitivity to warfarin.

are no reported cases of aprothrombinemia, which may not be compatible with life. FV deficiency, also called Owren's disease or parahemophilia, is usually a type 1 deficiency. Only one case of type 2 FV deficiency has been described. FVII deficiency is the most common of the rare bleeding disorders. Two-thirds are missense mutations. One-third are null mutations that decrease or abolish the expression of FVII. Most mild cases have missense mutations. Most severe cases have null mutations (deletions, insertions, splicing, and promoter mutations). FVII deficiency may be combined with other coagulation factor deficiencies [29]. FX deficiency is caused by missense mutations in about 75% of cases, and most cases have measurable levels of FX. Complete absence of FX is probably not compatible with life. There are no reported nonsense mutations. FXI deficiency (hemophilia C) may be caused by a nonsense mutation in exon 5 (p.Glu117Stop), HGVS: c403G<T,pGlu which is frequent in Ashkenazi and Iraqi Jews. The mutation causes very low

or undetectable levels of FXI in plasma in homozygotes. Another mutation, frequent in Ashkenazi Jews, is a missense mutation in exon 9 (p.Phe283Leu) that leads to a defective secretion, with plasma levels of FXI low but detectable at approximately 10%. Compound heterozygosity for both mutations is the most common cause of FXI deficiency among Jews [30]. Other missense mutations have been described in some European non-Jewish populations. A dominant negative effect through heterodimer formation has been described for some missense mutations. In FXIII deficiency, most mutations are located in the gene that encodes the A subunit, and only a minority in the B subunit. The mutations are spread throughout the gene and most mutations are unique.

Patients with combined FV and FVIII deficiency have a type 1 deficiency, with levels of the respective factor usually between 5% and 20%. The disorder is caused by a dysfunction in a reciprocal intracellular transport mechanism. A lectin mannose-binding protein (*LMAN1*, also called *ERGIC-53*) binds both FV and FVIII in the endoplasmic reticulum/Golgi intermediate compartment (ERGIC) and functions as chaperone in their intracellular transport. Mutations in the *LMAN1* gene cause the combined deficiency in most cases. Some cases are caused by deficiency of a cofactor to LMAN1, encoded by a gene called multiple coagulation factor deficiency 2 gene (*MCFD2*).

Multiple deficiencies of vitamin K-dependent coagulation factors can be caused by mutations that affect the gamma-glutamyl carboxylation of vitamin K-dependent proteins. This involves not only the coagulation factors II, VII, IX, and X, but also the coagulation inhibitors protein C and protein S together with some bone proteins, all of which are vitamin K dependent. The molecular basis of the multiple deficiencies is missense mutations in the gamma-glutamyl carboxylase gene (*GGCX*), or in the gene vitamin K epoxide reductase complex subunit 1 (*VKORC1*), which lead to the production of a dysfunctional enzyme [25].

Genotypic diagnosis of rare bleeding disorders is not performed routinely. There are generally no high-frequency mutations. This implies that screening the whole gene is necessary in most cases.

Internal quality control

Every PCR amplification should include a water blank to ensure that there is no contamination of PCR reagents by exogenous DNA. No amplified product should be visible from this reaction. Whenever any product is seen, all simultaneously amplified PCR products should be discarded.

PCR primers should be designed using a software program as "Primer Design-Exon Primer" (http://ihg.gsf.de/ihg/ExonPrimer.html) and checked for possible single nucleotide polymorphisms within the primer annealing sequence (https://ngrl.manchester.ac.uk/SNPCheckV3/snpcheck.htm).

When setting up analyses for the two common inversions positive controls should always be included. If possible DNA from patients and female carriers should be included.

The sequencing of an amplicon in which a candidate mutation has been identified must always be repeated, preferably by another method, for example, restriction enzyme analysis. A second scientist should independently check sequences, nucleotide number and base change, and its predicted effect on the protein. When analyzing family members for a previously identified mutation, a familial positive control plus a normal control lacking the familial mutation should be included.

When a sequence alteration is identified, use relevant databases to see if the mutation has been described before. If the mutation is new it should be named according to Human Genome Variation Society (HGVS) nomenclature (http://www.hgvs.org/mutnomen/). Nucleotide numbering should follow these rules that "A" in initiation codon ATG = +1. To convert HGVS-type amino acid numbering in FVIII (where initiator Met = +1) to the more common and universal numbering add 20 to negative numbers and 19 to positive numbers, for example, Met−19 becomes Met + 1 but Arg + 3 becomes Arg + 22.

For FIX add 47 to negative numbers and 46 to positive numbers, for example, Arg−4 becomes Arg43, but Gly + 4 becomes Gly50.

If a sequence alteration is suspected to have an effect on mRNA splicing, a number of prediction tools are available and the use of a number of these tools in combination is recommended before suggesting that an effect on splicing is likely; these include Fruit Fly (http://www.fruitfly.org/seq_tools/splice.html), NetGene2 (http://www.cbs.dtu.dk/services/NetGene2/) and Splice Site Finder (http://www.umd.be/HSF/). Where an effect on splicing is likely, follow-up by cDNA analysis can often confirm the prediction, but this usually is not possible in a routine setting up.

External quality assessment

Among the few external quality assessment (EQA) schemes available for molecular testing in hemophilia, the UK NEQAS for Blood Coagulation on Haemophilia Genetics is one example. This scheme runs twice yearly exercises that alternate between hemophilia A, hemophilia B, and VWD. As with other molecular genetic EQA schemes, the three areas of clerical accuracy, genotyping, and interpretation are examined (http://www.ukneqasbc.org/content/PageServer.asp?S=932234149&C=1252&ID=32).

Marks are lost for errors in each of these three areas.

Reporting

Develop standard templates for commonly used report types to avoid missing essential information. Reports should be written so that they can follow the patient and be interpreted by a number of different healthcare professionals.

Nomenclature

Nucleotide and amino acid numbering and nomenclature for sequence alterations should follow HGVS recommendations (http://www.hgvs.org/mutnomen/). GenBank reference sequences with version numbers should be stated for both cDNA and protein. Ref.seq: NM_000132 (F8) and ref.seq: NM_000133 (F9). Include version numbers.

References

1. Saenko EL, Ananyeva NM, Tuddenham EG, Kemball-Cook G. Factor VIII – novel insights into form and function. *Br J Haematol.* 2002;119:323–331.
2. Schmidt AE, Bajaj SP. Structure-function relationships in factor IX and factor IXa. *Trends Cardiovasc Med.* 2003;13:39–45.
3. Oldenburg J, Pavlova A. Genetic risk factors for inhibitors to factors VIII and IX. *Haemophilia.* 2006;12 (suppl 6):15–22.
4. DiMichele D. Inhibitor development in haemophilia B: an orphan disease in need of attention. *Br J Haematol.* 2007;138:305–315.
5. Peerlinck K, Arnout J, Di Giambattista M, et al. Factor VIII inhibitors in previously treated haemophilia A patients with a double virus-inactivated plasma derived factor VIII concentrate. *Thromb Haemost.* 1997;77:80–86.
6. Hoots WK. Urgent inhibitor issues: targets for expanded research. *Haemophilia.* 2006;12(suppl 6):107–113.
7. Hay CR. The epidemiology of factor VIII inhibitors. *Haemophilia.* 2006;12(suppl 6):23–28; discussion 28–29.
8. Gitschier J, Wood WI, Goralka TM, et al. Characterization of the human factor VIII gene. *Nature.* 1984; 312:326–330.
9. Kurachi K, Davie EW. Isolation and characterization of a cDNA coding for human factor IX. *Proc Natl Acad Sci U S A.* 1982;79:6461–6464.
10. Antonarakis SE, Rossiter JP, Young M, et al. Factor VIII gene inversions in severe hemophilia A: results of an international consortium study. *Blood.* 1995;86:2206–2212.
11. Bagnall RD, Waseem N, Green PM, Giannelli F. Recurrent inversion breaking intron 1 of the factor VIII gene is a frequent cause of severe hemophilia A. *Blood.* 2002;99:168–174.
12. Cumming AM. The factor VIII gene intron 1 inversion mutation: prevalence in severe hemophilia A patients in the UK. *J Thromb Haemost.* 2004;2:205–206.
13. Jayandharan G, Shaji RV, Chandy M, Srivastava A. Identification of factor IX gene defects using a multiplex PCR and CSGE strategy – a first report. *J Thromb Haemost.* 2003;1:2051–2054.
14. Habart D, Kalabova D, Novotny M, Vorlova Z. Thirty-four novel mutations detected in factor VIII gene by multiplex CSGE: modeling of 13 novel amino acid substitutions. *J Thromb Haemost.* 2003;1:773–781.
15. Frusconi S, Passerini I, Girolami F, et al. Identification of seven novel mutations of F8C by DHPLC. *Hum Mutat.* 2002;20:231–232.
16. Jayandharan G, Shaji RV, Baidya S, Nair SC, Chandy M, Srivastava A. Identification of factor VIII gene mutations in 101 patients with haemophilia A: mutation analysis by inversion screening and multiplex PCR and CSGE and molecular modelling of 10 novel missense substitutions. *Haemophilia.* 2005;11:481–491.
17. Schouten JP, McElgunn CJ, Waaijer R, Zwijnenburg D, Diepvens F, Pals G. Relative quantification of 40 nucleic acid sequences by multiplex ligation-dependent probe amplification. *Nucleic Acids Res.* 2002;30:e57.
18. Bowen DJ, Keeney S. Unleashing the long-distance PCR for detection of the intron 22 inversion of the factor VIII gene in severe haemophilia A. *Thromb Haemost.* 2003;89:201–202.
19. Liu Q, Nozari G, Sommer SS. Single-tube polymerase chain reaction for rapid diagnosis of the inversion hotspot of mutation in hemophilia A. *Blood.* 1998; 92:1458–1459.
20. Peyvandi F. Carrier detection and prenatal diagnosis of hemophilia in developing countries. *Semin Thromb Hemost.* 2005;31:544–554.
21. Peake IR, Lillicrap DP, Boulyjenkov V, et al. Haemophilia: strategies for carrier detection and prenatal diagnosis. *Bull World Health Org.* 1993;71:429–458.
22. Gigarel N, Frydman N, Burlet P, et al. Single cell co-amplification of polymorphic markers for the indirect preimplantation genetic diagnosis of hemophilia A, X-linked adrenoleukodystrophy, X-linked hydrocephalus and incontinentia pigmenti loci on Xq28. *Hum Genet.* 2004;114:298–305.
23. Michaelides K, Tuddenham EG, Turner C, Lavender B, Lavery SA. Live birth following the first mutation specific pre-implantation genetic diagnosis for haemophilia A. *Thromb Haemost.* 2006;95:373–379.
24. Peyvandi F, Jayandharan G, Chandy M, et al. Genetic diagnosis of haemophilia and other inherited bleeding disorders. *Haemophilia.* 2006;12(suppl 3):82–89.

25. Mannucci PM, Duga S, Peyvandi F. Recessively inherited coagulation disorders. *Blood*. 2004;104:1243–1252.

26. Acharya SS, Coughlin A, Dimichele DM. Rare Bleeding Disorder Registry: deficiencies of factors II, V, VII, X, XIII, fibrinogen and dysfibrinogenemias. *J Thromb Haemost*. 2004;2:248–256.

27. Peyvandi F, Duga S, Akhavan S, Mannucci PM. Rare coagulation deficiencies. *Haemophilia*. 2002;8:308–321.

28. Asselta R, Duga S, Tenchini ML. The molecular basis of quantitative fibrinogen disorders. *J Thromb Haemost*. 2006;4:2115–2129.

29. Girolami A, Ruzzon E, Tezza F, Allemand E, Vettore S. Congenital combined defects of factor VII: a critical review. *Acta Haematol*. 2007;117:51–56.

30. Franchini M, Veneri D, Lippi G. Inherited factor XI deficiency: a concise review. *Hematology*. 2006;11:307–309.

12 Detecting and quantifying acquired functional inhibitors in hemostasis

Bert Verbruggen[1], Myriam Dardikh[2], &
Britta Laros-van Gorkom[3]

[1]Laboratory of Clinical Chemistry and Haematology, Jeroen Bosch Hospital's-Hertogenbosch, The Netherlands
[2]Department of Laboratory Medicine, Laboratory of Haematology, Radboud University Nijmegen Medical Centre, Nijmegen, The Netherlands
[3]Department of Haematology, Radboud University Nijmegen Medical Centre, Nijmegen, The Netherlands

Introduction

Acquired functional inhibitors of hemostasis are immunoglobulins of allogeneic or autologous origin that arise either spontaneously or as a reaction to neoantigens and which interfere with blood coagulation. Most frequent inhibitors are lupus anticoagulants (LA), a subgroup of antiphospholipid antibodies, which bind to a complex of phospholipids and phospholipid-binding proteins ($ß_2$ glycoprotein-1, prothrombin, and others) resulting in prolongation of clotting times [1]. Antiphospholipid antibodies, especially the lupus positive ones, are well-recognized risk factors for venous and arterial thrombosis. However, LA-positive patients may occasionally exhibit hemorrhagic diathesis when one or more coagulation factors are decreased. The latter may be caused by elevated clearance of coagulation proteins–phospholipids complexes that are bound to nonneutralizing lupus antibodies [2]. Lupus inhibitors are outside the scope of this chapter and will be discussed elsewhere.

The other group of inhibitors recognizes functional epitopes of one of the individual coagulation proteins thereby inhibiting the functionality of that specific protein. Two different types have been described: autologous and allogeneic inhibitors.

Autologous inhibitors may develop in patients with previously normal hemostasis by a deregulation of the immune system. The most frequent spontaneous autologous inhibitor is directed against factor VIII (FVIII). The reported incidence is 1:1.48 million/year [3]. Autologous FVIII inhibitors, mostly affecting elderly people, are in a 40–50% of cases associated with underlying disorders such as an autoimmune disease, malignancy, or with pregnancy, but frequently have no underlying associated disease. It is a serious complication with a mortality of about 10% mostly due to bleeding problems [3]. Autoimmune factor IX (FIX) inhibitors [4] and factor XI (FXI) inhibitors, which are mainly associated with systemic lupus erythematosus [5], have a much lower incidence compared to autoimmune FVIII inhibitors.

Autologous inhibitors against each of the clotting factors V, XII and the vitamin K-dependent proteins are described but are very rare [6].

Allogeneic inhibitors against individual coagulation factors may develop in patients with congenital factor deficiency because of treatment with the missing factor or in patients otherwise treated with clotting products [7]. Among these inhibitors, FVIII inhibitors in hemophilia A patients who are treated with FVIII products are most frequent. The overall inhibitor incidence is 25–30% with the highest reported incidence in severely affected patients with genotypes that completely lack FVIII. The lowest incidence is reported in mild hemophiliacs [8]. The development of FVIII inhibitors usually occurs early after the beginning of therapy (less than 50 exposure days) and for this reason generally occurs during childhood.

Quality in Laboratory Hemostasis and Thrombosis, Second Edition. Edited by Steve Kitchen, John D. Olson and F. Eric Preston.
© 2013 John Wiley & Sons, Ltd. Published 2013 by Blackwell Publishing Ltd.

FIX inhibitors in patients with hemophilia B are much less common (1.5–3%) than FVIII inhibitors [9]. Patients with complete deletions or rearrangements of the FIX gene have a risk of inhibitor development of about 50%, whereas in patients with nonsense or frameshift mutations this risk is about 20% and for missense mutations the inhibitor risk is very low (<1%) [10]. Immune tolerance induction (ITI) therapy is successful in only 40% or less of hemophilia B patients with inhibitors [11–13]. In this patient group, the treatment with FIX concentrates unfortunately is greatly complicated by anaphylaxis [10]. FXI inhibitors may occur in the severe type of FXI deficiency (FXI:C <0.01 IU/mL), which is almost exclusively described in Ashkenazi and Iraqi Jews. The frequency of inhibitors in severe patients following plasma infusion is >30% [14]; most cases are detected at routine screening because these patients mostly do not bleed spontaneously.

Allogeneic inhibitors against other hemostasis factors have a low to very low frequency and will be discussed later.

Clinical manifestations of hemostasis inhibitors

Autologous inhibitors in individuals with previously normal hemostasis manifest themselves clinically by an unexpected moderate-to-severe bleeding tendency. Especially in the case of FVIII autoantibodies, the disease may be life threatening and the appropriate medical intervention is a prerequisite for survival.

Allogeneic inhibitors in patients with a pre-existing hemorrhagic disorder who are treated preventively or therapeutically for bleeding complications manifest themselves by excessive bleeding, bleeding in unusual parts of the body, or a low recovery and/or half-life of infused hemostatic products. However, the latter findings are not pathognomonic of the presence of an inhibitor since antibodies without inhibitor activity may also decrease clotting factor concentrations as a result of an increased clearance rate of the antigen–antibody complex [15]. Moreover, increased clearance of infused FVIII concentrate may also be caused by low von Willebrand factor (vWF) concentrations [16] or additional unknown factors [17]. Therefore, the clinical suspicion of an inhibitor has to be confirmed by objective laboratory tests. Laboratory

investigation of inhibitors always starts with screening tests followed, if necessary, by more specific tests to identify the exact nature of the inhibitor.

Screening tests for inhibitor detection

Inhibitors of the classic hemostasis pathway invariably are detected by one or more prolonged basic clotting tests like activated partial thromboplastin time (aPTT), prothrombin time (PT), and thrombin time (TT). Prolonged clotting times may be an accidental finding when screening a patient for a bleeding problem. However, these tests are also the first to be performed when a patient presents with the suspicion of an inhibitor.

In order to discriminate between true factor deficiencies, which also prolong clotting tests, and inhibitors, it is necessary to perform mixing tests with normal pooled plasma, preferably in a ratio 1:1. A prolonged clotting time that is not corrected in the mixing study is an indication for the presence of an inhibitor. However, the presence of heparin and/or other therapeutically administered direct anti-IIa and anti-Xa inhibitors (e.g., Argatroban, Dabigatran, Rivaroxaban) has to be excluded. Some coagulation factor inhibitors have a progressive mode of action. This means that inhibitors can only be detected when applying a prolonged incubation time of the mixture (≥60 minutes). Ideally, mixing studies should be performed both with short (≤1 minute) and long incubation times in order to discriminate between fast-acting inhibitors and slow-acting ones. However, this does not give additional information on the nature of the inhibitor because both types are described for LAs and individual clotting factor inhibitors [18].

An LA is suspected in case of failure to correct a prolonged aPTT in a 1:1 mixture within 5 seconds of normal pooled plasma [19]. However, such a general agreement neither exists for the other basic coagulation tests for detecting LA, nor for other types of inhibitors like FVIII inhibitors. Therefore, each laboratory has to build up its own experience and include appropriate control samples in the assay in order to draw conclusions on mixing tests.

The presence of an inhibitor can be confirmed by treating the plasma with sepharose-bound Protein A, Protein G, or 2-mercaptopyridine. Protein A and Protein G are surface proteins of streptococci that bind the Fc-part of IgG immunoglobulins, whereas it has been suggested that the interaction of IgM and 2-mercaptopyridine results from combined electron donating and accepting action of the ligand or, alternatively, a mixed mode hydrophilic–hydrophobic interaction. In our laboratory HiTrap™ Protein A HP, HiTrap™ Protein G HP, and HiTrap™ IgM Purification HP columns from Amersham Biosciences are used to remove immunoglobulins IgG (Protein A and G) or IgM from plasma and additionally purify the immune inhibitor. Purified plasma samples result in normal mixing studies when immunoglobulins are responsible for the abnormal mixing study. Eventually, the purified immunoglobulins may be used to confirm the inhibitor activity.

Differential classification of inhibitors

Differentiation between LA and inhibitors against coagulation factors is of clinical relevance because of the different therapeutic strategies for the two abnormalities (i.e., antithrombotic agents for LA and hemostatic agents for the factor inhibitors) [20]. However, both thrombosis and bleeding may occur in patients with LA and in patients with individual factor inhibitors making differential diagnosis of the nature of inhibitors by clinical observations unreliable.

Concerning laboratory diagnosis, the presence of LA in plasma may prolong the aPTT clotting times and may, therefore, interfere with factor inhibitor assays and result in falsely positive inhibitor titers [21]. Alternatively, inhibitors against individual coagulation factors can interfere with lupus testing and may cause falsely positive lupus confirmation tests [22, 23]. A further common laboratory finding in patients with these different types of inhibitors is one or more low-factor activities when assayed with the one-stage coagulation factor assay according to a parallel line bioassay [24]. Parallelism of the curves of patient and reference plasmas is a prerequisite for reliability of these assays. It was demonstrated that nonparallelism could only be detected in the presence of high-titer LAs with the use of lupus sensitive assays [25]. This finding may be useful in the differential laboratory diagnosis of the different types of inhibitors. Additional methods to improve the specificity of inhibitor testing are described in the section "*Pitfalls and limitations of the inhibitor assay.*"

Assay of inhibitors against individual coagulation factors

Assay principle

All functional assays to confirm and quantify inhibitors of individual coagulation factors are based on a universal method of measuring the decrease of clotting factor activity in a mixture of an exogenous source of the clotting factor (e.g., normal pooled plasma) and the putative inhibitor plasma in a certain time period. A reference measurement needs to be performed with the same method substituting the patient plasma by a control plasma sample that does not contain an inhibitor. Residual factor activities in the assay mixtures are measured by one-stage clotting assays (mostly aPTT) or chromogenic ones.

Immunologic assays are not suitable for inhibitor detection because they do not discriminate between antibodies with and without inhibitor activity [26–28]. However, in FVIII inhibitor-positive samples good correlations were found between enzyme-linked immunosorbent assay (ELISA) and inhibitor methods but variable results have been reported on specificity and sensitivity of the immunologic methods compared to the inhibitor activity assays [29–31].

Available methods

Initially all inhibitor assays were focused on the measurement of FVIII inhibitors.

The first assay to measure FVIII inhibitor activity was described by Biggs and Macfarlane [32] using the thromboplastin generation test followed by the Oxford method [33] using bovine FVIII concentrate (cryoprecipitate) in a mixing test with patient plasma. Later Kasper et al. [34] described the Bethesda assay and introduced a more uniform measurement of FVIII inhibitors by using normal pooled plasma as FVIII source in a 1:1 mix with patient plasma and imidazole buffer as control sample. The sensitivity and specificity of the assay was further improved in the Nijmegen assay by buffering the normal pooled plasma and replacing the imidazole buffer by inhibitor-free deficient plasma [35]. A variant of this assay has been described in the Osaka modified Bethesda assay [36] that differs from the Nijmegen assay in three points: buffering the test plasma instead of the pool plasma, using buffer as control sample, and using an algorithm to correct for the residual intrinsic FVIII activity instead of heating of the plasma. Compared to the Nijmegen assay, the method is more complicated and less specific due to the use of buffer as reference sample. The Nijmegen assay focuses on FVIII but can also be used for measuring other clotting factor inhibitors by replacing FVIII-deficient plasma by the appropriate factor-deficient plasma and assaying the residual activity of the appropriate factor. The method is recommended by the International Society on Thrombosis and Haemostasis Factor VIII/IX Scientific Subcommittee [37] for FVIII inhibitor testing. For this reason, the main points of this assay are described here in detail.

Reagents

• aPTT reagent
• Inhibitor-free plasma deficient for the factor to be measured (factor activity <0.01 IU/mL)
• Normal pooled plasma with an assigned factor level of 1 IU/mL
• 0.1 mol/L imidazole buffered normal pooled plasma. Preparation: add one volume of buffered 4 mol/L imidazole pH 7.4 to 39 volumes of a pool of citrated plasma of at least 50 healthy blood donors. Adjust pH to 7.4.
• 33 mmol/L calcium chloride

Equipment

• Plastic tubes, pipettes, and normal medical laboratory equipment
• Citrate-containing vacuum blood collection tubes
• Incubator or water bath of 37°C
• Coagulometer

The assay can be carried out using semi-automated or manual techniques. However, in order to get more reliable results, it is advisable to use fully automated devices to measure clotting times.

Method

The method is schematically shown in Figure 12.1.

To inactivate residual factor activity before testing, patient- and factor-deficient control plasma samples are heated at 58°C for at least 1.5 hours. In order to remove any debris caused by the heating process, the samples have to be centrifuged at 4000 g for 2 minutes (Eppendorf centrifuge). The inhibitor that has already been complexed with FVIII will not dissociate from the complex during heating and therefore, only free circulating inhibitor will be measured. [38].

Heated test plasma as well as factor-deficient control plasma are mixed with equal volumes of imidazole-buffered normal pooled plasma pH 7.4 and incubated for 2 hours at 37°C. Subsequently, the remaining factor activity in both test and control

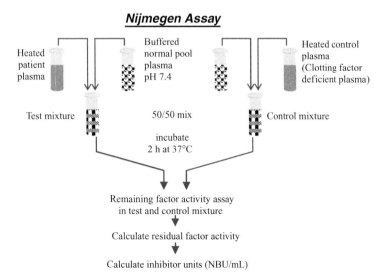

Nijmegen Assay

Heated patient plasma — Buffered normal pool plasma pH 7.4 — Heated control plasma (Clotting factor deficient plasma)

Test mixture — 50/50 mix incubate 2 h at 37°C — Control mixture

Remaining factor activity assay in test and control mixture

Calculate residual factor activity

Calculate inhibitor units (NBU/mL)

Figure 12.1 Schematic methodology of the Nijmegen–Bethesda assay for the quantification of inhibitors.

mixtures is determined by a one-stage factor assay or a chromogenic factor assay.

Evaluation of test results

The "residual factor activity" is defined as the relative percentage factor activity of the test mixture compared to the control mixture. One Nijmegen Bethesda unit (NBU) is defined as the amount of inhibitor that results in 50% residual factor activity. Inhibitor activity of patient samples is read in NBU/mL from a semilogarithmic plot representing the correlation between residual factor activity (logarithmic) and inhibitor activity (linear) [34]. The regression line is fully defined by 100% residual factor activity with 0 NBU/mL inhibitor and 50% residual activity with 1 NBU/mL inhibitor (Figure 12.2). Alternatively, the inhibitor titer may be calculated by the algorithm: Inhibitor titer (BU/mL) = (2-log residual activity)/0.3010. Dose-response curves of test plasma need to show parallelism with this calibration curve. If not, inhibitor data are not reliable and an alternative strategy needs to be followed (e.g., type II FVIII inhibitors).

When the residual factor activity of undiluted sample is below 25%, retesting of more diluted samples is recommended because of nonlinearity of inhibitor concentration and residual activity with high inhibitor titers. Dilutions have to be made with deficient plasma.

Expected values

Until now the only data on FVIII inhibitor assays have been published. In most reference laboratories 0.6 BU/mL is used as the cut-off value. This value has been derived from the results with the classic Bethesda assay and is a reflection of the low specificity of this method. However, the sensitivity and specificity, including the cut-off value, have been improved in the Nijmegen assay [35]. In fact every individual laboratory has to assign the laboratory-specific cut-off value by assaying positive and negative inhibitor samples from hemophilia patients. This may be difficult to perform as most laboratories do not have these samples available. An alternative is to dilute one or more inhibitor-positive samples with inhibitor-free FVIII-deficient plasma to low and very low inhibitor levels, compare the data of the inhibitor assays of these dilutions with a set of inhibitor-negative plasma samples, and establish the methodological cut-off value.

Improved sensitive assay

Recently, a more sensitive method has been described showing a cut-off value as low as 0.03 BU/mL [39]. Before analysis the test plasma is concentrated by selective protein filtration using a centrifugal technique. Thereafter the inhibitor activity is quantified similar to the Nijmegen assay, except for the incubation step in which a different ratio of normal pool plasma/test plasma (ratio 1:3) has to be used. The assay of residual FVIII activity should be performed chromogenically because of the small sample volume and the viscosity of the sample. The low titer assay is about 20-fold more sensitive for FVIII inhibitors than the Nijmegen assay with a cut-off value <0.03 NBU/mL.

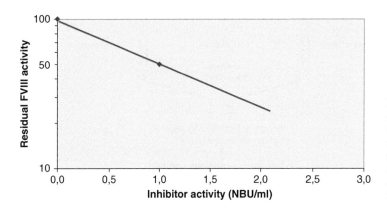

Figure 12.2 Calibration curve for quantification of inhibitors. On the y axis the residual factor activity expressed as the relative percentage factor activity of the test mixture compared to the control mixture (logarithmic). Inhibitor activity is plotted on the x axis the in Nijmegen–Bethesda unit/mL (linear).

The clinical relevance of the method is demonstrated in seven post ITI patients with shortened FVIII half-life (<5 hours) or low 12–16 hours recovery after FVIII administration. Unlike the Nijmegen assay, the new low titer assay showed increased inhibitor titers in these seven post ITI patients that may explain the abnormal FVIII pharmacokinetics in these patients and may explain the frequent occurrence of bleeding in post ITI patients. The method has to be validated more extensively in future.

Assay characteristics

A number of variables can influence the assay and may contribute to an undesirably high intra- and interlaboratory coefficient of variation of the results.

Buffered normal pooled plasma is used as a clotting factor source in the incubation mixture with patient and reference sample. The FVIII activity of the pool plasma may influence the measured inhibitor activity. As an example, increased FVIII content of the pooled plasma will need more inhibitor to inactivate a certain percentage of FVIII and thus, will lower the inhibitor titer. However, decreased FVIII content of the pooled plasma will need less inhibitor to inactivate a certain percentage of FVIII and will increase the inhibitor titer. Thus, increased factor activity in the pooled plasma will under note the inhibitor activity when compared with a pooled plasma of lower factor activity. A plasma pool of at least 50 healthy donors is necessary to guarantee a level as close as possible to 1IU FVIII/mL. Yet it is advisable to calibrate the FVIII content of the pool against an international standard for FVIII to ensure the potency [40]. Less than 50 donors in the pool may result in more deviation from 1 IU/mL and calibration with an external standard is then essential. A pool of at least 20 donors is needed to guarantee acceptable levels for the other clotting factors.

The residual factor activity measurements will only minimally be influenced by aberrations in the factor content of the pool for this is a relative measure that is not influenced by factor variations.

The pH stability of the incubation mixtures is an essential feature of the Nijmegen assay. During incubation at 37°C, the pH in nonbuffered mixtures increases resulting in uncontrolled and nonspecific

Table 12.1 Activity of clotting factors in normal pooled plasma before and after heating at 58°C for 90 minutes

	Native activity (IU/mL)	Activity after heating (IU/mL)
Factor II	1	0.008
Factor V	1	0.009
Factor VII	1	0.009
Factor X	1	0.008
Factor VIII	1	0.007
Factor IX	1	0.009
Factor XI	1	0.004

inactivation of labile coagulation factors [35]. pH stabilization of the incubation mixture by buffering the normal pooled plasma will overcome this problem and increase the specificity and sensitivity of the method.

Residual FVIII activity in the patient plasma can interfere with the inhibitor assay by increasing the remaining factor activity after incubation with normal pooled plasma leading to falsely low inhibitor titers. This problem can be overcome by heating the test and control plasma at 58°C for 90 minutes. This will destroy all the clotting factors (Table 12.1) whereas immunoglobulins are heat resistant leaving the inhibitor data unchanged.

The physiological binding of FVIII with vWF prevents rapid complex formation of an inhibitor with FVIII since only free FVIII can be bound. Therefore, the inhibition of FVIII is a time-dependent process that is determined by dissociation/association kinetics of FVIII and vWF. An *incubation time* of 2 hours is sufficient to bind all the inhibitors to the active site of the protein. However, there is a special group of FVIII inhibitors that inactivate the protein by proteolytic cleavage of the active site. These so-called proteolytic inhibitors can also be measured with the Nijmegen assay but need an incubation time that must be extended in order to fully exhibit the inhibitory action [41]. However, there is no simple test available to discriminate between proteolytic and neutralizing antibodies. Time dependency of the inhibitor titer may be useful but is in fact only described for purified anti-FVIII IgG [41].

Inhibitors against the other coagulation factors (e.g., FIX, V, XI) have a direct mode of action and therefore, a short incubation with the substrate is sufficient when assaying these inhibitors.

Pitfalls and limitations of the inhibitor assay

Quality assessment of inhibitor assays is still a problem for individual laboratories because *standard and control samples* are not (yet) available. Intralaboratory day-to-day quality assessment can be performed by assaying negative and positive inhibitor samples that are stored at −80°C. Interlaboratory surveys of FVIII inhibitor assays have been organized since 2005 by the External quality Control of Assays and Tests Foundation (ECAT) and by the UK National External Quality Assessment Scheme (NEQAS). The results of the surveys of the ECAT show a rather high interlaboratory coefficient of variation of about 30% for the Nijmegen assay and more than 40% for the original Bethesda method and do not improve in time. In order to address this phenomenon, a workshop was organized with the aim to investigate assay components that contribute to the high interlaboratory variation and to establish minimal assay conditions for a reliable FVIII inhibitor test. [42]. It appeared that, besides buffering of normal pool substrate plasma and the use of FVIII-deficient plasma as reference sample, the sample diluting procedure and the use of FVIII-deficient plasma as diluent is extremely important. Implementation of these assay conditions by the participants may reduce the interlaboratory variation to acceptable levels (ca. 10%).

Unfortunately, tests that fully *discriminate between LA and coagulation factor inhibitors* are still lacking. In order to ascertain the presence or absence of LA, it is strongly advised to use at least two tests of different design [21]. The diluted Russell's viper venom test should be included as it is hardly influenced by inhibitors of the intrinsic factors (e.g., FVIII, FIX) [21]. Alternatively, the interference of LA in the measurement of factor inhibitors, especially FVIII inhibitors, can be bypassed by measuring the residual activity in the Nijmegen assay with chromogenic substrates. Chromogenic substrate assays are not influenced by LA and are, therefore, more specific than aPTT-based assays [18, 43, 44].

FVIII inhibitors can be characterized as either *type I or type II* according to their kinetic behavior. Type I

inhibitors mostly occur as alloantibodies in FVIII-treated hemophiliacs and have second-order inactivation kinetics resulting in complete inhibition of FVIII activity at high plasma concentrations.

Type II inhibitors, mostly autologous antibodies, are defined as being unable to inactivate FVIII:C completely, even at maximum antibody concentration, and the lack of linearity between the logarithm of residual FVIII activity and the antibody concentration [45]. How to define inhibitors as type I or II can best be investigated by measuring the effect of varying concentrations of the inhibitor on the FVIII inactivation [31].

The lack of linearity between FVIII residual activity and inhibitor concentration with type II in the inhibitor test will result in dilution-dependent inhibitor data. Therefore, in order to obtain reliable results when monitoring a patient with type II FVIII inhibitor, typical dilutions of the patient plasma have to be used that give residual activities that are as close to 50% as possible.

The *type of deficient plasma* used as control sample and as substrate plasma in the residual activity assay greatly influences the FVIII inhibitor test results. As vWF is the natural carrier protein for FVIII, the vWF concentration is essential for its stability during the incubation process. It was shown by our group [46] that inhibitor titers, derived from assays with vWF-free immune depleted FVIII-deficient plasma as control sample and as substrate in the FVIII activity assay were 30–50% lower than to titers of assays using vWF containing deficient plasma (Table 12.2).

Aberrant results were also found when using heterogeneous systems with chemically depleted plasma (CDP) as control sample and immune-depleted or congenital-deficient plasma as substrate plasma. The production process can generate activated factor V in the CDP, cause shortening of the clotting times in the control mixture and thus overestimation of the inhibitor titer [46].

Finally, during the process of immune-depletion, anti-FVIII can be co-eluted from the column into the FVIII-deficient plasma resulting in falsely low inhibitor titers [46].

In conclusion, it is strongly recommended that vWF-containing FVIII-deficient plasma be used, either congenital or immune-depleted, in a homogenous system and to check each commercial immune-depleted FVIII-deficient plasma for FVIII antibodies before use.

Table 12.2 FVIII inhibitor activities of an inhibitor-positive sample (1 NBU/mL) analyzed with different combinations of deficient plasma in the control mixture and as substrate plasma in the FVIII assay

Type of control sample	Type of substrate plasma in factor VIII assay		
	Chemically depleted plasma	Immune-depleted	Congenital-deficient plasma
Chemically depleted plasma	0.94	1.66	1.66
Immune-depleted	0.97	0.58	1.10
Congenital-deficient plasma	0.99	0.87	1.16

In order to decrease the costs of the assay, albumin can also be used as a control sample in combination with von Willebrand containing substrate plasma [47].

Inhibitors against other clotting factors

Probably the most frequently occurring coagulation inhibitor besides FVIII and FIX inhibitors are *inhibitors against Factor V* (FV). Until 2002, 126 cases have been reported in literature of which 87 have been reported in the decade before 2002 [48]. An annual incidence of 0.29 cases per million was reported in an Australian region [49] and of 0.09 per million per year in Singapore [50].

In two-thirds of the patients described by Streiff [48], the FV inhibitors were caused by exposure to bovine thrombin. This thrombin, which is widely used for hemostatic control in surgery patients, is contaminated with FV and this may induce antibodies to bovine FV that cross-react with human FV [7, 51]. Patients will present with both an abnormal PT and aPTT and low or very low FV activity. Mixing studies have to be used to confirm the presence of the inhibitor that can be quantified using the Nijmegen assay.

Thrombin inhibitors are reported much less frequently than FV inhibitors although most of them also arise, like FV antibodies, from treatment with bovine thrombin products [52]. Thrombin inhibitors are extremely rare in patients without an underlying disease and are mostly related to autoimmune diseases.

Thrombin inhibitors cause a broad window of abnormal clotting assays both in native plasma and in mixing studies including abnormal PT, aPTT, TT, fibrinogen assays, and clotting factor assays because thrombin is the final protease activity in all assays

[53]. These inhibitors may be difficult to distinguish from LAs that exhibit similar abnormal results except for the TT that is normal in lupus plasma. Furthermore, one has to be aware of the fact that acquired abnormal fibrinogen molecules with increased sialylation of carbohydrate side chains may also present with abnormal TT mixing studies [54]. These abnormal molecules, usually synthesized in diseases of the liver or the biliary tract, inhibit fibrin clot formation of normal fibrinogen. The TT of these plasma samples mixed with normal plasma normalizes after defibrination at 56°C. Confirmation of the presence of an inhibitor can be performed by treating the plasma with Protein A and/or Protein G, which will result in normal TT in immune-mediated TT prolongation.

There are rare publications on *inhibitors of fibrinogen function*. The mechanisms of these inhibitors include direct inhibition of fibrin monomer aggregation due to paraproteins [55, 56], delay of fibrinopeptide B release [57], and of fibrinopeptide A release [58]. Most commonly these patients have a prolonged TT both in the native patient plasma and in a 1:1 mixture with normal plasma. The presence of acquired abnormal fibrinogen protein, as described in the previous paragraph, can be excluded by normalization of TT of a mix of defibrinated patient plasma with normal plasma. Confirmation of the presence of an inhibitor can be obtained by treating the plasma with Protein A and/or Protein G that will result in normal TT in immune-mediated TT prolongation and when possible characterization of the immunoglobulin [57].

Acquired deficiency of factor XIII (FXIII) has been described both with and without the presence of inhibitors with an incidence that equals that of acquired hemophilia [59]. *Inhibitors of FXIII* have been described in association with drugs, chronic renal failure, hepatic cirrhosis, and lymphoproliferative disorders, although about half of the patients does not have an underlying disease [59, 60]. In only a minority of cases the presence of FXIII inhibitors is complicated by serious hemorrhagic conditions. Inhibitors to FXIII cannot be detected with baseline coagulation screening tests such as aPTT, PT, or TT, as these tests are not FXIII sensitive. FXIII inhibitors are classified into three types:

1 Those that interfere with FXIII activity by preventing activation of FXIII.
2 Inhibitors that interfere with the function of FXIIIa.
3 Inhibitors altering the reactivity of the fibrin substrate [61].

All types of inhibitors strongly interfere with activity assays and can be diagnosed by mixing studies with normal plasma using quantitative photometric assays. The widely used ammonium release assay is hampered by a high background value of about 10% rendering the assay insensitive for abnormal low results [62]. Once an inhibitor is suspected its presence has to be confirmed by an immunoblot test or an ELISA for antibodies against different domains of FXIII.

Patients with *ADAMTS 13 deficiency* present with life-threatening microvascular thrombotic complications and the syndrome is known as thrombotic thrombocytopenic purpura (TTP). In most cases, both children and adolescents, a functional inhibitor causes the deficiency to ADAMTS 13 [63, 64]. The inhibitor cannot be detected with usual baseline tests and so for detection of these inhibitors mixing tests have to be performed. Of the four tests that are currently available (multimeric analysis, collagen-binding assay, FRETS-vWF 73, and GST-vWF 73 assay), the FRETS-vWF 73 assay appears to be superior in detecting and quantifying auto-inhibitors to the cleaving protease [65]. The test is based on the cleavage of a 73-aminoacid protein fragment derived from vWF containing the substrate for ADAMTS 13. This results in increased fluorescence over time with normal plasma while ADAMTS 13-deficient plasma and/or inhibitor plasma has no effect [65].

Acquired von Willebrand factor deficiency (AvWD) is a heterogeneous syndrome with clinical features similar to congenital von Willebrand disease but no prior history of personal or familiar bleeding tendency [66]. It is mainly associated with lymphoproliferative and myeloproliferative disorders, solid tumors, and immunologic and cardiovascular disorders. Three main mechanisms can be differentiated:

1 The presence of circulating antibodies.
2 Selective adsorption of vWF to abnormal cells.
3 Increased vWF proteolysis.

The syndrome is characterized by decreased vWF activity and antigen, decreased collagen-binding capacity, low FVIII activity, mostly type II like multimeric patterns because of loss of high multimers, and increased aPTT. Unlike the congenital form, the plasma vWF propeptide concentration is normal but the vWF clearance from circulation after DDAVP treatment is increased. FVIII inhibitors cannot be detected in these patients and in only 30% of the patients with inhibitors to vWF can be shown in a mixing assay [67, 68]. Quantification of inhibitors can be performed by a modified Nijmegen inhibitor assay using the ristocetin cofactor activity assay to measure the residual vWF activity in a mixture with normal plasma. An ELISA may be more sensitive but may also detect noninhibiting antibodies [69]. Confirmation of the presence of an inhibitor can be obtained by investigation of the inhibitory effect of patient IgG on the binding of ^{125}I–vWF to platelets [67].

Conclusion

Functional inhibitors to proteins involved in the coagulation process must always be considered when a patient presents with unexpected bleeding, thrombotic complications, or with abnormal clotting assays. Although mixing studies with patient and normal plasma are the first choice of laboratory investigation, they will not always result in the detection of the inhibitor or render an explanation for the coagulation abnormality. Specific tests have to be performed to identify the nature of the putative inhibitor. Sometimes noninhibiting antibodies, analyzed with immunologic assays, are the cause of the underlying abnormality. The ultimate confirmation of the presence of an inhibitor mostly needs advanced methods (e.g., IgG purification, radiolabeling of proteins), which unfortunately are usually not available in standard diagnostic laboratories.

References

1. Arnout J. Antiphospholipid antibody syndrome: diagnostic aspects of lupus anticoagulants. *Thromb Haemost.* 2001;86(1):75–82.

2. Urbanus RT, Derksen RH, de Groot PG. Current insight into diagnostics and pathophysiology of the antiphospolipid syndrome. *Blood Rev.* 2008;22(2):93–105.

3. Collins PW, Hirsch S, Baglin TP, et al. UK Haemophilia Centre Doctors' Organisation. Acquired hemophilia A in the United Kingdom: a 2-year national surveillance study by the United Kingdom Haemophilia Centre Doctors' Organisation. *Blood.* 2007;109(5):1870–1877.

4. Krishnamurthy P, Hawche C, Evans G, Winter M. A rare case of an acquired inhibitor to factor IX. *Haemophilia.* 2011;17(4):712–713.

5. Bortoli R, Monticielo OA, Chakr RM, et al. Acquired factor XI inhibitor in systemic lupus erythematosus–case report and literature review. *Semin Arthritis Rheum.* 2009;39(1):61–65.

6. Scott-Timperley LJ, Haire WD. Autoimmune coagulation disorders. *Rheum Dis Clin North Am.* 1997;23(2):411–423.

7. Bomgaars L, Carberry K, Fraser C, West A, Teruya J. Development of factor V and thrombin inhibitors in children following bovine thrombin exposure during cardiac surgery: a report of three cases. *Congenit Heart Dis.* 2010;5(3):303–308.

8. Oldenburg J, El-Maarri O, Schwaab R. Inhibitor development in correlation to factor VIII genotypes. *Haemophilia.* 2002;8(suppl 2):23–29.

9. DiMichele D. Inhibitor development in haemophilia B: an orphan disease in need of attention. *Br J Haematol.* 2007;138(3):305–315.

10. Thorland EC, Drost JB, Lusher JM, et al. Anaphylactic response to factor IX replacement therapy in haemophilia B patients: complete gene deletions confer the highest risk. *Haemophilia.* 1999;5(2):101–105.

11. Warrier I. Factor IX antibody and immune tolerance. *Vox Sang.* 1999;77(suppl 1):70–71.

12. Lusher JM. Inhibitors in young boys with haemophilia. *Baillieres Best Pract Res Clin Haematol.* 2000;13(3):457–468.

13. Chitlur M, Warrier I, Rajpurkar M, Lusher JM. Inhibitors in factor IX deficiency a report of the ISTH-SSC international FIX inhibitor registry (1997-2006). *Haemophilia.* 2009;15(5):1027–1031.

14. Salomon O, Zivelin A, Livnat T, et al. Prevalence, causes, and characterization of factor XI inhibitors in patients with inherited factor XI deficiency. *Blood.* 2003;101(12):4783–4788.

15. Dazzi F, Tison T, Vianello F, et al. High incidence of anti-FVIII antibodies against non-coagulant epitopes in haemophilia A patients: a possible role for the half-life of transfused FVIII. *Br J Haematol.* 1996;93(3):688–693.

16. Vlot AJ, Mauser-Bunschoten EP, Zarkova AG, et al. The half-life of infused factor VIII is shorter in hemophiliac patients with blood group O than in those with blood group A. *Thromb Haemost.* 2000;83(1):65–69.

17. Mondorf W, Klinge J, Luban NL, Bray G, Saenko E, Scandella D. Recombinate PUP Study Group. Low factor VIII recovery in haemophilia A patients without inhibitor titre is not due to the presence of anti-factor VIII antibodies undetectable by the Bethesda assay. *Haemophilia.* 2001;7(1):13–19.

18. Blanco AN, Alcira Peirano A, Grosso SH, Gennari LC, Pérez Bianco R, Lazzari MA. A chromogenic substrate method for detecting and titrating anti-factor VIII antibodies in the presence of lupus anticoagulant. *Haematologica.* 2002;87(3):271–278.

19. Brandt JT, Barna LK, Triplett DA. Laboratory identification of lupus anticoagulants: results of the Second International Workshop for Identification of Lupus Anticoagulants. on behalf of the subcommittee on lupus anticoagulants/antiphospholipid antibodies of the ISTH. *Thromb Haemost.* 1995;74(6):1597–1603.

20. Triplett DA. Simultaneous occurrence of lupus anticoagulant and factor VIII inhibitors. *Am J Hematol.* 1997;56(3):195–196.

21. Tripodi A, Mancuso ME, Chantarangkul V, et al. Lupus anticoagulants and their relationship with the inhibitors against coagulation factor VIII: considerations on the differentiation between the 2 circulating anticoagulants. *Clin Chem.* 2005;51(10):1883–1885.

22. Favaloro EJ, Bonar R, Duncan E, et al. RCPA QAP in Haematology Haemostasis Committee. Identification of factor inhibitors by diagnostic haemostasis laboratories: a large multi-centre evaluation. *Thromb Haemost.* 2006;96(1):73–78.

23. Favaloro EJ, Bonar R, Duncan E, et al. Mis-identification of factor inhibitors by diagnostic haemostasis laboratories: recognition of pitfalls and elucidation of strategies. A follow up to a large multicentre evaluation. *Pathology.* 2007;39(5):504–511.

24. Kirkwood TB, Snape TJ. Biometric principles in clotting and clot lysis assays. *Clin Lab Haematol.* 1980;2(3):155–167.

25. Ruinemans-Koerts J, Peterse-Stienissen I, Verbruggen B. Non-parallelism in the one-stage coagulation factor assay is a phenomenon of lupus anticoagulants and not of individual factor inhibitors. *Thromb Haemost.* 2010;104(5):1080–1082.

26. Klinge J, Auerswald G, Budde U, et al. Paediatric inhibitor study group of the german society on thrombosis and haemostasis. Detection of all anti-factor VIII antibodies in haemophilia A patients by the Bethesda assay and a more sensitive immunoprecipitation assay. *Haemophilia.* 2001;7(1):26–32.

27. Martin PG, Sukhu K, Chambers E, Giangrande PL. Evaluation of a novel ELISA screening test for detection of

factor VIII inhibitory antibodies in haemophiliacs. *Clin Lab Haematol.* 1999;21(2):125–128.

28. Blanco AN, Peirano AA, Grosso SH, Gennari LC, Bianco RP, Lazzari MA. An ELISA system to detect anti-factor VIII antibodies without interference by lupus anticoagulants. Preliminary data in hemophilia A patients. *Haematologica.* 2000;85(10):1045–1050.

29. Sahud MA, Pratt KP, Zhukov O, Qu K, Thompson AR. ELISA system for detection of immune responses to FVIII: a study of 246 samples and correlation with the Bethesda assay. *Haemophilia.* 2007;13(3):317–322.

30. Shetty S, Ghosh K, Mohanty D. An ELISA assay for the detection of factor VIII antibodies—comparison with the conventional Bethesda assay in a large cohort of haemophilia samples. *Acta Haematol.* 2003;109(1):18–22.

31. Ling M, Duncan EM, Rodgers SE, et al. Classification of the kinetics of factor VIII inhibitors in haemophilia A: plasma dilution studies are more discriminatory than time-course studies. *Br J Haematol.* 2001;114(4):861–867.

32. Biggs R, Macfarlane RG. *Human Blood Coagulation and its Disorders.* 2nd ed. Oxford: Blackwell Scientific Publications.

33. Biggs R, Bidwell E. A method for the study of anti-haemophilic globulin inhibitors with reference to six cases. *Br J Haematol.* 1959;5:379–395.

34. Kasper C, Aledort L, Counts R, et al. A more uniform measurement of factor VIII-inhibitors. *Thromb Diath Haemorrh.* 1975;34:869–872.

35. Verbruggen B, Novakova I, Wessels H, et al. The Nijmegen Modification of the Bethesda Assay for Factor VIII:C Inhibitors: Improved Specificity and Reliability. *Thromb Haemost.* 1995;73(2):247–251.

36. Torita S, Suehisa E, Kawasaki T, et al. Development of a new modified Bethesda method for coagulation inhibitors: the Osaka modified Bethesda method. *Blood Coagul Fibrinolysis.* 2011;22(3):185–189.

37. Giles AR, Verbruggen B, Rivard GE, Teitel J, Walker I. A Detailed comparison of the performance of the standard versus the Nijmegen modification of the Bethesda assay in detecting factor VIII:C inhibitors in the haemophilia A population of Canada. Association of Hemophilia Centre Directors of Canada. Factor VIII/IX Subcommittee of Scientific and Standardization Committee of International Society on Thrombosis and Haemostasis. *Thromb Haemost.* 1998;79(4):872–875.

38. Verbruggen B, van Heerde WL, Laros-van Gorkom BA. Improvements in factor VIII inhibitor detection: from Bethesda to Nijmegen. *Semin Thromb Hemost.* 2009;35(8):752–759.

39. Dardikh M, Thilo A, Masereeuw R, et al. Low-titre inhibitors, undetectable by the Nijmegen assay, reduce

40. Mannucci PM, Tripodi A. Factor VIII clotting activity.In: *Laboratory Techniques in Thrombosis-A manual.* 2nd revised ed. of ECAT Assay Procedures. 1999;107–113.

41. Lacroix-Desmazes S, Wootla B, Dasgupta S, et al. Catalytic IgG from patients with hemophilia A inactivate therapeutic factor VIII. *J Immunol.* 2006;177(2):1355–1363.

42. Verbruggen B, Dardikh M, Polenewen R, van Duren C, Meijer P. The factor VIII inhibitor assays can be standardized: results of a workshop. *J Thromb Haemost.* 2011;9(10):2003–2008.

43. Chandler WL, Ferrell C, Lee J, Tun T, Kha H. Comparison of three methods for measuring factor VIII levels in plasma. *Am J Clin Pathol.* 2003;120(1):34–39.

44. Blanco AN, Cardozo MA, Candela M, Santarelli MT, Pérez Bianco R, Lazzari MA. Anti-factor VIII inhibitors and lupus anticoagulants in haemophilia A patients. *Thromb Haemost.* 1997;77(4):656–659.

45. Gawryl MS, Hoyer LW. Inactivation of factor VIII coagulant activity by two different types of human antibodies. *Blood.* 1982;60(5):1103–1109.

46. Verbruggen B, Giles A, Samis J, Verbeek K, Mensink E, Nováková I. The type of factor VIII deficient plasma used influences the performance of the Nijmegen modification of the Bethesda assay for factor VIII inhibitors. *Thromb Haemost.* 2001;86(6):1435–1439.

47. Verbruggen B, van Heerde W, Nováková I, Lillicrap D, Giles A. A 4% solution of bovine serum albumin may be used in place of factor VIII:C deficient plasma in the control sample in the Nijmegen modification of the Bethesda factor VIII:C inhibitor assay. *Thromb Haemost.* 2002;88(2):362–364.

48. Streiff MB, Ness PM. Acquired FV inhibitors: a needless iatrogenic complication of bovine thrombin exposure. *Transfusion.* 2002;42(1):18–26.

49. Favaloro EJ, Posen J, Ramakrishna R, et al. Factor V inhibitors: rare or not so uncommon? A multi-laboratory investigation. *Blood Coagul Fibrinolysis.* 2004;15(8):637–647.

50. Ang AL, Kuperan P, Ng CH, Ng HJ. Acquired factor V inhibitor. A problem-based systematic review. *Thromb Haemost.* 2009;101(5):852–859.

51. Ortel TL, Mercer MC, Thames EH, Moore KD, Lawson JH. Immunologic impact and clinical outcomes after surgical exposure to bovine thrombin. *Ann Surg.* 2001;233(1):88–96.

52. Savage WJ, Kickler TS, Takemoto CM. Acquired coagulation factor inhibitors in children after topical bovine thrombin exposure. *Pediatr Blood Cancer.* 2007;49(7):1025–1029.

53. La Spada AR, Skålhegg BS, Henderson R, Schmer G, Pierce R, Chandler W. Brief report: fatal hemorrhage in a patient with an acquired inhibitor of human thrombin. *N Engl J Med.* 1995;333(8):494–497.

54. Cunningham MT, Brandt JT, Laposata M, Olson JD. Laboratory diagnosis of dysfibrinogenemia. *Arch Pathol Lab Med.* 2002;126(4):499–505.

55. Dear A, Brennan SO, Sheat MJ, Faed JM, George PM. Acquired dysfibrinogenemia caused by monoclonal production of immunoglobulin lambda light chain. *Haematologica.* 2007;92(11):111–117.

56. Saif MW, Allegra CJ, Greenberg B. Bleeding diathesis in multiple myeloma. *J Hematother Stem Cell Res.* 2001;10(5):657–660.

57. Llobet D, Borrell M, Vila L, Vallvé C, Felices R, Fontcuberta J. An acquired inhibitor that produced a delay of fibrinopeptide B release in an asymptomatic patient. *Haematologica.* 2007;92(2):e17–e19.

58. Gris JC, Schved JF, Branger B, et al. Autoantibody to plasma fibrinopeptide A in a patient with a severe acquired haemorrhagic syndrome. *Blood Coagul Fibrinolysis.* 1992;3(5):519–529.

59. Ichinose A. Hemorrhagic acquired factor XIII (13) deficiency and acquired hemorrhaphilia 13 revisited. *Semin Thromb Hemost.* 2011;37(4):382–388.

60. Nijenhuis AV, van Bergeijk L, Huijgens PC, Zweegman S. Acquired factor XIII deficiency due to an inhibitor: a case report and review of the literature. *Haematologica.* 2004;89(5):ECR14.

61. Thomas F. Gregory and Barry Cooper. Case report of an acquired factor XIII inhibitor: diagnosis and management. *Proc (Bayl Univ Med Cent).* 2006;19(3):221–223.

62. Ajzner E, Muszbek L. Kinetic spectrophotometric factor XIII activity assays: the subtraction of plasma blank is not omissible [corrected]. *J Thromb Haemost.* 2004;2(11):2075–2077.

63. Furlan M, Robles R, Galbusera M, et al. von Willebrand factor-cleaving protease in thrombotic thrombocytopenic purpura and the hemolytic-uremic syndrome. *N Engl J Med.* 1998;339(22):1578–1584.

64. McDonald V, Liesner R, Grainger J, Gattens M, Machin SJ, Scully M. Acquired, noncongenital thrombotic thrombocytopenic purpura in children and adolescents: clinical management and the use of ADAMTS 13 assays. *Blood Coagul Fibrinolysis.* 2010;21(3):245–250.

65. Shelat SG, Smith P, Ai J, Zheng XL. Inhibitory autoantibodies against ADAMTS-13 in patients with thrombotic thrombocytopenic purpura bind ADAMTS-13 protease and may accelerate its clearance in vivo. *J Thromb Haemost.* 2006;4(8):1707–1717.

66. Franchini M, Lippi G. Acquired von Willebrand syndrome: an update. *Am J Hematol.* 2007;82(5):368–375.

67. Mohri H, Motomura S, Kanamori H, et al. Clinical significance of inhibitors in acquired von Willebrand syndrome. *Blood.* 1998;91(10):3623–3629. Erratum in: *Blood.* 1999;93(1):413.

68. Nitu-Whalley IC, Lee CA. Acquired von Willebrand syndrome–report of 10 cases and review of the literature. *Haemophilia.* 1999;5(5):318–326.

69. Siaka C, Rugeri L, Caron C, Goudemand J. A new ELISA assay for diagnosis of acquired von Willebrand syndrome. *Haemophilia.* 2003;9(3):303–308.

13 Standardization of D-dimer testing

Guido Reber & Philippe de Moerloose

Haemostasis Unit, Department of Internal Medicine, University Hospital and Faculty of Medicine, Geneva, Switzerland

Introduction

The rationale of D-dimer measurement as an indicator of coagulation activation and fibrin digestion was provided by the studies of Gaffney more than 30 years ago [1]. Until monoclonal antibodies were available, fibrin and fibrinogen degradation products were measured in serum, mainly with either polyclonal antifibrinogen antibodies or with the staphylococcal clumping test. The results of these tests were obscured by many artifacts [2]. In the early eighties, monoclonal antibodies obtained by immunization with D-dimer were raised and this was the milestone of a novel area in hemostasis [3]. Indeed, the monoclonal antibodies allow the measurement of soluble fibrin fragments (even in the presence of fibrinogen and its degradation products), opening new insights in the coagulation and fibrinolysis fields. In particular, D-dimer measurement provided an important contribution to the diagnostic work-up of venous thromboembolic disease (VTE) [4] and disseminated intravascular coagulation (DIC) [5, 6]. The test is now widely used in clinical laboratories and there are more than 30 assays available designed in various assay formats, using more than 20 monoclonal antibodies. The numerical assay results may vary widely among assays because: in patient plasmas the analyte is highly heterogeneous, the specificity of the monoclonal antibodies differs depending on the mixture of fragments in the sample, the calibrators are different [7]. Since the efforts for the standardization of the assays were unsuccessful [8], harmonization procedures have been proposed [9–12]. This is an important issue particularly because each commercial assay has its own cut-off value for VTE exclusion that may confuse clinicians. In DIC field, clinical scores have been proposed by the International Society of Thrombosis and Haemostasis (ISTH) [5] and the Japanese Ministry of Health and Welfare for overt DIC [6] in which a D-dimer value is included. However, as shown by a recent study, the numerical value of a patient's sample may differ by about 20 times depending on the assay used [11]. As a consequence, the amount of points related to D-dimer value computed in the patient's DIC score may range from zero to three [5, 6].

Heterogeneity of D-dimer containing fragments

After thrombin removal of the fibrinopeptide A, the N-terminal sequence of the α-chain becomes the site of polymerization in fibrinogen domain E. This polymerization site interacts with a corresponding site located in the D-domain of another fibrin or fibrinogen molecule [13]. The double-stranded fibrin polymer grows and results in a protofibril. The lateral association of the protofibrils forms fibrin fibrils. Each γ-chain contains two binding sites in the appendage linked to the D-domain. Thrombin activation of factor

Quality in Laboratory Hemostasis and Thrombosis, Second Edition. Edited by Steve Kitchen, John D. Olson and F. Eric Preston.
© 2013 John Wiley & Sons, Ltd. Published 2013 by Blackwell Publishing Ltd.

XIII is catalyzed by polymerized fibrin. Upon factor XIII action, two covalent bonds form between adjacent D-domains that result in cross-linked fibrin. The velocity of the polymerization process, which is a function of fibrinogen and thrombin concentrations, governs the structure of the polymers. Because the presence of two cross-linking sites per γ-chain, in addition to D-dimers, D-trimers, and D-tetramers are formed, which ensure the branching between adjacent fibrin fibrils [14].

Fibrin catalyzes plasminogen conversion to plasmin by tissue plasminogen activator, which results in localized fibrinolytic activity. Therefore, fibrin formation and breakdown occur concomitantly and part of the fibrin measured consists of soluble plasmin degraded fibrin. Patients' plasma samples contain a mixture of intravascular and extravascular clot-derived fibrin as well as circulating soluble fibrin including D-dimer, D-trimers, and D-tetramer motifs [15]. The terminal product of plasmin digestion is the fragment D-dimer whose molecular weight is about 195 kDa. In the circulation, it is found as a complex with fragment E (DD/E) [16, 17]. Due to variable degrees of plasmin proteolysis, patients' plasma samples contain a mixture of fibrin fragment complexes containing one or several D-dimer motifs whose molecular weights range from 228 kDa (DD/E) to several thousand kDa (X-olimers) [8]. In addition, fibrinogen (as shown by the presence of fibrinopeptide A) is also found in high-molecular weight fibrin (HMWF) fragments [18]. As shown in Figure 13.1, the current "D-dimer measurement" means, in fact, a mixture of D-dimer containing fibrin fragments' measurement.

Specificity of monoclonal antibodies directed to D-dimer motif

The first monoclonal antibody (3B6/22) was reported by Rylatt et al. in 1983 [3]. Since then, more than 20 monoclonal antibodies have been developed. In theory, they should react minimally with fibrinogen or fibrinogen degradation products. In addition, they should not react with fibrin and fibrinogen fragments from elastase proteolysis [19]. The assay format is important since proper combination of two monoclonal antibodies (catcher and tag) displaying some cross-reactivity with fibrinogen degradation products

may paradoxically result in an ELISA specific for cross-linked fibrin degradation products [20].

The characterization of differences among the commercial tests concerning analyte reactivity has been studied in depth in the FACT study [10]. In this study, 23 quantitative D-dimer assays were evaluated in order to develop common calibrators. The 39 patients' samples were measured with six ELISA, 15 latex-enhanced photometric immunoassays, and two membrane-based immunoassays. Depending on the assay, the mean values for the 39 samples varied from 0.63 μg/mL (range 0.01–3.42 μg/mL) to 13.35 μg/mL (range 0.07–258 μg/mL). Increasing amounts of t-PA digested cross-linked fibrin diluted into normal plasma were measured with all assays. The slope of the response differed widely between assays (from 1 to 48). When replacing cross-linked fibrin by fibrinogen degradation products, two assays gave a high response indicating marked cross-reactivity with fragment D. Slopes of dilutions of plasma pools from DIC and deep venous thrombosis (DVT) patients into normal plasma differed between assays and for some assays between the two pools. To evaluate the response of assays to the type of fibrin species, high-molecular weight fibrin (HMWF) was extracted from DIC pool and diluted into normal plasma. The slopes obtained varied from one to five. This HMWF material was digested with plasmin in order to obtain low-molecular weight cross-linked fibrin (LMWF) and was tested in the same way. The ratio of the slopes (native HMWF/plasmin-treated HMWF) showed that some assays react better to HMWF whereas others perform better with LMWF. This suggests that plasmin treatment may reveal additional epitopes that are the preferred target of some assays, especially ELISA-type. Conversely, longer fibrin fragments could better favor particle agglutination in latex-enhanced immunoassays because of the distance between latex particles [10].

Calibrators for D-dimer assays

Manufacturers of D-dimer assays choose the type of calibrator that fits best with their assay. The majority of assays are calibrated with material obtained by controlled lysis of fibrin clots. Accordingly, calibrators' concentrations are often expressed as the amount of fibrinogen present in the mixture used to prepare

D-dimer-containing fragments	D-trimer-containing fragments	D-tetramer-containing fragments	Size kDa*	Generic formula
D-D or D dimer	—	—	190	D_2
DY or D-DE	—	—	240	D_2E
—	D-D-D or D trimer	—	285	D_3
YY or ED-DE	—	—	290	D_2E_2
XD or DED-D	D-D-DE	—	335	D_3E
—	—	D-D-D-D or D tetramer	380	D_4
XY or DED-DE	ED-D-DE	—	385	D_3E_2
DXD or D-DED-D	—	D-D-D-DE	430	D_4E
—	E ED-D-DE	—	435	D_3E_3
DXY or D-DED-DE	—	ED-D-D-DE	480	D_4E_2
YXY or ED-DED-DE	—	E ED-D-D-DE	530	D_4E_3

* Assumed sizes for monomolecular core constituents: E [—●—], 50 kDa; D [—Ⓓ], 95 kDa; Y [—●—Ⓓ], 145 kDa; X [Ⓓ—●—Ⓓ], 240 kDa

Figure 13.1 Macromolecular fragments from plasmic digests of cross-linked fibrin. From reference 15.

the calibrator material. Results thus may be expressed as fibrinogen equivalent units (FEU, µg/L). Experimental conditions have to be carefully controlled in order to ensure the reproducibility of the mixture (HMWF and LMWF) in the final product. Some assays are calibrated with purified fibrin fragment D-dimer equivalents. Again, the experimental conditions of the purification have to be carefully controlled to avoid variability in antibody response [21]. According to their respective molecular weight (340 and 195 kD), D-dimer values expressed in FEU should be theoretically about twice as high as those expressed in D-dimer units. However, it has to be taken into account that fibrin digests do not contain D-dimer fragments only but also HMWF depending on the lysis procedure. One assay is calibrated with plasma pools with different D-dimer levels prepared from DIC patients' samples [22].

In the FACT study [10], all assays were calibrated with (a) terminal fibrin fragments, (b) HMWF fragments, or (c) dilutions of DIC patients' plasma pools in normal plasma. Individual patients' plasma ($n =$ 39) was measured with the three calibration curves. With terminal fibrin fragments, one assay could not be calibrated and two others overestimated patients' samples. Calibration with HMWF fragments resulted in either underestimation (three assays) or overestimation (three assays) of sample values. Calibration with DIC patients' plasma resulted in a better uniformity. In case DIC plasma cannot be used, calibration with HMWF fragments should be preferred because they mirror better than the mixture contained in the patients' samples as compared with terminal fibrin fragments.

Standardization of D-dimer assays

The first attempt towards D-dimer assays standardization was conducted by the National Institute for Biological Standards and Control (NIBSC) [8]. Purified D-dimer preparations from three laboratories as well as a preparation of HMWF fragments were tested with three monoclonal antibodies. If the same epitopes were present on the different fragments, then binding would be similar and the standardization of measurements might be easier. Two antibodies bound similarly to all preparations immobilized on polyvinyl chloride wells whereas the binding of the third one

varied widely depending on the preparation. When tested as catcher antibodies in an ELISA format, two of them showed marked differences in the response to the four preparations whereas the responses of the third one were more comparable. These data ruled out the possibility that the same epitopes would be present irrespective of the type of fibrin fragments.

From a formal perspective, a standardization process has to meet some requirements. The analyte to be measured has to be fully characterized. Obviously, this cannot be the case for D-dimer assays since the analyte in plasma samples is a mixture of fibrin degradation products containing different structures and a wide range of molecular weights. Therefore, this heterogeneity precludes the preparation of a primary standard. This heterogeneity and the various responses of monoclonal antibodies (and their combinations) impede the establishment of a reference method. That is why a less stringent approach was tested, known as harmonization procedure. This approach was, for example, applied successfully to the prothrombin time for monitoring oral anticoagulation and resulted, despite some limitations, in the worldwide accepted international normalized ratio (INR).

Harmonization of D-dimer assays

Harmonization relies on the use of a mathematical model in order to render more comparable results obtained with different assays.

The first attempt was conducted in the framework of the Scientific and Standardization Committee of the ISTH [9]. The goal was to investigate whether it was possible to establish an international reference material (not a standard) for the harmonization of D-dimer assays. Two plasma pools from 20 patients with various diseases (i.e., not only patients with VTE or DIC) were prepared. A third pool was prepared by mixing equal volumes of the two pools. These pools were tested with five D-dimer assays (four microplate ELISA and one microlatex) from four manufacturers. For each pool, the average of the numerical values obtained by each assay was computed and assigned as "pool consensus" value (Table 13.1). For each assay, the numerical result obtained with each pool was divided by the corresponding "pool consensus" value, and the three values (corresponding to the three pools) were averaged (Table 13.2). To ascertain whether this

Table 13.1 Reported values (mean ± SD) per assay (in μg/mL) and consensus values of the pools

Pool	Assay					Consensus
	1	2	3	4	5	
A	6.22 ± 0.21	1.24 ± 0.30	7.80 ± 0.01	1.46 ± 0.04	1.21 ± 0.04	3.60
B	2.15 ± 0.06	0.31 ± 0.02	2.31 ± 0.02	0.63 ± 0.01	0.48 ± 0.01	1.24
C	3.94 ± 0.04	0.65 ± 0.14	5.24 ± 0.05	1.20 ± 0.06	0.88 ± 0.01	2.46

Adapted from reference 9.

model, based on pool measurements, was applicable at the individual level, the 40 samples used to prepare the pools were measured. Results were processed with the same model, that is, 40 "sample consensus" values were computed and each sample result was divided by the corresponding "sample consensus" value. For each assay, these 40 "individually harmonized values" were plotted against the values obtained by dividing the 40 original results by the mean value of the three pools ("pool harmonized values"). The squared regression coefficient values ranged from 0.7 to 0.92. From this study, it was concluded that a conversion factor, computed from patients' plasma pools, rendered comparable individual D-dimer numerical results obtained with different assays and that this conversion factor was independent of a pool [9].

Table 13.2 Ratio of the consensus over the reported values

Assay	Pool	Ratio	Mean ± SD
1	A	0.58	
	B	0.58	0.59 ± 0.02
	C	0.62	
2	A	2.90	
	B	4.00	3.56 ± 0.48
	C	3.78	
3	A	0.46	
	B	0.54	0.49 ± 0.04
	C	0.47	
4	A	2.47	
	B	1.97	2.16 ± 0.22
	C	2.05	
5	A	2.98	
	B	2.18	2.79 ± 0.16
	C	2.80	

Adapted from reference 9.

A second attempt of harmonization has been reported in the framework of the FACT study [10]. The approach differed somewhat from that of Nieuwenhuizen since no plasma pools but individual samples were used. In addition, median instead of mean values were used for the computation of conversion factors. As already mentioned, 39 samples were tested with 23 assays, including ELISA, microlatex-enhanced and membrane-based D-dimer assays. A conversion factor was computed using the median of the median values obtained for each sample with all assays, and for each assay the median value obtained with all samples. Multiplication of the individual sample assay result with the assay-specific conversion factor led to an adjustment of the scales of the assays. The median values of these converted values for each individual sample were used as a single sample consensus value (SSCV). As shown in Table 13.3, the correlation of the between-individual assay results and the corresponding SSCV was analyzed by regression analysis and by Spearman rank correlation. Good correlations were observed with most assays, especially when Spearman rho coefficient was considered because it attenuated the influence of outliers and ceiling effects in some assays.

A third procedure for D-dimer results harmonization has been proposed [11]. This model takes into account the possible variation among test results and consensus values at different D-dimer levels. It relies on the transformation of an assay-specific regression line to a reference regression line, both obtained by measuring a set of five samples. These samples were prepared by dilutions of a patients' plasma pool ($n = 50$) into normal plasma. These samples were distributed to participants ($n = 502$) of the external quality control surveys of the European Concerted Action on Thrombosis Foundation and the German INSTAND Institute. After outlier exclusion,

Table 13.3 Mean, median, minimum, and maximum values of 39 clinical samples. Conversion factor, linear correlation with median of converted values of samples, including Y-intercept, slope and numerical coefficient of correlation, and Spearman rank correlation rho of individual assay results with the single sample consensus value (SSCV)

Assay	Mean (µg/mL)	Median (µg/mL)	Min (µg/mL)	Max (µg/mL)	Conversion factor	Linear correlation with SSCV			Spearman rank correlation coefficient rho
						y-intercept	Slope	Regression coefficient R^2	
AGEN dimertest gold	0.63	0.41	0.01	3.42	4.95	0.260	0.106	0.842	0.963
Biomerieux Vidas D-dimer	3.52	3.54	0.09	30.00	0.57	3.256	0.660	0.353	0.843
Biopool TintElize D-dimer	3.49	0.91	0.04	50.56	2.10	−0.890	1.278	0.970	0.969
DadeBehring Enzygnost D-dimer	1.31	0.49	0.01	19.73	3.99	−0.339	0.489	0.947	0.892
Organon Teknika Fibrinostika FbDP	8.42	2.29	<0.22	98.02	0.90	−1.908	3.017	0.962	0.883
Stago Asserachrom D-dimer	9.76	4.17	0.13	86.95	0.49	1.160	2.513	0.864	0.802
AGEN Autolatex D-dimer	1.22	0.81	<0.065	>2.00	2.48	0.635	0.170	0.579	0.955
Biopool AutoDimer LPIA	3.43	1.09	0.02	50.00	1.89	−0.834	1.247	0.964	0.984
Biopool Miniquanr d-dimer	3.53	1.54	0.01	57.98	1.32	−0.264	1.108	0.687	0.968
DadeBehring D-dimer PLUS	1.06	0.46	0.06	12.04	4.29	−0.005	0.312	0.982	0.916
DadeBehring Advanced D-dimer	9.20	4.18	0.53	103.00	0.48	0.104	2.657	0.981	0.921
DadeBehring Turbiquant D-dimer	1.13	0.65	<0.20	6.28	3.03	0.537	0.173	0.695	0.963
Diamed d-dimer LPIA	3.61	1.59	<0.10	43.50	1.30	−0.217	1.117	0.980	0.963
Helena D-dimer LPIA	1.47	1.1	0.01	5.58	1.82	1.091	0.107	0.233	0.972
Iatron D-dimer LPIA	11.35	5.15	0.10	123.80	0.33	1.983	2.677	0.816	0.938
Instrumentation Laboratories IL-Test D-dimer ACL	3.77	1.62	0.16	40.24	1.25	−0.211	1.164	0.991	0.993
Instrumentation Laboratories IL-Test D-dimer TurbILab	4.87	1.32	0.01	63.87	1.46	−1.081	1.737	0.988	0.978
AGEN Autolatex D-dimer LPIA, Organon Teknika Thrombolyzer	0.99	0.89	0.05	2.97	2.35	0.690	0.088	0.557	0.975
Organon Teknika MDA d-dimer	13.35	1.52	0.07	258.00	1.34	−8.927	6.508	0.941	0.928
Roche Diagnostics TINAquant d-dimer	5.95	3.01	0.10	35.69	0.57	2.107	1.122	0.877	0.948
Stago STA LIATest d-dimer	9.06	3.37	<0.22	89.50	0.60	−0.003	2.648	0.915	0.794
Nycomed Nycocard d-dimer	3.08	1.40	<0.10	30.00	1.49	0.309	0.809	0.963	0.975
Roche Diagnostics Cardiac Reader D-dimer	4.12	3.20	<0.10	10.00	0.55	3.629	0.188	0.064	0.815

Adapted from reference 10.

Table 13.4 Method-specific consensus values (ng/mL ± SEM) of eight different D-dimer methods of five different samples (A–E)

Method/Sample	n	A	B	C	D	E
bioMérieux Vidas D-dimer	52	321 ± 8.2	655 ± 11.2	942 ± 14.7	2409 ± 32.3	4118 ± 44.8
bioMérieux Latex	25	64 ± 12.8	212 ± 38.8	251 ± 12.0	978 ± 112.8	1235 ± 24.9
Dade Behring D-dimer Plus	75	28 ± 3.5	56 ± 3.0	88 ± 3.0	230 ± 2.9	421 ± 5.7
Dade Behring Turbiquant	16	11 ± 6.2	35 ± 7.9	89 ± 9.4	328 ± 26.4	638 ± 41.6
Diagnostica Stago	50	40.2 ± 11.2	945 ± 11.0	1336 ± 14.8	2863 ± 34.7	5551 ± 202
IL D-dimer	35	118 ± 9.3	269 ± 9.8	413 ± 52.9	1197 ± 52.9	2159 ± 97.4
Nycomed Nycocard D-dimer	60	212 ± 29.7	246 ± 33.9	454 ± 57.7	1089 ± 71.5	2004 ± 105
Roche Tinaquant	65	522 ± 11.7	1155 ± 13.9	1677 ± 18.0	4282 ± 42.0	7480 ± 76.5
Overall median value		252	425	736	1733	2816

Adapted from reference 11.

seven methods were analyzed. The mean value for each sample with each method was computed (Table 13.4). For each sample, the median values of the mean values obtained with the seven assays were plotted against the amount of pool added in order to obtain the reference line. For each assay, the mean values of each sample were also plotted against the amount of pool added in order to obtain the assay-specific line (Figure 13.2). Using the slope (b), the intercept (a) of the assay-specific line (A), and the reference line (H), the harmonized results (Y_H) can be computed from the measured result (Y_A) with the following equation:

$$Y_H = a_H \left(\frac{Y_A - b_A}{a_A} \right) b_H$$

Using this model, the between-assays coefficient of variations of the five plasma measured showed a dramatic decrease (Table 13.5). This model applies to the whole measuring range of the assays provided that a linear relationship is obtained. Further validation of this model with more assay systems is necessary.

Another procedure for D-dimer results harmonization has been tested in the framework of the UK National External Quality Assessment Scheme (NEQAS) external quality surveys [12]. Five samples

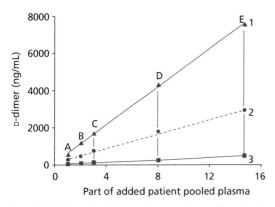

Figure 13.2 Example of harmonization by transforming the regression line through the method-specific consensus values (1 = Roche Tinaquant; 3 = Dade Behring D-dimerPlus to the regression line through the overall median values (2), using the residual slope and intercept of both regression equations). A to E = calibrator samples. Adapted from reference 11.

Table 13.5 Coefficients of variation for the method-specific consensus values of all methods included before and after harmonization for the five different plasma samples

Sample	Overall median value (ng/mL)	Before harmonization (%)	After harmonization (%)
A	252	91.0	18.2
B	425	92.3	7.4
C	736	86.8	6.1
D	1733	83.6	5.9
E	2816	82.3	1.5

Adapted from reference 11.

Table 13.6 Improvement in between-centre agreement after calibration. Overall results

	Sample D6			Sample D7		
	N	Median (ng/mL)	CV (%)	N	Median (ng/mL)	CV (%)
FEU						
Original data	118	1252	25.9	116	950	22.4
Original data (outliers removed)	118	1252	25.9	115	960	22.0
All calibrated data	118	1162	11.6	116	918	8.9
Calibrated data, $r > 0.95$	118	1162	11.6	116	918	8.9
Calibrated data, $r > 0.95$, outliers removed	118	1161	11.6	115	920	7.7
Non-FEU						
Original data	302	411	45.3	302	348	40.8
Original data (outliers removed)	293	412	45.3	294	350	39.8
All calibrated data	302	427	34.3	302	356	111.5
Calibrated data, $r > 0.95$	299	426	22.7	299	356	13.0
Calibrated data, $r > 0.95$, outliers removed	293	427	21.6	284	358	11.6

Adapted from reference 12.

were distributed to more than 500 participants. For statistical reasons, only assays ($n = 9$) used by more than 10 participants were taken into account; the results of three assays being expressed in FEU and the others in ng/mL. Three of the samples served as calibrators and two served as test samples. For these three samples, individual laboratory results were plotted against the median values obtained with all methods. All but three laboratories had correlation coefficients $r > 0.95$. The values obtained with the two test samples by each laboratory were converted in harmonized values using the laboratory's own regression line. As shown in Table 13.6, this model resulted in an important decrease in coefficients of variation as compared to those obtained with the original values. Unfortunately, the model was applied separately to assays calibrated in D-dimer ng/mL and to assays calibrated in FEU and, therefore, it cannot be ascertained whether this model can be generalized to all kinds of assays.

New studies on harmonization of D-dimer results are ongoing.

Problems in daily practice

The lack of standardization/harmonization of D-dimer results may be misleading in daily laboratory and clinical practice due particularly to the different cut-off values and units among assays. In a survey in Europe, nearly 90% of laboratories used D-dimer assay for the exclusion of VTE, 52% for diagnosis and monitoring of DIC, this test being available 24 hours per day in 81% of laboratories [23]. A recent D-dimer proficiency testing by the College of American Pathologists showed that many laboratories were unclear about the units they reported (8% of laboratories did not know the type of units they were using) [24]. The cut-off value for VTE exclusion is also a matter of concern; in this survey, more than one-third of laboratories (488/1506) reported VTE cut-off values above that recommended by the manufacturer or by the literature (from 10% to 71% of the recommended value), which probably results in erroneous exclusion of VTE in patients. In the European survey, 55% of participants reported higher VTE cut-off values and 24% lower than the recommended cut-off. This can be explained in part by the fact that some manufacturers recommend the assessment of a local cut-off, although such a task is usually above the possibilities of small hospitals and private laboratories. In addition, for several assays, prospective validation studies are not available because in some countries such trials are not a precondition for launching tests into the market [23]. Depending on the prevalence of VTE in the population referred to the diagnostic centre, several hundreds of patients suspected of VTE have to be tested in order to determine the VTE exclusion cut-off. The established cut-off has then to be validated in a prospective study, with a similar number of patients, based on the local diagnostic decision scheme; patients in whom anticoagulation is withheld on the basis of D-dimer (and possibly other criteria) have to be followed during several months to exclude an ulterior VTE. When testing D-dimer with closed assay systems (such as VIDAS, Stratus, AxSYM, and others) or with the couple reagent/device from the same manufacturer, cut-off values indicated in the reagent insert should be used, provided that there is no significant batch-to-batch variability and that accurate validation studies have been conducted to assess it. When using reagent and device from different manufacturers, the recommended cut-off should be carefully checked because of the possible effect of the device on assay results. With closed systems, within- and between-laboratories coefficients of variation, as found in reports of external quality control surveys, are useful tools to estimate the analytical performances of the assays.

For DIC categorization and monitoring, the absence of standardization/harmonization of D-dimer results obscures the adequate use of clinical scores. In both the ISTH and Japanese scores, D-dimer values contribute from zero to three points [5, 6]. No point is added for D-dimer values less than or equal to 1.0 μg/mL in the ISTH score and for less than 10 μg/mL in the Japanese one. In the Japanese score, one point is added for D-dimer values greater than or equal to 10 μg/mL and less than or equal to 25 μg/mL, but two points in the ranges 1.0–5.0 μg/mL in the ISTH one. Three points correspond to values greater than 5.0 μg/mL in the ISTH and 25 μg/mL in the Japanese scores, respectively. It has to be noted that for both the scores, no precision is given about the test to be used, which is critical when we know that numerical D-dimer values may vary as many as 20 times depending on the assay used [11]. Therefore, users of assay systems yielding relatively low D-dimer values are likely to underscore the Japanese score and users of assays yielding high values will overestimate the ISTH one. Harmonization of D-dimer results would provide some uniformity to D-dimer contribution in DIC scores even if the mathematical model used yields up to 20% variability in numerical values.

Reference material for D-dimer assays

During the last decade, many efforts have been made by the members of the Science and Standardization Committee (SSC) of the ISTH in order to design a reference material for D-dimer assays. Many data presented in this section can be found in the minutes of the SSC meetings (http://www.isth.org/default/index.cfm/ssc1/ssc-minutes/).

Since D-dimer antigen is not a homogenous analyte, a primary reference standard cannot be formulated. As already mentioned, fragment D-dimer represents only a part of fragments' mixture and complexes found in the patients' plasma. Therefore, purified D-dimer fragment is not a good candidate for a reference material. In clinical samples, D-dimer assays detect mainly fibrin degradation products as well as high-molecular weight cross-linked fibrin complexes. D-dimer assays display differences in reactivity toward high-molecular weight fragments and complexes or toward terminal products of plasmin digestion. Depending on the particular reactivity of the assay, the results obtained with clinical samples may be over or underestimated. *In vitro* analysis of the products released by a clot perfused with plasmin reveals that their average molecular weight is about 6,000,000 Da and range from 250,000 to 10,000,000.

Results of the fourth Fibrin Assay Comparison Trial (FACT) demonstrated that pooled plasma from patients with DIC serially diluted in pooled plasma from healthy volunteers gave similar results with 28 different D-dimer assays tested. Therefore the reference material should contain a pattern of D-dimer containing fragments as close as possible as those present in clinical samples.

A consensus definition of D-dimer antigen was accepted by SSC members: "D-dimer antigen indicates antigenic material detected by the use of monoclonal antibodies generated by immunization with fibrin fragment D-dimer and related compounds. The minimal structure detected is fibrin fragment D-dimer, but larger compounds containing dimerized D-domains are detected as well." Because of the heterogeneity of patients' plasma pools and fibrin preparations, a method for measuring D-dimer concentration was proposed by the members of the FACT group: "Aliquots of the plasma pool or fibrin preparation are incubated with a high concentration of plasmin in presence of calcium and a thrombin inhibitor. Both fibrin, and fibrinogen in the sample are degraded, resulting fibrin fragment D-dimer/E complex as main terminal breakdown product of the crosslinked fibrin. Proteolysis of fibrinogen, in contrast, yields fibrinogen fragments D and E. After insuring that proteolysis is complete by SDS-polyacrylamide gel electrophoresis and immunoblotting, using polyclonal antifibrinogen antiserum for detection, concentration of fibrin fragment D-dimer is measured. For the measurement of fibrin fragment D-dimer, several D-dimer assays are used which are not influenced by the presence of fibrinogen degradation product D (FDP-D) and show good reactivity with fibrin fragment D-dimer. These assays are calibrated with purified fibrin fragment D-dimer. The resulting concentration levels of fibrin fragment D-dimer reflect the total concentration of D-dimer antigen (dimerized D-domains) in the original plasma samples."

This procedure yields the amount of dimerized D-dimer independently of the size distribution of the complexes and/or fibrin derivatives present in the original material. The measured D-dimer value is then assigned to the original material. This procedure allows to prepare successive lots of reference material having the same level of D-dimer antigen. This type of reference material should be used for harmonization trials of D-dimer assays.

In the FACT 5 reference, laboratories of the manufacturers tested a set of 50 pooled samples with various levels of D-dimer antigen as well as a pool containing high levels of D-dimer antigen to prepare calibrators upon dilution with assay-specific diluents. Assay results from the 30 assays were well correlated (mean regression coefficient 0.946 ± 0.054, range 0.703–0.999). Calibration with this common material decreased CV from about 60% to about 20%.

A similar trial was organized in 2008 by the Standardization Committee of the Japanese Society of Laboratory Hematology, the Japanese Society of Laboratory Medicine, and the Japanese Society of Thrombosis and Hemostasis including 13 D-dimer assays from 11 manufacturers. Five calibrators were prepared by diluting a pool of 80 patients' samples into normal plasma. For harmonization, a reference method was chosen and results were recalculated using regression curves with the reference method. Sixteen patients' samples were tested and the CV fell from 34% to 9.9% after harmonization.

At the SSC meeting held in Cairo in 2010, it was reported in the SSC Fibrinolysis Subcommittee that a large pool from patients with high D-dimer levels had been prepared for lyophilization at the National Institute of Biological Standards and Controls to assist standardization initiatives.

Conclusion

The availability of assays able to measure cross-linked fibrin fragments in the presence of fibrinogen and its degradation products has been an important step for clinical laboratories and a useful tool for diagnostic purposes. Unfortunately, the numerical results of D-dimer measurements obtained with various assays are different due to the nature of the analyte to be measured, the diversity of monoclonal antibodies, and the calibration process. For these reasons, standardization of D-dimer assay is unlikely. In order to attain a better comparability of results, harmonization procedures appear as valuable surrogates. However, it is important to keep in mind that they carry some inherent imprecision and that the assessment of unique cut-off values for VTE exclusion for all assays seems more particularly difficult due to the potential consequences of a false-negative result that may be life-threatening. In contrast, the relative imprecision of harmonization procedures seems more acceptable for clinical scores such as those used for DIC patients. With the present assays, the values measured in a high positive sample may vary from 2.97 to 258 μg/mL (Table 13.3); even if harmonization induces a variation as high as 20%, this is far better than any result obtained without harmonization.

These harmonization procedures have to be validated with a large number of samples. This should be performed in collaboration with the manufacturers. If scientists and manufacturers agree on the suitability of one of the models, manufacturers should provide a chart with the correspondences between measured and harmonized values. Finally, this has to be endorsed by scientific authorities such as ISTH.

References

1. Gaffney PJ. Distinction between fibrinogen and fibrin degradation products in plasma. *Clin Chim Acta.* 1975;65:109–115.

2. Gaffney PJ, Perry MJ. Unreliability of current serum fibrin degradation product (FDP) assays. *Thromb Haemost.* 1985;53:301–302.

3. Rylatt DB, Blake AS, Cottis LE, et al. An immunoassay for human D-dimer using monoclonal antibodies. *Thromb Res.* 1983;31:767–778.

4. Bounameaux H, de Moerloose P, Perrier A, Miron MJ. D-dimer testing in suspected venous thromboembolism: an update. *QJM.* 1997;90:437–442.

5. Taylor FB Jr, Toh CH, Hoots WK, Wada H, Levi M. Scientific Subcommittee on Disseminated Intravascular Coagulation (DIC) of the International Society on Thrombosis and Haemostasis (ISTH). Towards definition, clinical, and laboratory criteria, and a scoring system for disseminated intravascular coagulation. *Thromb Haemost.* 2001;86:1327–1330.

6. Wada H, Gabazza EC, Asakura H, et al. Comparison of diagnostic criteria for disseminated intravascular coagulation (DIC): diagnostic criteria of the International Society of Thrombosis and Hemostasis and of the Japanese Ministry of Health and Welfare for overt DIC. *Am J Hematol.* 2003;74:17–22.

7. Reber G, de Moerloose P. D-dimer assays for the exclusion of venous thromboembolism. *Semin Thromb Hemost.* 2000;26:619–624.

8. Gaffney PJ, Edgell T, Creighton-Kempsford LJ, Wheeler S, Tarelli E. Fibrin degradation product (FnDP) assays: analysis of standardization issues and target antigens in plasma. *Br J Haematol.* 1995;90:187–194.

9. Nieuwenhuizen W. A reference material for harmonisation of D-dimer assays. Fibrinogen Subcommittee of the Scientific and Standardization Committee of the International Society of Thrombosis and Haemostasis. *Thromb Haemost.* 1997;77:1031–1033.

10. Dempfle CE, Zips S, Ergül H, Heene DL. Fibrin Assay Comparative Trial study group. The Fibrin Assay Comparison Trial (FACT): evaluation of 23 quantitative D-dimer assays as basis for the development of D-dimer calibrators. FACT study group. *Thromb Haemost.* 2001;85:671–678.

11. Meijer P, Haverkate F, Kluft C, de Moerloose P, Verbruggen B, Spannagl M. A model for the harmonisation of test results of different quantitative D-dimer methods. *Thromb Haemost.* 2006;95:567–572.

12. Jennings I, Woods TA, Kitchen DP, Kitchen S, Walker ID. Laboratory D-dimer measurement: improved agreement between methods through calibration. *Thromb Haemost.* 2007;98:1127–1135.

13. Olexa SA, Budzynski AZ. Effects of fibrinopeptide cleavage on the plasmic degradation pathways of human cross-linked fibrin. *Biochemistry.* 1980;19:647–651.

14. Mosesson MW, Siebenlist KR, Meh DA. The structure and biological features of fibrinogen and fibrin. *Ann N Y Acad Sci.* 2001;936:11–30.

15. Mosesson MW. Terminology for macromolecular derivatives of cross-linked fibrin. On behalf of the Subcommittee on Fibrinogen of the Scientific and Standardization Committee of the ISTH. *Thromb Haemost.* 1995;73:725–726.

16. Gaffney PJ, Lane DA, Kakkar VV, Brasher M. Characterisation of a soluble D-dimer–E complex in cross-linked fibrin digests. *Thromb Res.* 1975;7:89–99.

17. Marder VJ, Budzynski AZ, Barlow GH. Comparison of the physicochemical properties of fragment D derivatives of fibrinogen and fragment D–D of cross-linked fibrin. *Biochim Biophys Acta.* 1976;427:1–14.

18. Pfitzner SA, Dempfle CE, Matsuda M, Heene DL. Fibrin detected in plasma of patients with disseminated intravascular coagulation by fibrin-specific antibodies consists primarily of high-molecular weight factor XIIIa—cross-linked and plasmin-modified complexes partially containing fibrinopeptide A. *Thromb Haemost.* 1997;78:1069–1078.

19. Francis CW, Marder VJ. Degradation of cross-linked fibrin by human leukocyte proteases. *J Lab Clin Med.* 1986;107:342–352.

20. Pittet JL, de Moerloose P, Reber G, et al. VIDAS D-dimer: fast quantitative ELISA for measuring D-dimer in plasma. *Clin Chem.* 1996;42:410-415.

21. Wylie FG, Walsh TP. Variable immunoreactivity of D-dimer preparations for monoclonal antibody DD-3B6/22. *Blood Coagul Fibrinolysis.* 1995;6:738–742.

22. Adema E, Gebert U. Pooled patient samples as reference material for D-dimer. *Thromb Res.* 1995;80:85–88.

23. Spannagl M, Haverkate F, Reinauer H, Meijer P. The performance of quantitative D-dimer assays in laboratory routine. *Blood Coagul Fibrinolysis.* 2005;16:439–443.

24. Olson J, Cunningham M, Brandt J, et al. Use of the D-dimer for exclusion of VTE: difficulties uncovered through the proficiency testing program of the College of American Pathologists (CAP). *J Thromb Haemost.* 2005;3(suppl 1): OR303 (abstract)

14 Point-of-care testing in hemostasis

Chris Gardiner[1,2], Dianne Kitchen[3], Samuel Machin[1,4], & Ian Mackie[1,4]

[1]Haematology Department, University College London Hospitals NHS Trust
[2]Nuffield Department of Obstetrics and Gynaecology, John Radcliffe Hospital, Oxford, UK
[3]UK NEQAS Blood Coagulation, Sheffield, UK
[4]Haemostasis Research Unit, Haematology Department, University College London, London, UK

Introduction

Point-of-care testing (POCT) and near-patient testing (NPT) are used synonymously to describe analytical testing undertaken by a health care professional or a non-medical person in a setting distinct from a conventional hospital laboratory. In principle, locating test equipment near to the patient provides a more rapid service than that which may be achieved in the hospital laboratory. This may be useful in a life-threatening situation, where the test may indicate an urgent therapeutic choice, in the management of long-term conditions, where the results can inform the consultation, influence a procedure, or where the patient may have heightened concern about the outcome of the test [1].

At present, the main applications of POCT in hemostasis are:
• Vitamin K antagonist therapy (prothrombin time/international normalized ratio (PT/INR)
• High-dose heparin management (activated clotting time (ACT), whole blood thrombin time)
• Global assessment of hemostasis during major surgery or in the intensive care unit (thrombelastography, thromboelastometry)
• Monitoring of therapy with certain coagulation factor concentrates in haemophilia
• Platelet function testing
• D-dimer testing to exclude a diagnosis of venous thromboembolism

The devices differ in complexity from small, hand-held coagulation monitors intended for patient self testing (PST), to small desktop analyzers designed for use by health care professionals in a clinic or hospital environment. They are mostly used with whole blood samples, sometimes making it difficult to compare the results with those from hospital laboratories using plasma. There are a wide range of platelet function POCT devices [2]; these are mostly used for research purposes and there is little clinical validation except in the setting of antiplatelet drug therapy. Quality control (QC) of these devices is difficult since platelet function deteriorates on storage in currently used anticoagulants and is affected by fixation processes. Many users test a healthy normal control blood sample with each batch of tests as a quality check. Platelet POCT devices will not be discussed further in this review.

Monitoring of oral anticoagulation

Oral anticoagulant therapy (OAT) using vitamin K antagonists (VKA) is commonly used in the treatment and long-term prevention of thromboembolic events, with an estimated 0.95 million patients using warfarin in the UK and 3 million in the USA [3, 4]. These patients require regular prothrombin time/international normalized ratio (PT/INR) determination. An ageing population and the continuing expansion of clinical indications for VKA have led to further increases in demand [5]. Consequently, several new models of patient care, involving various degrees of decentralization and POCT of PT/INR, have been

Quality in Laboratory Hemostasis and Thrombosis, Second Edition. Edited by Steve Kitchen, John D. Olson and F. Eric Preston.
© 2013 John Wiley & Sons, Ltd. Published 2013 by Blackwell Publishing Ltd.

Table 14.1 POCT devices for oral anticoagulant control (available in UK)

Device	Manufacturer	Blood sample	Sample volume (μL)	Available for self-testing	Calibration method	QC material	Data handling
CoaguChek XS	Roche Diagnostics, Basel, Switzerland	Capillary or venous blood, non-citrated	8	Yes	Code chip; user must check	Strip integrity check	No data handling, but connection to home PC available.
CoaguChek XS Plus/Pro	Roche Diagnostics, Basel, Switzerland	Capillary or venous blood, non-citrated	8	No	Code chip, automatic	Liquid QC; strip integrity check	Alphanumeric input; bi-directional interface. XS Pro has bar code reader.
Hemochron Jr Signature +	ITC, Edison, NJ, USA	Venous or capillary blood	50	No	Barcode on cuvette, automatic	Internal QC and liquid QC	Numerical input; bi-directional interface
INRatio	Hemosense Inc., San Jose, CA, USA	Capillary blood	10	Yes	Manual entry of five digit code	Internal QC only	No data handling; RS232 interface
Protime 3	ITC, Edison, NJ, USA	Capillary or venous blood, non-citrated	27	Yes	Barcode on cuvette, automatic	Internal QC and liquid QC	No data handling; RS232 interface

implemented [6–9]. Since the introduction of POCT PT/INR monitors in the 1990s [10], the volume of blood required for testing has gradually decreased (now 8–50 μL), as well as the size and cost of devices (for details see Table 14.1). The reliability and precision of POCT devices for INR has improved considerably in recent years, largely due to the development of new technologies and QC procedures. These improvements have alleviated initial concerns [11]. There is increasing disparity between different methods at INR values above 4.5, regardless of whether POCT devices or large laboratory analyzers are used, due to the method of International Sensitivity Index (ISI) assignment (which utilizes only normal subjects and stabilized VKA patient samples) and INR calculation, as well as differences in thromboplastin sensitivity to vitamin K-dependent factors [12–14]. The upper limit of the measuring range therefore varies between POCT devices. A recent study has suggested that POCT methods can yield comparable results to

laboratory analyzers in samples with high INR values, particularly if a similar thromboplastin is used [15].

There are several POC devices available for coagulation testing, which fall broadly into one of two types: devices for professional use and devices for use by the patients themselves. Relatively few patients are self testing in the UK, but numbers are increasing and in some parts of Europe there are many tens of thousands of patients who are successfully self testing and self managing their VKA therapy. The high cost of professional devices effectively rules out their use for PST.

Coagulation monitors intended for PST should satisfy certain requirements:

• There is a consensus of opinion, backed by proficiency testing data, that low ISI thromboplastins (ISI 0.9–1.7 and ideally close to 1.0) should be used for INR determination (see also Chapters 9 and 22). The higher ISI reagents are associated with a high degree of imprecision and may give less-dependable INR values

during the induction period of OAT with VKA and in poorly stabilized patients [16–18].
• The INR result must be accurate and reproducible. Ideally, when compared to a reference method, >85% of samples within the therapeutic range should give an INR value within 0.5 INR units [19].
• The result should be clearly and simply displayed in suitably large character size and be easily read.
• A suitable QC system must exist to ensure the validity of results.
• The operation should be simple, with minimal user-definable steps, and should not require a high degree of dexterity.
• It must be small enough to be easily portable, ideally handheld and low weight.
• Stored patient and QC results should be readily distinguishable.
• The sample volume requirement should be <30 μL with no requirement for accurate blood volume measurement.
• The sample application point must be easily accessible for patients with poor dexterity.
• Connectivity to a laboratory information system via an ethernet link and data management system is an advantage.

Quality assurance of point-of-care INR monitors

As with any other diagnostic test, quality assurance of POCT devices is required to ensure that the results are reliable. All POCT devices have a system verification procedure that is performed automatically when the instrument is switched on. Some instruments also have an electronic QC cartridge that simulates a test endpoint. However, electronic QC does not assess the performance of the test strip/cuvette and does not represent a valid alternative to conventional QC procedures. The Hemochron Jr. II series has an electronic tester that should be used daily to check the electrical circuits of the devices before any testing. The latest model, the Hemochron Elite, has this electronic check built in, thus removing the extra process. Some devices have an internal QC system built into each test strip/cuvette and this helps to ensure the validity of each test, although a QC system independent from the manufacturer is preferred, since both device and internal QC could be miscalibrated. POCT coagulometers for professional use, that perform tests on citrated plasma, can use the same quality assurance

programs as laboratory analyzers (with lyophilized plasmas) and will not be discussed further. Whole blood POCT coagulation monitors operate on several different measurement principles and it is these that dictate the type of QC that can be used.

In the US, the FDA states that a QC check should be performed with each test sample. Consequently, POCT monitors that use onboard controls are widely used. In Europe, the preference is for liquid QC and the type of POCT monitors in common use reflects this. Some devices offer both options.

Optical clot-detection uses LED detectors to measure the motion of a blood sample as it is pumped back and forth within a cuvette containing freeze-dried thromboplastin. As clot formation begins, the movement decreases below a predetermined rate and the endpoint is detected. Instruments using this principle (Protime III and Hemochron Jr. II series, International Technidyne Corporation) cannot detect clot formation in plasma samples and the presence of red cells is required. Lyophilized whole blood controls, containing dried fixed red cells with buffered plasma are reconstituted in a diluent containing calcium ions. This is usually achieved by crushing a glass ampoule containing the diluent, within a plastic vial and mixing the contents by inversion. The reconstituted blood is then tested in the same way as a patient sample. EQA programmes are available for these devices but the material must have red blood cells present in order for the devices to register that a sample has been applied.

Some monitors use the amperometric (electrochemical) measurement of thrombin activity as a surrogate measure of clot detection (CoaguChek XS/XS Plus/XS Pro, Roche Diagnostics). In principle, lyophilized plasma QC materials may be used with this system, but at present the manufacturer using this technique does not offer a QC preparation for use with all of their instruments. However, in the UK, EQA schemes using lyophilized controls are available for all such instruments.

The electrogenic test method employs a marker that is generated when a substrate, included in the reagent and mixed with the test sample, reacts with thrombin. As coagulation progresses, the marker concentration increases and is detected by a sensing electrode. This system is used in the i-STAT device (Abbott Point-of-Care) that is able to analyze many parameters using different test cartridges. This system has liquid

149

QC available and EQA is available in some areas of Europe, including the UK.

The electrical impedance method measures the change in electrical current flow that occurs when fibrinogen is converted to fibrin. These test strips contain thromboplastin reagent and electrodes within layered plastic. The only instrument currently using this detection method (INRatio, Hemosense Inc) has an onboard QC but no commercial or external liquid QC material is currently available. An alternative EQA system for this device is available in some European countries whereby the test strips are distributed from the EQA program and a patient INR is measured. The results of the onboard QC values (generated in the same test strip as the patient sample and at the same time as the patient sample as mentioned below) are returned to the EQA provider for assessment. Although this does not assess the whole system, it may be a way of assessing some aspects of the device and could be useful if suitably interpreted.

Integral onboard controls (sometimes referred to as in-built), contained within the test strip/cuvette are available for some POCT coagulation monitors. Some test strips (CoaguChek XS/XS Plus) have an incorporated QC function that assesses integrity in the measuring channel after sample application. Resazurin is incorporated and this chemical is sensitive to ambient factors such as light, humidity, and temperature and is transformed into Resorufin. The concentration of Resorufin is measured electrochemically and can be considered as a measure of strip damage. However, the device does not show the results of these tests or the range, but simply displays a "tick" to indicate that the onboard QC has passed. The manufacturer states that any test strip that fails the onboard QC would not display a result.

Other POCT monitors using onboard QC (Protime III and INRatio) use cuvettes where one or more channels containing lyophilized plasma plus other additives become activated when mixed with the test sample. Typically the controls are formulated to clot in ranges equivalent to normal (low) and a therapeutic (high) INR values. Onboard controls are designed primarily to detect test strip degradation and do not always display numerical values but do state whether the control result meets the acceptable criteria set by the manufacturer.

An alternative approach is to assess the POCT monitor normally used by the patient self testers in a center

that participates satisfactorily in an accredited EQA program. In this case, the patient should test their blood on their monitor and test strip system and the monitor and test strip system belonging to the clinic; INR results between 2.0 and 4.5 should be within 0.5 INR units of each other. A paired venous sample may also be collected at the same time as the capillary blood sample for the POCT INR; the venous sample is then analyzed in an appropriate hospital laboratory. INR results of stabilized patients should be within 0.5 INR units of each other. If this "split sample" approach is used, the procedure must be repeated at least once every 6 months. One published study that used a single reference laboratory reported that satisfactory quality assurance could be achieved using this method [20]. However, there are difficulties with this approach because the quality of hospital laboratory INR results is variable and sometimes discrepancies will occur. Consequently, differences between the laboratory and the POCT method may not be due to problems with the POCT device. Discrepancies between INR methods are known to be increased when OAT is unstable, especially at INR values >4.5. It should also be remembered that other factors may cause discrepant results, including: the presence of lupus anticoagulant, high or low haematocrit, and elevated bilirubin levels. It is not usually feasible to use a single reference laboratory, especially if the postal service is poor, the distances involved are large, or if the ambient temperature is high, as these factors could all adversely affect sample stability. The quality of the initial test sample may affect the INR result obtained by either method and the laboratory method can be influenced by many other preanalytical variables. Another UK study [21] reported a high degree of discrepancy between POCT and laboratory INR values when ten general practitioner (GP) practices providing a POCT service sent paired, citrated venous blood samples to their local hospital laboratory (this involved six different hospital laboratories). Results varied greatly with some GP practices and their local laboratory showing reasonable agreement, but others showing discrepancies (some due to systematic errors in laboratory methods) [21].

Patient self-monitoring of oral anticoagulation

Some patients receiving vitamin K antagonists can control their own anticoagulation, either by PST or patient self-monitoring (PSM). In fact, it is often a natural progression from PST to PSM where the health care provider is supportive of this change. Several studies have shown that PSM of oral anticoagulation is a reliable and effective alternative to hospital based anticoagulant clinics. Patients who self-monitor tend to have fewer thromboembolic events or major haemorrhages and lower mortality rates than those attending hospital anticoagulant clinics. The potential benefit of self-monitoring depends very much on the existing quality of anticoagulation. Where patients are managed by dedicated anticoagulation clinics, and the time in target therapeutic range is ≥60%, an improvement in the quality of anticoagulation may not always be discernable [22]. However, where anticoagulation management is conducted in the physician's office, the time in target therapeutic range may be considerably less than 60% and in this setting, substantial improvements in the quality of anticoagulation may be achieved. Not all patients are suitable to self-monitor and the process requires careful selection of candidates as well as a program of education and training for the individual before implementation [23]. After the exclusion of patients on account of alcoholism, intravenous drug abuse, visual impairment dexterity problems etc., approximately 50% of patients receiving long-term warfarin in an OAT clinic of a UK hospital were suitable for PST [24].

The British Committee for Standards in Haematology [25] and the International Self-Management Association for Oral Anticoagulation [26] have produced guidelines for patient self-monitoring based on the available evidence. The main recommendations are summarized below:

• Under normal circumstances, only patients with long-term indications for OAT/VKA should be considered for self-monitoring.
• Previous stability of INR is not a prerequisite to self-monitoring as patients with poor control may benefit from increased independence and increased frequency of testing.
• Patients (or carers) must give informed consent to undertake self-monitoring. This should include agreement to record results accurately.
• Education and training on the theoretical and practical aspects of INR testing and anticoagulation is essential for all patients undergoing self-monitoring.

• Competence to perform a POCT INR must be assessed by a trained health care professional before allowing home testing.
• Competence to correctly interpret an INR result must be assessed by a health care professional before allowing self management.
• Patients being considered for self-monitoring must have a documented INR target in line with accepted guidelines and clinical practice.
• Contraindications for self-monitoring include previous non-compliance in relation to clinic attendance or taking warfarin as instructed.
• Patients undertaking self-monitoring must retain contact with a named health care professional and be reviewed at least every 6 months by the responsible clinician.
• QC should be performed on a regular basis. The type of QC will be dependent on the type of monitor used and the institution.
• Self-monitoring patients should participate in some form of external QC/proficiency testing.
• Any INR result between 4.0 and 8.0 should be repeated with the POCT device to ensure that the prolonged result is not a consequence of poor sample quality.
• If an INR of >8.0 or sample error is obtained, a venous sample should be collected the same day and analyzed in an appropriate hospital laboratory.

aPTT testing

POCT for aPTT is not widely used in the UK and many methods have been withdrawn worldwide, although methods are still available for the Hemochron series. Several semi-automated coagulometers are suitable for use in hospital clinics and intensive care units, but require sample and reagent preparation as well as a certain degree of skill in pipetting technique and so are only suitable for experienced, trained users. POCT aPTT only has clinical utility for heparin monitoring and is not advised when screening for inherited or acquired coagulation defects. As with all aPTT methods, the reagents and devices vary in their sensitivity to heparin, coagulation factors, and the lupus anticoagulant. Studies comparing POCT aPTT tests with traditional hospital laboratory tests have shown poor agreement in surgical patients, although the correlation was better for healthy volunteers [27, 28]. Liquid

QC plasmas are available for the semi-automated and Hemochron methods and these should be run daily or with every batch of tests.

aCT

The activated clotting time (aCT) is widely used for monitoring heparin anticoagulation during cardiopulmonary bypass (CPB) procedures [29]. The aCT is most frequently used to demonstrate that there is sufficient heparin anticoagulation to fully anticoagulate the patient and avoid blockage of the extracorporeal circuit. The required accuracy and precision of the test does not therefore have to be particularly high, that is, it is sufficient to demonstrate that the clotting time is prolonged to within a relatively wide therapeutic range. aCT tests are sometimes performed at the end of cardiac bypass to ensure that suitable amounts of protamine have been used to reverse the heparin anticoagulation.

The sensitivity of the aCT to aprotinin (which is sometimes given in difficult CPB procedures or during further cardiac surgery) appears to differ depending on the analyzer used and the formulation of the activator. Some reports have suggested that kaolin aCT is less affected by aprotinin than the celite aCT [30], which probably reflects the weaker contact activation activity of celite.

Several POCT devices are available for aCT, the most widely used are the Hemochron series and the Medtronic series, although others including the i-STAT (Abbott) are also available. The Hemochron Response is a two-channel analyzer that can measure aCT as well as a variety of other parameters (aPTT, PT, thrombin time, fibrinogen assay). The reagents are pre-loaded in the reaction tubes, with color-coded tops for different types of test. Blood is placed in the tube, which also contains a plastic paddle that rotates when the tube is inserted into the analyzer. Clot detection is by a mechanical principle. The aCT tubes are generally designed to take 2 mL blood and the thrombin time tubes 1 mL. The Hemochron Junior Signature analyzer can measure aCT, aPTT, and PT. Reagents are contained in test cuvettes, which require addition of approximately 15 μL blood. Clot detection is by an optical method, monitoring cessation of movement of blood along a capillary. The Medtronic ACT Plus analyzer can measure aCT only, although a similar instrument (ACT II) can measure a variety of clotting times. Reagents are pre-loaded in plastic cuvettes and contain plastic paddles, which facilitate mechanical clot endpoint detection. Less than 1 mL blood is required for each test.

Liquid QC samples are available for aCT methods and should be performed on each day that the method is used. EQA schemes have recently been introduced in the UK for certain devices and cuvettes. aCT testing is only performed on whole blood so that the provision of an EQA material with similar properties to the usual test sample is difficult and specific materials must be designed for each system. In the UK, an EQA program is currently available for the Hemochron cuvette system for the high-range aCT tests.

Thrombin time

The thrombin clotting time can be performed on citrated plasma or whole blood. The latter may be used during surgery for detecting the presence of heparin, investigating fibrinogen function in the presence and absence of heparin, and for monitoring heparin anticoagulation. The test is not affected by aprotinin. Various modifications of the test exist, using different concentrations of thrombin and with the addition of protamine sulfate to neutralize heparin.

The Hemochron Response analyzer may be used with three different reagent tubes:
1 TT tubes—containing low concentrations of human thrombin (with the manufacturer's currently predicted normal range being 39–53 s), is intended for the investigation of fibrinogen function and presence of heparin. 1 mL blood is required.
2 HNTT tubes—containing human thrombin and protamine sulfate (the manufacturer's currently predicted normal range is 33–58 s), is intended for the investigation of abnormal fibrinogen function and presence of heparin (in combination with the TT tubes). 1 mL blood is required.
3 HiTT tubes—containing high concentrations of human thrombin, protamine, and snake venom (which is not affected by heparin and aids clot formation). These are used for monitoring high levels of heparin anticoagulation during CPB surgery. 1.5 mL blood is required.

The thrombin time is not affected by aprotinin and therefore offers a potential means of assessing anticoagulation during CPB. The HiTT tubes can be used during CPB to ensure that the clotting time is prolonged and sufficient heparin has been given. If required, TT and HNTT tubes can be used to assess fibrinogen function in patients who are bleeding and to investigate whether prolonged clotting times are due to heparin. The varying sensitivity to heparin of each tube type allows each situation to be covered. Liquid QC samples are available from the manufacturer.

Low molecular weight heparin monitoring

At present, there is only one POCT device available for monitoring low-molecular-weight heparin (LMWH). The clot-based test (Hemonox, ITC) measures the anticoagulant effect of LMWH in non-citrated fresh blood and is a modified dilute thromboplastin time. The manufacturers provide a lyophilized whole blood control but currently no EQA schemes are available. One study demonstrated sensitivity to therapeutic levels of intravenous enoxaparin [31], but the test currently has limited clinical application.

D-dimer

There are a variety of POCT D-dimer methods available for use in the exclusion of venous thromboembolism (VTE) [32, 33]. Their sensitivity to VTE is variable and some may not be as sensitive as the best laboratory tests [34].

The earliest, widely used test was a red cell agglutination assay (SimpliRED, Agen), and due to the principle of the method, appropriate EQA is difficult. Most of the other assays are based on enzyme-linked or turbidometric immunoassays. The Miniquant (Biopool, Trinity Biotech Ltd), Nycocard (Axis Shield POC, Oslo, Norway) and Cobas H 232 (Roche) methods all have liquid QC products available and these should be used on any days where patient samples are analyzed. The CARDIAC D-dimer assay (Roche Diagnostics) and Triage D-dimer (Biosite Inc) have built in QC systems that check the performance of the analyzer and lyophilized plasma controls are also available. EQA programs for D-dimer POCT are under trial in the UK to establish a sample that will be suitable for the

various devices and to produce a user friendly report for participating centers

Thrombelastography

Thrombelastography was first described by Hartet in 1948 [35]. The technology has been incorporated into two types of hemostasis analyzer, the Thrombelastograph (TEG, Haemoscope) and the rotation thromboelastometer (ROTEM, Diagnostica Stago) (see also Chapter 9). These devices measure viscoelastic changes during coagulation, and provide information on the time taken for the initiation of clot formation, the rate of clot formation, the tensile strength of the clot and its rate of dissolution. Thus, the test is influenced by the levels and activity of clotting factors, rate of fibrin polymerization, fibrinogen level, presence of inhibitors, platelet function, and fibrinolysis [36, 37]. Although the system may be used with plasma, it is more commonly used with whole blood and a variety of activators and reagents are available depending on the clinical application.

The most common applications of TEG/ROTEM are during cardiac surgery and liver transplant procedures, in order to detect excess heparin and coagulopathies. Data are rapidly obtained and indicate the type of therapeutic intervention required (protamine, plasma, cryoprecipitate, platelets, aprotinin). The analyzers have also been used in the assessment of hypercoagulability and in the evaluation of new haemostatic agents (e.g., recombinant factor VIIa) and platelet inhibitor compounds, but these are mainly research applications.

The TEG and ROTEM provide similar haemostatic information, but use slightly different technologies to achieve this and so the results are not directly interchangeable and require separate reference ranges. Differences in measurement variables also occur depending on whether non-anticoagulated or citrated blood is used and depending on the time from blood collection. With respect to the latter, some authors recommend that citrated blood is not tested during the first 30 minutes from collection. During major surgery, results are often required rapidly and non-anticoagulated blood is usually tested immediately. Citrated blood should certainly be tested within 4 hours from collection, but standardization of the time is recommended. Before use each day, the analyzer setup software should be run and baseline determination/adjustment performed. This verifies and maintains the electronic function of the analyzer. Lyophilized QC plasmas are available from the manufacturers and should be used daily (when test are performed) and with each new batch of reagents. Lyophilized plasma EQA samples have been provided for both of these technologies, although they have limitations due to the lack of red blood cells and platelets, which, together with fibrinogen level in the sample, all have an impact on the results [38].

Management of POCT services

There may often be several types of POCT instrument in different departments of the same institution with similar clinical applications. In some countries, these issues are addressed by POCT committees, which may include: a haematologist, a physician, nursing staff, laboratory managers, quality assurance managers, pharmacy managers, and others who are needed to train and implement the service. A specific POCT coordinator is recommended for larger institutions. In the UK, guidance is available concerning the establishment and management of a haematology POCT service [39].

Before a POC coagulation test is introduced, it is first necessary to be clear about the purpose of the test, that is, diagnosis, monitoring, or treatment of disease. A quality manual should be prepared and requirements related to POCT reviewed [40]. Standard operating procedures must be written and regularly reviewed. They should include full details of how to use the POCT device and manage the service, what actions to take on generation of a result and what to do in the event of a fault on the instrument. Safety regulations recognizing potential hazards should also be documented. Training protocols must be established and all potential operators must achieve an adequate level of competence; a list of authorized users should be drawn up and approved by the service director. Staff must have a clear understanding that they must not allow others access to tests without undergoing a documented formal training process. Some devices have security features which only allow access to accredited operators, via a personal access code. Retraining intervals and a continuing education program should be established and POCT operator performance monitored as part of the quality assurance programme.

Quality assurance requires the satisfactory recording of analytical data and it is essential that the POCT results are documented with operator identification. Ideally, results and patient/sample identification details should be transferred electronically from the POCT device to a computer, to avoid potential transcription errors, but this is not available on all devices (Table 14.1). In the absence of appropriate computer systems, results must be documented in a logbook, which also identifies reagent batch Lot numbers and the name of the operator; as well as the Lot numbers of any calibrants and IQC materials. The POCT results should be permanently stored in the patients' medical records. Where computers are available, the record should distinguish between POCT results and those obtained from the central laboratory [40]. All computerized results should be password protected. Unfortunately, these standards are often not achieved and potentially significant clinical errors may occur. Regular effective QC procedures, as outlined above, are essential to allow POCT to become widely accepted, proven clinical practice.

Conclusion

POCT has the advantage of decentralization and reduced turnaround times, since no transport of blood samples or return of results is required. The type of analysis (e.g., thrombelastography) will, in some cases, provide different types of information to that available from traditional hemostasis laboratory tests, and, according to some, will lead to improved health outcomes. However, POCT methods have historically suffered from poor quality assurance procedures and a lack of standardization of methods. It is not uncommon for untrained operators to perform POCT, particularly in the operating theatre. Devolving POCT to the community has been expected by many to reduce the overall costs of service delivery. Identifying true costs in health care is complicated but the higher costs per test in reagents, external QC and consumables actually tend (at least in the UK) to lead to increased costs in assessments to date.

References

1. Perry DJ, Fitzmaurice DA, Kitchen S, Mackie IJ, Mallett S. Point-of-care testing in haemostasis. *Br J Haematol.* 2010;150:501–514.

2. Harrison P. Platelet function analysis. *Blood Reviews.* 2005;19:111–123.

3. Baglin TP, Cousins D, Keeling DM, Perry DJ, Watson HG. Recommendations from the British committee for standards in haematology and national patient safety agency. *Br J Haematol.* 2007;136:26–29.

4. Gregoratos G. Perspectives: oral anticoagulant therapy: current issues. *Prev Cardiol.* 2000;3:178–182.

5. Fitzmaurice DA. Oral anticoagulation control: the European perspective. *J Thromb Thrombolysis.* 2006;21:95–100.

6. Cromheecke ME, Levi M, Colly LP, et al. Oral anticoagulation self-management and management by a specialist anticoagulation clinic: a randomised cross-over comparison. *Lancet.* 2000;356:97–102.

7. Gardiner C, Williams K, Mackie IJ, Machin SJ, Cohen H. Can oral anticoagulation be managed using telemedicine and patient self-testing? A pilot study. *Clin Lab Haematol.* 2006;28:122–125.

8. Fitzmaurice DA, Murray ET, McCahon D, et al. Self management of oral anticoagulation: randomised trial. *BMJ.* 2005;331:1057.

9. Beyth RJ, Quinn L, Landefeld CS. A multicomponent intervention to prevent major bleeding complications in older patients receiving warfarin. A randomized, controlled trial. *Ann Intern Med.* 2000;133:687–695.

10. Machin SJ, Mackie IJ, Chitolie A, Lawrie AS. Near patient testing (NPT) in haemostasis—a synoptic review. *Clin Lab Haematol.* 1996;18:69–74.

11. Tripodi A, Arbini AA, Chantarangkul V, Bettega D, Mannucci PM. Are capillary whole blood coagulation monitors suitable for the control of oral anticoagulant treatment by the international normalized ratio? *Thromb Haemost.* 1993;70:921–924.

12. Panneerselvam S, Baglin C, Lefort W, Baglin T. Analysis of risk factors for over-anticoagulation in patients receiving long-term warfarin. *Br J Haematol.* 1998;103:422–424.

13. Testa S, Morstabilini G, Fattorini A, Galli L, Denti N, D'Angelo A. Discrepant sensitivity of thromboplastin reagents to clotting factor levels explored by the prothrombin time in patients on stable oral anticoagulant treatment: impact on the international normalized ratio system. *Haematologica.* 2002;87:1265–1273.

14. Horsti J, Uppa H, Vilpo JA. Poor agreement among prothrombin time international normalized ratio methods: comparison of seven commercial reagents. *Clin Chem.* 2005;51:553–560.

15. Lawrie AS, Hills J, Longair I, et al. The clinical significance of differences between INR methods in over-anticoagulated patients. *Thromb Res.* 2011;130:110–114.

16. Moriarty HT, Lam-Po-Tang PR, Anastas N. Comparison of thromboplastins using the ISI and INR system. *Pathology.* 1990;22:71–76.

17. British Committee for Standards in Haematology. *Guidelines on Oral Anticoagulation: third edition. Br J Haematol.* 1998;101:374–387.

18. Baglin TP, Keeling DM, Watson HG. For the British Committee for Standards in Haematology. *Guidelines on Oral Anticoagulation (Warfarin): third edition–2005 Update. Br J Haematol.* 2005;132:277–285.

19. Gardiner C, Adcock DM, Carrington LR, et al. *H57-A Protocol for the Evaluation, Validation and Implementation of Coagulometers*; Proposed Guideline. *CLSI*, 2007. (ISBN 1-56238-642-5).

20. Solvik UO, Stavelin A, Christensen NG, Sandberg S. External quality assessment of prothrombin time: the split-sample model compared with external quality assessment with commercial control material. *Scand J Clin Lab Invest.* 2006;66:337–349.

21. Kitchen DP, Murray ET, Jennings I, et al. Comparison of Coaguchek S INRs with hospital laboratory citrated plasma INRs. What is the truth? *Br J Haematol.* 2005;129(suppl 1):18.

22. Gardiner C, Williams K, Longair I, Mackie IJ, Machin SJ, Cohen H. A randomised control trial of patient self-management of oral anticoagulation compared with patient self-testing. *Br J Haematol.* 2005;132:598–603.

23. Heneghan C, Alonso-Coello P, Garcia-Alamino JM, Perera R, Meats E, Glasziou P. Self-monitoring of oral anticoagulation: a systematic review and meta-analysis. *Lancet.* 2006;367:404–411.

24. Gardiner C, Longair I, Pescott MA, et al. Self-monitoring of oral anticoagulation: does it work outside trial conditions? *J Clin Pathol.* 2009;62:168–171.

25. Fitzmaurice DA, Gardiner C, Kitchen S, Mackie I, Murray ET, Machin SJ; British Society of Haematology Taskforce for Haemostasis and Thrombosis. An evidence-based review and guidelines for patient self-testing and management of oral anticoagulation. *Br J Haematol.* 2005;131:156–165.

26. Ansell J, Jacobson A, Levy J, Völler H, Hasenkam JM. Guidelines for implementation of patient self-testing and patient self-management of oral anticoagulation. International consensus guidelines prepared by International Self-Monitoring Association for Oral Anticoagulation. *Int J Cardiol.* 2005;99:37–45.

27. Ferring M, Reber G, de Moerloose P, Merlani P, Diby M, Ricou B. Point of care and central laboratory determinations of the aPTT are not interchangeable in surgical

intensive care patients. *Can J Anaesth*. 2001;48:1155–1160.

28. Choi TS, Greilich PE, Shi C, Wilson JS, Keller A, Kroll MH. Point-of-care testing for prothrombin time, but not activated partial thromboplastin time, correlates with laboratory methods in patients receiving aprotinin or epsilon-aminocaproic acid while undergoing cardiac surgery. *Am J Clin Pathol*. 2002;117:74–78.

29. Despotis GJ, Gravlee G, Filos K, Levy J. Anticoagulation monitoring during cardiac surgery: a review of current and emerging techniques. *Anesthesiology*. 1999;91:1122–1151.

30. Despotis GJ, Filos KS, Levine V, Alsoufiev A, Spitznagel E. Aprotinin prolongs activated and nonactivated whole blood clotting time and potentiates the effect of heparin in vitro. *Anesth Analg*. 1996;82:1126–1131.

31. El Rouby S, Cohen M, Gonzales A, et al. The use of a HEMOCHRON JR. HEMONOX point of care test in monitoring the anticoagulant effects of enoxaparin during interventional coronary procedures. *J Thromb Thrombolysis*. 2006;21:137–145.

32. Geersing GJ, Janssen KJM, Oudega R, et al. Excluding venous thromboembolism using point of care D-dimer tests in outpatients: a diagnostic meta-analysis. *BMJ*. 2009;339:b2990.

33. Geersing GJ, Toll DB, Jannsen KJ, et al. Diagnostic accuracy and user-friendliness of 5 point-of-care D-dimer tests for the exclusion of deep vein thrombosis. *Clin Chem*. 2010;56:1758–1766.

34. Heim SW, Schectman JM, Siadaty MS, Philbrick JT. D-dimer testing for deep venous thrombosis: a metaanalysis. *Clin Chem*. 2004;50:1136–1147.

35. Hartert H. Blutgerrinnungsstudien mit der thrombelastographie, einem neuen untersuchungsverfahren. *Klinische Wochenschrift*. 1948;26:577–583.

36. Mallett SV, Cox DJ. Thrombelastography. *Br J Anaesth*. 1992;69:307–313.

37. Luddington RJ. Thrombelastography / Thrombelastometry. *Clin Lab Haem*. 2005;27:81–90.

38. Kitchen DP, Kitchen S, Jennings I, Woods T, Walker I. Quality assurance and quality control of thrombelastography and rotational Thromboelastometry: the UK NEQAS for blood coagulation experience. *Semin Thromb Hemost*. 2010;36:757–763.

39. Briggs C, Guthrie D, Hyde K, et al. Guidelines for point of care testing: Hematology. British Committee for Standards in Haematology (BCSH) General Haematology Task Force. *Br J Haematol*. 2008;142:904–915.

40. International Standards Organisation; ISO 22870:2006. Point-of-care testing (POCT)—Requirements for quality and competence. www.iso.org.

PART 3

Quality in Testing for Platelet Function and von Willebrand Disease

15 Diagnostic assessment of platelet function

Paquita Nurden[1], Alan Nurden[1], & Martine Jandrot-Perrus[2]

[1]Centre de Référence des Pathologies Plaquettaires, Plateforme Technologique d'Innovation Biomédicale, Hôpital Xavier Arnozan, Pessac, France
[2]INSERM U698 and Paris 7 University, Paris, France

Platelets are small anucleate blood cells produced in large numbers in the bone marrow by mature megakaryocytes (MKs) [1]. In the event of blood vessel injury, platelets are rapidly recruited to the area of damage where they accumulate to prevent blood loss. In this way they are essential elements in the arrest of bleeding and hemostasis. Included in this process are platelet adhesion, aggregation, thrombin generation with the formation of a clot, and wound healing.

Adhesion is the process whereby platelets attach through membrane receptors to cellular and extracellular matrix constituents of the subendothelial tissue. For example, the GPIb-IX-V complex binds to multimers of vWF exposed within the injured vessel wall [2]. This step occurs at high shear and is responsible for transient platelet tethering. It is followed by the activation-dependent stable attachment of platelets to collagen and other extracellular matrix constituents. The $\alpha2\beta1$ integrin and GPVI are the principal receptors involved in the platelet–collagen interaction promoting platelet spreading and activation including secretion [3]. Platelet aggregation occurs through the interaction of soluble proteins such as vWF and fibrinogen (Fg) with the $\alpha IIb\beta3$ integrin and the cross-linking of adjacent platelets [4]. Aggregation is promoted by soluble cofactors or metabolites released from platelets such as ADP and thromboxane A_2 (TXA_2), and by thrombin formed on the newly procoagulant platelet surface [4, 5]. Thrombin initiates fibrin polymerization leading to clot formation and retraction, while released substances and α-granule stored proteins accelerate tissue repair [6].

All platelet functional responses must be tightly regulated to ensure that the newly formed blood clot is of sufficient size to seal off the damaged area whilst not disrupting blood flow to vital organs by causing vessel occlusion. The consequences of abnormal platelet regulation can be either bleeding or the development of arterial thrombosis. Bleeding develops when there are qualitative or quantitative defects in platelets. Thrombotic complications involving platelets are mostly seen in the context of cardiovascular-related diseases such as heart attack and stroke which are often associated with atherosclerosis [7].

Bleeding syndromes arising through an inherited defect of platelet production constitute a heterogeneous group of rare diseases [8, 9]. Some, including the Bernard–Soulier syndrome (BSS) and Wiskott–Aldrich syndrome (WAS), associate a low circulating platelet count with a deficiency in a functional protein. In many familial thrombocytopenias (FTs), platelet dysfunction is secondary and the cause of bleeding is the inability of MKs to produce platelets in sufficient numbers. Recent evidence on the way that platelet lifespan is regulated suggests the existence of FT with accelerated platelet destruction [10]. Other syndromes associate defects of platelet function with a normal platelet count. In Glanzmann's thrombasthenia (GT), an absence of aggregation is due to a deficiency or a functional abnormality of

Quality in Laboratory Hemostasis and Thrombosis, Second Edition. Edited by Steve Kitchen, John D. Olson and F. Eric Preston.
© 2013 John Wiley & Sons, Ltd. Published 2013 by Blackwell Publishing Ltd.

the αIIbβ3 integrin [11]. Other pathologies concern agonist receptors such as P2Y$_{12}$ (ADP), TPα (TXA$_2$) or GPVI (collagen). Intracellular defects include the storage pool deficiencies where defects in the biogenesis of dense granules or α-granules give rise to the Hermansky–Pudlak and Chediak–Higashi syndromes or the gray platelet syndrome [12, 13]. An emerging field concerns intracellular signaling pathways and/or enzymes essential for energy or active metabolite production [8].

Platelet adhesive properties are central to a variety of pathophysiological processes that extend from inflammation to host defense and cancer. Platelets are also causally implicated in many acquired conditions including autoimmune diseases such as idiopathic thrombocytopenic purpura (ITP) and drug-dependent thrombocytopenias [14, 15], major diseases (e.g., kidney and liver disease, diabetes, microbial, and viral infections, Alzheimer's disease) and the response to treatment with drugs or chemotherapy [16]. Tests are performed to explain the origin of a bleeding syndrome, to aid evaluate the risk of bleeding prior to surgery or during pregnancy, or to monitor the efficiency of antiplatelet treatment in thrombotic or inflammatory syndromes. The use of aspirin to prevent thrombosis has become generalized, while new more potent antiplatelet drugs have been developed such as the powerful αIIbβ3 inhibitors (abciximab, eptifibatide, or tirofiban) and prodrugs such as clopidogrel or prasugrel whose metabolites specifically block ADP-induced platelet aggregation and which can be used as long-term maintenance anticoagulation [17, 18]. Assessment of the clinical efficacy of such drugs is a new discipline.

Bleeding time

The skin bleeding time (BT) was introduced some 50 years ago as an *in vivo* test used for assessing primary hemostasis [19]. Historically, the Duke procedure was first used, the earlobe being pierced with a lancet. This was later replaced with the Ivy BT, where a small incision was made in the forearm. This was later modified into the template BT, in which the size and depth of the cut was standardized by placing a template on the skin. A spring-loaded blade within the device makes a cut through a slit in the template. Two such template devices are Surgicutt® (International Technidyne Corp) and Simplate® (Organon Teknika Corp). Cessation of bleeding is dependent on an adequate number of platelets and of the ability of platelets to form the hemostatic plug. Many variables influence the BT, including hematocrit, skin thickness, temperature, blood vessel anatomy, location of the incision, and the skill of the operator. No study has clearly established the ability of BT measurement to predict the risk of hemorrhage in individual patients; it is not sensitive for the diagnosis of Type I von Willebrand disease (type I-VWD) while neonates may react differently to adults. The establishment of a normal range and/or control values is essential. For practical reasons, the BT is being replaced by such tests as the PFA-100 (see below); we do not use it ourselves and do not include it in our recommended schema for diagnosing patients with inherited platelet disorders (Figure 15.1).

Prothrombin consumption

This simple procedure assesses residual prothrombin levels after coagulation is complete when whole blood is coagulated in a nonsiliconized glass tube at 37°C [20]. The test depends on platelets and, in particular, on the availability of membrane phospholipid (formerly called platelet factor 3). Expressed as a percentage, prothrombin consumption (PT) is abnormal in BSS and in the very rare Scott syndrome [7]. The test suffers from a lack of reproducibility but can highlight defects in hemostasis that are not detected by other procedures. We perform the test regularly.

Platelet counting and morphology

Platelet counting is mostly performed automatically with hematology analyzers. A normal platelet count ranges from 150 to 400 $\times$ 10^9/L in whole blood. Commercially available machines include: Act 8 or LH 780 from Beckman Coulter (Miami FL); Advia 1200, 1650, 2400 (Bayer Healthcare, Tarrytown, NY); Cell-Dyn 4000 or Sapphire (Abbott Laboratories, Santa Clara, CA); Sysmex KX21 and XE2100 (Sysmex Corporation, Kobe, Japan) [21]. Counting is usually performed in EDTA-anticoagulated blood. The analyzers

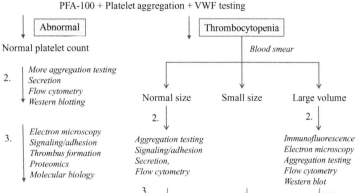

Figure 15.1 Simplified schema for the work-up of a patient with an inherited bleeding disorder. This is a personalized view in which the patient is examined three times and which requires that nonspecialized laboratories progressively establish networks with specialized centers perhaps through national societies or, as in France, by the national health ministry.

use impedance, optical, or immunological methods. A problem with impedance is to distinguish between small red cells and platelets (with an underestimation of large platelets). The use of analyzers identifying platelets with fluorochrome-labeled monoclonal antibodies (MoAbs) directed against markers of the MK lineage has been limited due to the high cost. It is recommended that an unexpected low platelet count is verified manually to look for agglutinates that the assay is repeated using a citrate-based anticoagulant to rule out pseudothrombocytopenia caused by natural antibodies acting after Ca^{2+}-chelation.

Platelet volume measurements can help diagnose the origin of a thrombocytopenia. Nevertheless, interpretation of results remains difficult since the analyzers are infrequently standardized, and a blood smear should also be examined. Coloration with Wright's or May-Grünwald–Giemsa (MGG) and examination using a light microscope will confirm the presence of large platelets; the absence of α-granules and a pale gray color identifies gray platelet syndrome, while the presence of platelet agglutinates can suggest type 2B VWD or the Montreal platelet syndrome [22, 23]. Of diagnostic importance for *MYH9*-related macrothrombocytopenias is the detection of abnormal inclusions, namely Döhle bodies, in leukocytes. A low platelet count and a small platelet volume is suggestive of X-linked thrombocytopenia and defects in the

WAS gene if the thrombocytopenia is isolated. WAS is to be considered if the major clinical signs include repeated infections and eczema.

Electron microscopy (EM), a sophisticated technique requiring special training, allows a precise ultrastructural analysis of platelet morphology and of the activation mechanisms including exocytosis [23, 24]. EM is very useful for characterizing certain inherited platelet disorders. A distinguishing feature of giant platelet syndromes (e.g., *MYH9*-related disease and BSS) is the presence of enlarged round platelets. Often they have a heterogeneous distribution of α-granules with zones enriched in membranes and/or the dense tubular system. In the gray platelet syndrome, EM shows how the α-granules in the somewhat enlarged platelets are replaced by vacuoles [25]. Fused α-granules are a characteristic of the Paris–Trousseau syndrome. Figure 15.2 shows a gallery of photographs obtained from patients with different types of thrombocytopenia. When required, EM can be combined with immunogold labeling (I-EM) to localize specific membrane or granular components [25]. Immunofluorescence or confocal microscopy can be used to specifically identify α-granules in platelets [26], while evaluating the distribution of nonmuscle myosin heavy chain IIA in leukocytes has become a standard test for *MYH9*-related disorders [22].

161

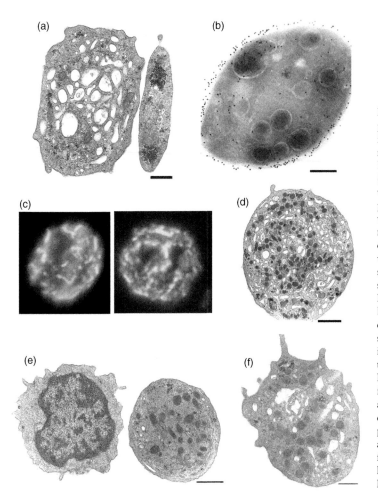

Figure 15.2 Inherited disorders of platelets: a gallery of photographs to illustrate different aspects of platelet morphology as seen by EM (a,b, d–f) or by immunofluorescence microscopy (c). In (a) are shown two platelets from a patient with the gray platelet syndrome [13]. One platelet is enlarged, round, and full of vacuoles, the second is discoid and of normal size. Neither platelet has α-granules. In (b) is a platelet from a variant form of Paris–Trousseau syndrome. Note the large vesicular structure composed of fused α-granules. I-EM has been performed, and the gold beads show the normal presence of the αIIbβ3 integrin. In (c), we illustrate the IF staining of leukocytes for the myosin-IIA isoform. The patch-like distribution is typical of the May–Hegglin anomaly [22]. In (d) is shown a typical enlarged platelet from a patient with the May–Hegglin anomaly. Note the nonuniform distribution of the α-granules and the presence of membrane complexes. In (e) and (f) are shown enlarged round platelets from two patients with type 2B vWD. A leukocyte is shown in (e) for comparison. Bars = 1 μm.

The platelet function analyzer

The platelet function analyzer (PFA-100) closure time (CT) provides a simple and rapid assessment of high shear-dependent platelet function [27, 28]. The apparatus is now commercially available from Siemens. Two types of cartridges are used: one containing an artificial membrane coated with collagen and epinephrine (C-EPI), the second is impregnated with collagen and ADP (C-ADP). Each membrane has a 150 μm central aperture. Platelet aggregates will block the central aperture when citrate-anticoagulated normal blood is aspirated across the membrane. Platelet dysfunction will prolong the CT or even prevent closure (defined as >300 second). Each laboratory should establish its own reference range. Like the BT, the PFA-100 CT is sensitive to changes in the platelet count or hematocrit. This test is particularly dependent on vWF and therefore is often used in screening for vWD. In congenital platelet disorders, the test lacks sensitivity and the CT varies with the severity and nature of the platelet defect [28]. Plug formation does not occur for patients with GT and BSS. For patients with P2Y$_{12}$ deficiency as well for patients with granule deficiencies the results are variable [28]; for aspirin-like defects and SPD the C-EPI cartridge is the most sensitive. Care must be taken with neonates who have shorter CT because of higher hematocrit and vWF levels.

The PFA-100 is often used to predict bleeding risk in patients about to undergo surgery (cardiopulmonary bypass, management of coronary syndromes) and to evaluate the efficacy of antiplatelet drugs in patients with cardiovascular disease [29, 30]. It is excellent for monitoring the action of the powerful anti-αIIbβ3 drugs that prolong or prevent closure of either cartridge. But it is less effective in monitoring milder-acting drugs such as aspirin where only the C-EPI cartridge is recommended. Controversy has arisen as to whether it will allow the so-called aspirin resistance seen in a significant proportion of patients [30, 31]. The PFA-100 is relatively insensitive for monitoring treatment with drugs blocking the action of ADP on platelets, a situation illustrated by the fact that the CT was normal for a patient with a total lack of P2Y$_{12}$ (Paquita Nurden, personal communication). It may be considered when monitoring therapy in patients undergoing bleeding (e.g., DDAVP, recombinant FVIIa, platelet, or vWF transfusions) although there is as yet no hard evidence linking changes in the PFA-100 CT with clinical outcome. In conclusion, this test offers the relative comfort of a rapid screening; nevertheless, all platelet abnormalities are not detected. In rare patients with a bleeding diathesis, a prolonged CT is seen in the absence of other indications (normal coagulation, normal platelet aggregation) suggesting that as yet unknown causes can contribute to alterations in CT and therefore bleeding.

The VerifyNow and point-of-care tests

Much effort has gone into producing machines that offer a rapid evaluation of bleeding risk. We have already dealt with the PFA-100, but other approaches are available. Excellent reviews of these technologies exist and the reader is referred to these for more detailed information [29, 30]. The VerifyNow (Accumetrics, San Diego, CA) (formerly called the Ultegra rapid PFA) is a cartridge-based whole blood assay designed to measure directly the effects of antiaggregants. It falls into the category of point-of-care tests designed for use at the patient's bedside. Different cartridges allow the evaluation of the efficacy of aspirin, thienopyridines or anti-αIIbβ3 drugs in a cardiovascular context. The device measures the agglutination of Fg-covered latex beads by platelets activated *in situ*. The percentage of drug inhibition for ADP or arachidonic acid is calculated relative to that obtained with a strong agonist, thrombin

receptor activating peptide (TRAP) [32, 33]. Plateletworks (Helena Laboratories, Beaumont, TX) compares platelet counts in whole blood anticoagulated with EDTA and citrate using ADP and collagen as agonists. It is mostly used to monitor antiplatelet therapy [34, 35]. The thromboelastograph PlateletMapping system (Haemoscope Corporation, Niles, IL) studies blood clotting in a rotating cup, the clot's strength being measured through force transmitted to a central pin. Addition of platelet agonists enhances clot strength. It has been used to evaluate antiplatelet therapy as well as the efficacity of transfused platelets to restore hemostatic function in patients [32, 35, 36]. Through its ability to provide information on clotting and fibrinolysis, it has been used in studies on the Quebec platelet syndrome where there is increased platelet expression of urokinase-type plasminogen activator [37]. Finally, there is the Impact Cone and platelet analyzer (Diamed Cressier, Switzerland) where blood is exposed to uniform shear by the spinning of a cone in a standardized cup. Platelet adhesion and thrombus formation are subsequently analyzed by computer software. Again, the monitoring of antiaggregant therapy has been the principle use [38].

Platelet aggregometry

Analysis of platelet aggregation in citrated platelet-rich plasma (PRP) has become the gold standard for platelet function testing and is a key part of any initial diagnosis of a platelet defect (Figure 15.3) [9]. Whole blood aggregometers working on the principles of electrical impedance or particle counting are available and while they have the advantage of testing the platelet response in the presence of other blood cells and of eliminating artifacts resulting from the preparation of PRP, their use has never become widespread [39].

For optical platelet aggregometry, venous blood is usually taken into vacutainers with trisodium citrate (3.2% or 3.8%) as anticoagulant; PRP is obtained by centrifuging the tubes at a low speed (150 to 180g for 10 or 15 minutes at room temperature). The PRP is aspirated from the tubes and platelet-poor plasma (PPP) prepared by subjecting the remaining blood to a new centrifugation at 1500 g for 10 minutes. Commercially available aggregometers often permit the analysis of multiple samples simultaneously. These include

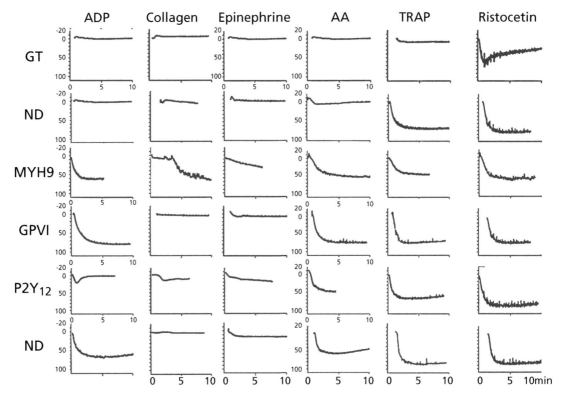

Figure 15.3 Illustrations of the use of aggregometry to study rare disorders of platelets. Citrated PRP has been challenged with the following agonists: ADP (10 μM), high dose collagen (2 μg/mL), epinephrine (4 μM), arachidonic acid (AA, 0.5 mg/mL), TRAP (50 μM), and ristocetin (1.5 mg/mL). Shown are tracings for a GT patient with no aggregation to all agonists except for ristocetin where aggregation was reversible. The response of the large platelets of a patient with *MYH9*-related disease was basically normal despite thrombocytopenia. A newly characterized patient with a GPVI deficiency specifically failed to respond to collagen while a patient lacking the P2Y$_{12}$ ADP receptor showed a characteristic reduced and rapidly reversible aggregation to ADP and a reduced response to collagen (under conditions where secreted ADP plays a major role). Also shown are the tracings for two nondiagnosed (ND) patients where purported defects in a signaling pathway affect the response to specific agonists but not TRAP.

the APACT 4004 (LABITec, Ahrensburg, Germany), Model 700 from Chrono-log (Havertown PA) or the PAP-8 aggregometer from Biodata Corporation (Horsham, PA). Light transmittance is measured in stirred suspensions at 37°C; the aggregation tracing is calibrated between 0% and 100%, 0% corresponding to the PRP and 100% to the PPP (Figure 15.2). As aggregation proceeds, the amount of light that passes across the stirred suspension is recorded. There is no consensus about the need for standardizing the platelet count before testing; indeed, platelet refractoriness may be induced by adding PPP to dilute the PRP [40]. The initial screening of platelet function disorders requires a panel of agonists that include: ADP (1–10 μM); fibrillar collagen (1–5 μg; equine type I Horm, Nycomed, Munich), epinephrine (5–10 μM), arachidonic acid (0.5–1 mg/ml), TRAP-6 mer or −14 mer (2–50 μM). Both high and low doses of collagen should be tested while care should be taken in establishing control values when using different commercial collagen preparations; they may show different reactivities depending on the type of collagen that is present. Ristocetin is also used at low and high concentrations (0.5 and 1.5 mg/mL); low doses are used to verify the absence of spontaneous GPIb/vWF interactions as in platelet-type vWD or type 2B vWD while an absent response at 1.5

mg/mL points to BSS [41]. Reference values need to be established for each agonist [42]. A biphasic response as seen with low doses of ADP consists of an initial aggregation that is supplemented by the release of storage pool ADP and newly synthesized TXA_2 [42]. An initial platelet shape change after the addition of an agonist is recognized by the presence of a prompt and brief increase of light transmittance. Shape change is not given by epinephrine. Figure 15.2 shows profiles that are characteristic for patients belonging to a series of well-characterized inherited disorders such as GT or $P2Y_{12}$ or GPVI deficiencies.

Initial results should be confirmed for a second blood sample taken at a later date. Other agonists can now be tested (Figure 15.2). For example, if the collagen response is abnormal and particularly when used at low doses, the snake venom protein, convulxin, or collagen-related peptides that directly activate platelets through the GPVI receptor should be included [25, 42]. An "aspirin-like" response suggests the use of the following: (i) the TXA_2 analogue U46619 that acts through the TPα receptor, (ii) phorbol 12-myristate 13-acetate (PMA) which interacts directly with protein kinase-C leading to diacylglycerol and inositol triphosphate formation, and (iii) the ionophore A23187 which directly mobilizes intracellular pools of Ca^2. Information gained from such agonists is particularly important if the defect concerns intracellular signaling or secretory pathways.

Platelet aggregation can also be performed using washed platelets separated from plasma by differential centrifugation and resuspended in buffers that maintain the platelet functional response [43, 44]. Gel filtration on Sepharose 2B and centrifugation on inert density gradients (albumin, stractan) are alternative procedures but are infrequently used. The use of washed platelets allows the concentration of platelets from thrombocytopenic patients and permits an evaluation of the platelet functional response at physiologic extracellular Ca^{2+} levels. The absence of plasma Fg facilitates an analysis of the aggregation response to thrombin. Typical doses are 0.05 U/mL for a low concentration of thrombin and 0.5 to 1 U/mL for maximal activation and secretion. For testing other agonists with washed platelets, the addition of Fg (300 μg/mL) is necessary. The use of washed platelets is a good way of controlling for the presence of plasma inhibitors of platelet aggregation. For example, antibodies in ITP patients reactive with surface receptors can block

the functional response as well as induce thrombocytopenia. Incubating the patient's plasma with washed control platelets prior to stimulation can confirm inhibitor activity. A rapid microtiter assay for screening potential drugs on platelet aggregation has been proposed [45].

Platelet secretion

Dense granules can be visualized using the fluorescent dye mepacrine and counted by fluorescence microscopy or by examining whole mounts by EM [46]. If a dense granule abnormality is suspected then the releasable and total platelet pools of ADP and ATP should be quantified and their ratio calculated. An alternative approach is to assess platelet capacity to take up and then release serotonin. As well as a qualitative storage pool deficiency, defects may concern a block in the secretory mechanism [8]. Dense granule secretion can be determined by measuring the release of ATP during platelet aggregation in a lumi-aggregometer (Chrono-log, Havertown, PA) by adding luciferin–luciferase reagent to the platelet samples [42]. Secretion is measured at 37°C with stirring, and step changes in the luminescence recording can be used to calculate the amount of ATP released by comparison to a calibration curve. Only the intragranular pool of ATP is secreted and measured; the metabolic pool remains in the cytoplasm. Incubation of platelets with agonists (e.g., ADP, collagen, thrombin) with or without stirring for different times will allow an evaluation of the kinetics of secretion. The release of selected α-granule proteins such as PF4 and PDGF can be quantified using commercial ELISA procedures or radioimmunoassay [25, 47]. The evaluation of platelet secretion by flow cytometry (FC) will be discussed in the next section.

Flow cytometry

FC is a powerful and often used tool that can provide much information on the functional status of platelets [48]. A large number of flow cytometers are commercially available: machines that adapt readily to platelets are the Cytomics FC500 from Beckman Coulter (Fullerton, CA) and the FACSCalibur or FACSarray TMcustom from Becton Dickinson

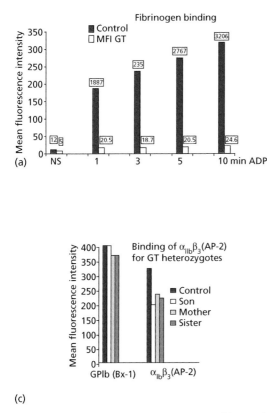

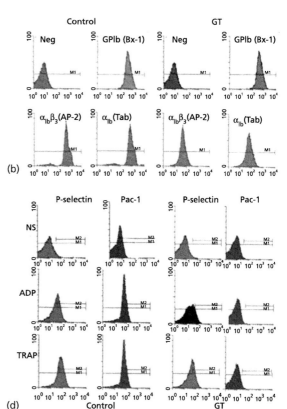

Figure 15.4 A series of analyses to show the usefulness of FC in diagnosing the platelet defect in a patient with a variant form of GT with a β3 L196P mutation. In the upper left quadrant is shown the inability of the platelets to bind FITC-labeled Fg after stimulation with ADP. In the upper right quadrant is shown the binding of a MoAb to GPIbα (Bx-1), to a complex-dependent determinant on the αIIbβ3 integrin (AP-2) and to the αIIb subunit (Tab). Note the normal presence of GPIb and the presence of small amounts of residual nonfunctional αIIbβ3. In the lower left quadrant is shown the ability of FC to detect reduced amounts of αIIbβ3 in family members shown to carry the mutation. In the lower right quadrant is illustrated the ability of the patient's platelets to express P-selectin when stimulated (ADP and TRAP) and the inability of the patient's residual αIIbβ3 to bind the conformation-dependent MoAb PAC-1—a result which agrees with the absence of Fg binding.

(San José, CA). FC assesses cell size and granularity within a large population of cells, while simultaneously quantifying the fluorescence emitted from cell-bound fluorochrome-labeled antibodies and ligands. It allows a precise assessment of the physical and antigenic properties of platelets (e.g., surface expression of receptors, bound ligands, secretion, platelet aggregates, leukocyte–platelet aggregates). It facilitates the diagnosis of inherited (e.g., BSS, GT, storage pool disease) or acquired platelet disorders (e.g., ITP). Studies on platelets of a GT variant are shown in Figure 15.4. FC also allows an assessment of the following: (i) the pathological activation state of platelets

(e.g., in the setting of acute coronary syndromes, cerebrovascular ischemia, peripheral vascular disease, cardiopulmonary bypass, diabetes), (ii) the efficacy of antiplatelet drugs to combat thrombosis, and (iii) the efficacy of platelet transfusion in the event of bleeding as well as controlling the functional state of stored platelets [49–51].

Using a panel of antibodies, the structure of membrane glycoprotein receptors can be studied in detail; for example, for αIIbβ3 there are not only MoAbs-recognizing epitopes on each subunit but also epitopes specific for the complex. The IgM MoAb, PAC-1 is able to recognize the activated form of the complex;

while to detect the binding of ligands; there are two categories of MoAbs, the anti-RIBS (receptor-induced binding site) and anti-LIBS (ligand-induced binding site) [49]. Another useful tool to detect functionally activated αIIbβ3 is fluorescein isothiocyanate (FITC)-coupled Fg. To quantify binding, antibodies can be conjugated directly with fluorochromes such as FITC or phycoerythrin (PE). Assessment can also be indirect with bound primary antibodies recognized by a species-specific second antibody coupled to one of a large panel of fluorochromes [48]. Results are printed in the form of histograms, with mean fluorescent intensity (MFI) (x axis) plotted against cell number (y axis). Prior fixation of platelets with paraformaldehyde stabilizes surface antigens and allows transport of samples. Analyses can be performed on PRP or in whole blood; in the latter the use of a double-labeling procedure can permit an evaluation of an antigen on MoAb-identified cells and on mixed cell aggregates [52]. Commercially available quantification kits (Biocytex, Marseille, France) allow a precise assessment of the number of bound MoAbs directed to the main platelet receptors (αIIbβ3, GPIb-V-IX, α2β1); the test could be adapted for the quantification of other receptors for which specific mouse IgG1 MoAbs are available such as for GPVI. Granule secretion is measured using anti-CD62P as a marker of α-granules and anti-CD63 as a marker of dense bodies and lysosomal granules. Access to cytoplasmic proteins and to storage organelles is achieved by fixing the platelets with paraformaldehyde, and permeabilizing them with agents such as Triton X-100 or saponin. The use of the membrane-permeable dye, mepacrine, allows an indirect assessment of the platelet dense granule content in suspected storage pool disease. The use of thiazole orange allows the analysis of reticulated platelets (newly released platelets), a technique that is proposed for evaluating platelet production and/or turnover [53].

A new application for drug surveillance involves the use of permeabilized PFA-fixed platelets to measure the phosphorylation state of VASP protein by way of a MoAb that specifically recognizes the phosphorylated form of this protein (kit commercialized by Biocytex). VASP is dephosphorylated after ADP activates P2Y$_{12}$. The assay uses prostaglandin E$_1$ to increase intraplatelet cAMP and fully phosphorylated VASP making the assay more sensitive and specific for the effects of ADP. Assuming that the degree of dephosphorylation reflects the interaction between ADP and its receptor, this test is used to evaluate the clinical efficacity of antiplatelet drugs such as clopidogrel and prasugrel [54]. In a patient with a total P2Y$_{12}$ deficiency, ADP was without effect on VASP phosphorylation (Paquita Nurden, personal communication).

Another application of FC is the study of platelet procoagulant activity. Phosphatidylserine (PS) is an essential platelet membrane phospholipid that is exposed at the platelet surface after activation and forming a procoagulant surface and promoting thrombin generation. The placental protein, annexin-V, binds specifically to PS and is used in FC to identify PS at the platelet surface. The mechanisms that induce the flip-flop phenomenon of PS during platelet activation also result in the liberation of microparticles (MPs) by a mechanism that involves the Ca^{2+}-dependent protease, calpain [55]. Annexin can bind PS only in the presence of Ca^{2+} meaning that activation is realized in vitro using washed platelets. To obtain maximal amounts of annexin-V binding, platelets need to be stimulated by a thrombin and collagen mixture or by the ionophore A23187. A total lack of surface PS expression and MP formation is seen in the Scott syndrome [8]. Others have called the procoagulant platelets, "coated-platelets" based on the presence of surface-bound and secreted proteins covalently bound by a mechanism that involves serotonin [56]. Platelet-derived MPs can be measured in plasma by ELISA as well as by FC [57]. By using cell-specific MoAbs during the analysis, the cells from which the MPs are derived can be identified [58]. The MPs are said to be prothrombotic, but they can also have major roles in the development of atherosclerotic plaques, in wound healing and in inflammation.

FC is especially useful in the diagnosis of inherited disorders of platelet function if combined with western blotting (WB). Suspensions of washed platelets are solubilized by the ionic detergent sodium dodecyl sulfate (SDS) and the soluble proteins separated by polyacrylamide gel electrophoresis in the presence of the detergent (SDS-PAGE). The transfer of proteins to nitrocellulose membrane followed by their renaturation with nonionic detergent permits their identification through antibody binding. Proteins suspected to be absent in platelets of diseases such as GT and BSS can be evaluated in this way, while alterations in protein structure (i.e., truncated proteins, degraded proteins) can also be identified provided that antibody-binding epitopes are retained [59]. With the use of chemiluminescent antibody detecting procedures this is a very sensitive assay that can be applied to minor platelet proteins.

Clot retraction

Blood coagulation is followed by clot retraction resulting from the association of fibrin fibers with activated platelets. The retraction is brought about by the platelet contractile system with surface receptors forming a bridge with the fibrin [60]. Clot retraction is essential for thrombus stability and proceeds through a $\beta 3$ and myosin IIA-dependent signaling pathway probably regulated by myosin light-chain phosphorylation itself under the control of RhoA. In the absence or nonfunctioning of $\alpha IIb\beta 3$, clot retraction does not occur; in some patients with GT with residual $\alpha IIb\beta 3$ receptors it occurs partially [11]. It may also be abnormal in *MYH9*-related diseases. Clot retraction can be measured by simply incubating nonanticoagulated blood in a nonsiliconized glass tube at $37°C$. Retraction is a slow process that can take several hours. It is more rapid when using calcification of citrated PRP as a mode of thrombin generation.

Signaling pathways

As we have seen, agonist binding to platelet receptors mediates functional responses such as adhesion, activation, secretion, and aggregation. The signaling network in platelets that brings about these processes is complex, involving multiple pathways that often converge. As well as being a receptor for vWF, GPIbα participates in thrombin-induced signaling [2]. GPVI and the $\alpha 2\beta 1$ integrin harmonize to assure a stable platelet adhesion to collagen. GPVI associates with the FcRγ-chain which signals through its immunoreceptor tyrosine-based activation motif (ITAM) via the adaptor LAT leading to the activation of phospholipase (PL) Cγ2 [3, 61]. Many of the primary agonists of platelets have more than one receptor belonging to the seven transmembrane domain receptor family: ADP, P2Y$_1$ and P2Y$_{12}$; thrombin, PAR-1, and PAR-4. Each receptor is linked to a specific G-protein

whose subunits (α, β/γ) can lead to bidirectional signaling [62]. Diverse signaling routes have been characterized, in particular those involving specific tyrosine kinases (Syk, Src, and Fyn), phospholipase A$_2$ (with TXA$_2$ generation), PLCγ2 (involving Cbl, LAT), PLC-β (adenylyl cyclase), protein kinase C (diacyl glycerol, ITP$_3$) and the PI 3-kinases often involving Akt [61, 63]. Studying these pathways requires collaborations with specialist laboratories. Phosphorylation on serine or threonine residues, or on tyrosine residues can be studied using immunological tools often involving immunoprecipitation and/or WB with the use of specific MoAbs reactive with the phosphorylated amino acids. These signaling routes converge and result in calcium mobilization that is an absolute requirement for normal platelet aggregation. The cytoplasmic Ca^{2+} concentration can be measured on limited volume samples by FC using fluorescent calcium dye such as Fluo3AM.

As well as involving newly bound secreted proteins such as thrombospondin-1, aggregate stability also appears to involve a whole new generation of membrane receptors such as the ephrins and eph kinases, semaphorin 4D [61]. Many patients with bleeding disorders where the platelet receptors are present and appear to act normally are suspected to have defects within a signaling pathway [8].

In vitro studies on thrombus formation

Requiring specialist procedures, this can be studied under static or flow conditions.

Platelet adhesion to collagen and other adhesive proteins under static conditions

The first approach is to quantify platelet adhesion in microtiter plates. Wells are coated with the protein of interest (collagen or convulxin as an example). After saturating the protein-free sites with BSA, platelets, washed or in PRP, are incubated in the wells for fixed (end point) or increasing times (kinetic). After careful washing without detergents, adherent platelets are quantified by an acid phosphatase assay and results are expressed relative to a standard curve. Coating with different proteins (fibrillar or soluble collagen or convulxin or CRP) and incubation in the presence of aggregation inhibitors (e.g., RGD peptide), or various divalent cation concentrations (Ca^{2+}/Mg^{2+}) facilitates the clarification of the role of given adhesion receptors such as GPVI, α2β1, or αIIbβ3.

A suggested approach to studying platelet adhesion in disease states is to analyze and compare platelet spreading on collagen, Fg, and vWF coated on glass coverslips [64–66]. After blocking protein-free sites with BSA, a drop containing a suspension of washed platelets is added and the platelets left in contact with the surface for 30 minutes prior to their observation by differential interference contrast (DIC) microscopy with a wide-field objective. Real-time imaging can also be performed. The procedure can be adapted to the use of fluorochrome-labeled probes whose localization is determined by confocal microscopy following PFA-fixation. Surface receptors can be visualized directly; while actin polymerization can be followed using fluorochrome-labeled phalloidin after cell permeabilization. The attachment of platelets to collagen first promotes the formation of long filopodia, while spreading is accompanied by secretion and the formation of distinct wave-like lamellipodia. Changes in intracellular Ca^{2+} can be followed using the calcium reporter dye Oregon Green-BAPTA 1-AM. Platelet adhesion and spreading on vWF, involves both GPIb and αIIbβ3; spreading is blocked by integrin inhibitors but can be restored by ristocetin or botrocetin where GPIb-mediated signaling now predominates [66]. This adhesion test is potentially very useful for detecting signaling defects in platelets and is recommended for thrombocytopenias where the platelet count is too low for aggregometry.

Thrombus formation on immobilized collagen under flow conditions

Many of the regulatory processes involved in thrombus growth are well assessed *in vitro* in flow assays. Various procedures have been developed in which anticoagulated blood from patients is perfused through flow chambers or glass capillaries containing surfaces that have been coated with an adhesive protein, often type I collagen from equine tendon but also vWF and Fg [67–69]. Initially restricted to some laboratories using customized perfusion chambers, this method has become more accessible with the development of commercial systems such as Bioflux or Venaflux. The blood is perfused in the device with a

pump at flow rates adapted to create venous or arterial rheological conditions. Platelets can be labeled with a fluorescent dye such as DiOC6, rhodamine 6G, or mepacrine, allowing direct evaluation by epifluorescent videomicroscopy. Alternatively, evaluation is by light microscopy and computer analysis after fixation of the thrombi. Flow chambers have been designed to allow direct visualization of the platelet adhesion and aggregation process by, for example, reflexion interference contrast microscopy that is recorded with a video camera [68]. Image sequencing of the time-lapse recording and analysis of surface coverage and thrombus volume can be compared from controls and patients and at controlled shear rates. After fixation, the use of fluorochrome-labeled antibodies and confocal microscopy can provide information on the localization and role of specific proteins [68]. The use of such dyes as Oregon green 488 BAPTA-1 and FURA Red AM, allows the study of calcium signaling during aggregation and thrombus build up [69].

Platelet procoagulant activity

The optimal rate of clotting is attained through the procoagulant function of activated platelets; surface exposure of PS and the secretion of procoagulant factors such as FV and polyphosphates contribute to the assembly of the enzymatic complexes tennase and prothrombinase and to the activation of the intrinsic pathway that sustain procoagulant response. Calibrated automated thrombin generation in PRP provides a global assessment of platelet procoagulant potential. It consists of measuring, in real time, the concentration of thrombin in clotting PRP preactivated or not with selected agonists by monitoring the splitting of a chromogenic substrate in a microwell titration plate. The lag time preceding thrombin generation, the maximal (peak height), and total (peak surface) concentrations of formed thrombin are informative parameters on platelet function.

New technologies

Proteomics and genomics

These are powerful tools for studying platelets. Proteomics allows a large-scale study of the platelet proteome. It involves the separation of detergent-soluble platelet extracts by high-resolution two-dimensional gel electrophoresis or by sophisticated chromatographic procedures. Proteins are often identified by mass spectroscopy, usually by the analysis of peptides obtained by proteolyic digestion. Upward of 641 proteins compose the platelet proteome [70]. While some groups have attempted to resolve the whole platelet proteome, others have confined themselves to specifically studying membrane glycoproteins, the secretome (i.e., proteins released from the storage pool), or the phosphoproteome (proteins involved in signaling pathways) [70–72]. Although anucleate, platelets retain sufficient mRNA to allow transcript profiling using microarray [73, 74]. In total, transcripts of 1526 genes were identified in one study [74]. In identifying pathological changes in a cell, profiling of mRNA levels has the potential to identify not only defective genes but also those abnormally regulated by a mutated protein. An example is the decreased platelet expression of myosin regulatory light-chain polypeptide (MYL9) and other genes associated with platelet dysfunction in a patient with FT and a CBFA2/RUNX1 mutation [75]. A major use of genomics and microarrays will be to study SNPs that affect virtually all genes [76]. Arguments can be put forward that a global assessment of the SNPs of platelet genes will provide much information to explain the biological functional activity of platelets and its variation from individual to individual.

Gene sequencing

Any diagnosis of an inherited platelet disorder is incomplete without knowledge of the molecular defect that is responsible for the disease. In more frequently encountered diseases such as GT, gene sequencing has become commonplace and population studies are being performed [77]. While in the past years pre-screening for gene defects using PCR-SSCP or DGGE was commonplace, the preference now is for direct sequencing of gene promoters, exons, and splice sites. BSS results from mutations affecting the *GPIBA*, *GPIBB, and GP9* genes; as these are single exon genes (except for *GPIBB* which has two exons) direct sequencing is the rule. Genotyping of human platelet alloantigens (HPA) associated with *ITGB3, ITGA2B,* and *GPIBA* as major immunological targets is

important in the diagnosis and treatment of neonatal alloimmune thrombocytopenic purpura, post-transfusion purpura, and refractoriness to platelet transfusion therapy [78]. Mutations in transcription factor genes are often responsible for FTs [23]. One example is the GATA-1 gene where morphologically enlarged platelets may have a decreased GPIbα and α-granule content, while some patients also show red cell defects typical of β-thalassemia [79]. Notwithstanding this progress, many of the molecular defects giving rise to FTs remain without a classification. There is a need for gene sequencing on a large scale.

References

1. Patel SR, Hartwig JH, Italiano JE Jr. The biogenesis of platelets from megakaryocyte proplatelets. *J Clin Invest.* 2005;115:3348–3354.
2. Andrews RK, Berndt MC, Lopez JA. The glycoprotein Ib-IX-V complex. In: Michelson A, ed. *Platelets.* 2nd ed. San Diego, CA: Academic Press; 2007:145–163.
3. Sarratt KL, Chen H, Zutter MM, Santoro SA, Hammer DA, Kahn ML. GPVI and α2β1 play independent critical roles during platelet adhesion and aggregate formation to collagen under flow. *Blood.* 2005;106:1268–1277.
4. Jackson SP. The growing complexity of platelet aggregation. *Blood.* 2007;109:5087–5095.
5. Balasubramanian Y, Grabowski E, Bini A, Nemerson Y. Platelets, circulating tissue factor, and fibrin colocalize in ex vivo thrombi: real-time fluorescence images of thrombus formation and propagation under defined flow conditions. *Blood.* 2002;100:2787–2792.
6. Nurden AT, Nurden P, Sanchez M, Andia I, Anitua E. Platelets and wound healing. *Front Biosci.* 2005;13:3532–3548.
7. Choudhury RP, Fuster V, Fayad ZA. Molecular, cellular and functional imaging of atherothrombosis. *Nat Rev Drug Discov.* 2004;3:913–925.
8. Nurden P, Nurden AT. Congenital disorders associated with platelet dysfunctions. *Thromb Haemost.* 2008;99:253–263.
9. Bolton-Maggs PHB, Chalmers EA, Collins PW, et al. A review of inherited platelet disorders with guidelines for their management on behalf of the UKHCDO. *Br J Haematol.* 2006;135:603–633.
10. Mason KD, Carpinelli MR, Fletcher JI, et al. Programmed anuclear cell death delimits platelet lifespan. *Cell.* 2007;128:1173–1186.
11. Nurden AT, George JN. Inherited abnormalities of the platelet membrane: Glanzmann Thrombasthenia, Bernard-Soulier syndrome, and other disorders.

In: Colman RW, Marder VJ, Clowes AW, George JN, Goldhaber S, eds. *Hemostasis and Thrombosis*. 5th ed. Philadelphia, PA: Lippincott, Williams & Wilkins;2006:987–1010.

12. Gunay-Ayqun M, Huizing M, Gahl WA. Molecular defects that affect platelet dense granules. *Semin Thromb Hemost*. 2004;30:537–547.

13. Nurden AT, Nurden P. The Gray platelet syndrome: clinical spectrum of the disease. *Blood Reviews*. 2007;21:21–36.

14. Bussel JB. Immune thrombocytopenic purpura. In: Michelson A ed. *Platelets*. 2nd ed. San Diego, CA: Academic Press; 2007:831–846.

15. Aster RH, Bougie DW. Drug-induced thrombocytopenia. *New Engl J Med*. 2007;357:580–587.

16. Rao AK. Acquired disorders of platelet function. In: Michelson A, ed. *Platelets*. 2nd ed. San Diego, CA: Academic Press; 2007:1051–1076.

17. Agah R, Plow EF, Topol EJ. αIIbβ3 (GPIIb-IIIa) antagonists. In: Michelson A, ed. *Platelets*. 2nd ed. San Diego, CA: Academic Press; 2007:1145–1163.

18. Jakubowski JA, Winters KJ, Naganuma H, Wallentin L. Prasugrel: a novel thienopyridine antiplatelet agent. a review of preclinical and clinical studies and the mechanistic basis for its distinct antiplatelet profile. *Cardiovasc Drug Rev*. 2007;25:357–374.

19. Rodgers RP, Levin J. A critical appraisal of the bleeding time. *Semin Thromb Haemost*. 1990;16:1–20.

20. Quick AJ, Favre-Gilly JE. The prothrombin consumption test: Its clinical and theoretic implications. *Blood*. 1949;1281–1289.

21. Briggs C, Harrison P, Machin SJ. Platelet counting. In: Michelson A, ed. *Platelets*. 2nd ed. San Diego, CA: Academic Press; 2007:465–483.

22. Balduini CL, Cattaneo M, Fabris F, et al. Italian Gruppo di Studio delle Piastrine. Inherited thrombocytopenias: a proposed diagnostic algorithm from the Italian Gruppo di Studio delle Piastrine. *Haematologica*. 2003;88:582–592.

23. Nurden P, George JN, Nurden AT. Inherited thrombocytopenias. In: Colman RW, Marder VJ, Clowes AW, George JN, Goldhaber S, eds. *Hemostasis and Thrombosis*. 5th ed. Philadelphia, PA: Lippincott, Williams & Wilkins; 2006:975–986.

24. White JG. Platelet structure. In: Michelson A ed. *Platelets*. 2nd ed. San Diego, CA: Academic Press; 2007:45–73.

25. Nurden P, Jandrot-Perrus M, Combrié R, et al. Severe deficiency of glycoprotein VI in a patient with gray platelet syndrome. *Blood*. 2004;104:107–114.

26. Italiano JE Jr, Richardson JL, Patel-Hett S, et al. Angiogenesis is regulated by a novel mechanism: pro- and anti-angiogenic proteins are organized into separate platelet α-granules and differentially released. *Blood*. 2008;111:1227–1233.

27. Harrison P. The role of PFA-100® testing in the investigation and management of haemostatic defects in children and adults. *Br J Haematol*. 2005;130:3–10.

28. Hayward CP, Harrison P, Cattaneo M, Ortel TL, Rao AK, Platelet Physiology Subcommittee of the Scientific and Standardization Committee of the International Society on Thrombosis and Haemostasis. Platelet function analyzer (PFA)-100 closure time in the evaluation of platelet disorders and platelet function. *J Thromb Haemost*. 2006;4:312–319.

29. Michelson AD, Frelinger AL 3rd, Furman MI. Current options in platelet function testing. *Am J Cardiol*. 2006;98:4N–10N.

30. Gurbel PA, Becker RC, Mann KG, Steinhubl SR, Michelson AD. Platelet function monitoring in patients with coronary artery disease. *JACC*. 207;50:1822–1834.

31. Podda GM, Bucciarelli P, Lussana F, Lecchi A, Cattaneo M. Usefulness of PFA-100 testing in the diagnostic screening of patients with suspected abnormalities of hemostasis: comparison with the bleeding time. *J Thromb Haemost*. 2007;5:2393–2398.

32. Steinbuhl SR, Talley JD, Braden GA, et al. Point-of-care measured platelet inhibition correlates with a reduced risk of an adverse cardiac event after percutaneous coronary intervention: results of the GOLD (AU-Assessing Ultegra) multicenter study. *Circulation*. 2001;103:2572–2578.

33. Jakubowski JA, Payne CD, Li YG, et al. The use of the VerifyNow P2Y12 point-of-care device to monitor platelet function across a range of P2Y12 inhibition levels following prasugrel and clopidogrel administration. *Thromb Hemost*. 2008;99:409–415.

34. Van Werkum JW, Gerritsen WB, Kelder JC, et al. Inhibition of platelet function by abciximab or high-dose tirofiban in patients with STEMI undergoing primary PCI: a randomized trial. *Neth Heart J*. 2007;15:375–381.

35. Craft RM, Chavez JJ, Snider CC, Muenchen RA, Carroll RC. Comparison of modified thromboelastograph and Plateletworks whole blood assays to optical platelet aggregation for monitoring reversal of clopidogrel inhibition in elective surgery patients. *J Lab Clin Med*. 2005;145:309–315.

36. Male C, Koren D, Eichelberger B, Kaufmann K, Panzer S. Monitoring survival and function of transfused platelets in Glanzmann thrombasthenia by flow cytometry and thromboelastography. *Vox Sang*. 2006;174–177.

37. Diamandis M, Adam F, Kahr WH, et al. Insights into abnormal hemostasis in the Quebec platelet disorder from analysis of clot lysis. *J Thromb Haemost*. 2006;4:1086–1094.

38. Osende JL, Fuster V, Lev EI, et al. Testing platelet activation with a shear-dependent platelet function test versus aggregation-based tests: relevance for monitoring long-term glycoprotein IIb/IIIa inhibition. *Circulation*. 2001;103:1488–1491.

39. Jarvis GE. Platelet aggregation in whole blood: impedence and particle counting methods. *Methods Mol Biol*. 2004;272:77–87.

40. Cattaneo M, Lecchi A, Zighetti ML, Lussana F. Platelet aggregation studies: autologous platelet-poor plasma inhibits platelet aggregation when added to platelet-rich plasma to normalize platelet count. *Haematologica*. 2007;92:694–697.

41. Federici AB, Mannucci PM. Management of inherited von Willebrand disease in 2007. *Ann Med*. 2007;39:346–358.

42. Dawood BB, Wilde J, Watson SP. Reference curves for aggregation and ATP secretion to aid diagnosis of platelet-based bleeding disorders: effect of inhibition of ADP and thromboxane A2 pathways. *Platelets*. 2007;18:329–345.

43. Cazenave J-P, Ohlmann P, Cassel D, Eckly A, Hechler B, Gachet C. Preparation of washed platelet suspensions from human and rodent blood. *Methods Mol Biol*. 2004;272:13–28.

44. Kim S, Jin J, Kunapuli SP. Akt activation in platelets depends on Gi signaling pathways. *J Biol Chem* 2004;279:4186–4195.

45. Moran N, Kiernan A, Dunne E, Edwards RJ, Shields DC, Kenny D. Monitoring modulators of platelet aggregation in a microtiter plate assay. *Analyt Biochem*. 2006;357:77–84.

46. Enders A, Zieger B, Schwartz K, et al. Careful clinical and molecular diagnosis is essential to discriminate between Griscelli syndrome and Hermansky-Pudlak syndrome type II. *Blood*. 2006;108:81–87.

47. Weiss HJ, Witte LD, Kaplan KL, et al. Heterogeneity in storage pool deficiency: Studies on granule-bound substances in 18 patients including variants deficient in α-granules, platelet factor 4, β-thromboglobulin, and platelet-derived growth factor. *Blood*. 1979;54:1296–1319.

48. Michelson AD, Linden MD, Barnard MR, Furman MI, Frelinger III AL. Flow cytometry. In: Michelson A, ed. *Platelets*. 2nd ed. San Diego, CA: Academic Press; 2007:545–563.

49. Bihour C, Durrieu-Jaïs C, Macchi L, et al. Expression of markers of platelet activation and the interpatient variation in response to abciximab. *Arterioscler Thromb Vasc Biol*. 1999;19:212–219.

50. Frelinger AL 3rd, Jakubowski JA, Li Y, et al. The active metabolite of prasugrel inhibits ADP-stimulated thrombo-inflammatory markers of platelet activation:

51. influence of other blood cells, calcium and aspirin. *Thromb Haemost*. 2007;98:192–200.

51. Linden MD, Furman MI, Frelinger AL 3rd, et al. Indices of platelet activation and the stability of coronary artery disease. *J Thromb Haemost*. 2007;4:761–765.

52. Barnard MR, Linden MD, Frelinger AL 3rd, et al. Effects of platelet binding on whole blood flow cytometry assays of monocyte and neutrophil procoagulant activity. *J Thromb Haemost*. 2005;3:2563–2570.

53. McCabe DJ, Harrison P, Sidhu PS, Brown MM, Machin SJ. Circulating reticulated platelets in the early and late phases after ischaemic stroke and transient ischaemic attack. *Br J Haematol*. 2004;126:861–869.

54. Aleil B, Ravanat C, Cazenave JP, Rochoux G, Heitz A, Gachet C. Flow cytometric analysis of intraplatelet VASP phosphorylation for the detection of clopidogrel resistance in patients with ischemic cardiovascular disease. *J Thromb Haemost*. 2005;3:85–92.

55. Dachary-Prigent J, Pasquet JM, Freyssinet JM, Nurden AT. Calcium involvement in aminophospholipid exposure and microparticle formation during platelet activation : a study using Ca2 + -ATPase inhibitors. *Biochemistry*. 1995;34:11625–11634.

56. Dale GL. Coated-platelets: an emerging component of the procoagulant response. *J Thromb Haemost*. 2005;3:2185–2192.

57. Lynch SF, Ludlam CA. Plasma microparticles and vascular disorders. *Br J Haematol*. 2007;137:36–48.

58. Morel O, Toti F, Hugel B, et al. Procoagulant microparticles. Disrupting the vascular homeostasis equation. *Arterioscler Thromb Vasc Biol*. 2006;26:2594–2604.

59. Milet-Marsal S, Breillat C, Peyruchaud O, et al. Glanzmann thrombasthenia secondary to a Glu[324] to Lys substitution in the αIIb subunit of the fibrinogen receptor: analysis of the amino acid requirement for a normal αIIbβ3 maturation. *Thromb Haemost*. 2002;88:655–662.

60. Schoenwaelder SM, Yuan Y, Cooray P, Salem HH, Jackson SP. Calpain cleavage of focal adhesion proteins regulates the cytoskeletal attachment of integrin αIIbβ3 (platelet glycoprotein IIb/IIIa) and the cellular retraction of fibrin clots. *J Biol Chem*. 1997;272:1694–1702.

61. Brass LF, Stalker TJ, Zhu L, Woulfe DS. Signal transduction during platelet plug formation. In: Michelson A ed. *Platelets*. 2nd ed. San Diego, CA: Academic Press; 2007:319–346.

62. Offermanns S. Activation of platelet function through G protein-coupled receptors. *Circ Res*. 2006;99:1293–1304.

63. Kahner BN, Shankar H, Murugappan S, Prasad GL, Kunapuli SP. Nucleotide receptor signaling in platelets. *J Thromb Haemost*. 2006;4:2317–2326.

64. Pula G, Schuh, K, Nakayama K, Nakayama KI, Walter U, Poole A. PKCδ regulates collagen-induced platelet aggregation through inhibition of VASP-mediated filopodia formation. *Blood*. 2006;108:4035–4044.

65. Thornber K, McCarty OJ, Watson SP, Pears CJ. Distinct but critical roles for integrin αIIbβ3 in platelet lamellipodia formation on fibrinogen, collagen-related peptide and thrombin. *FEBS Letts*. 2006;273:5032–5043.

66. McCarty OJT, Calaminus SDJ, Berndt MC, Machesky LM, Watson SP. Von Willebrand factor mediates platelet spreading through glycoprotein Ib and αIIbβ3 in the presence of botrocetin and ristocetin, respectively. *J Thromb Haemost*. 2006;4:1367–1378.

67. Goto S, Tamura N, Arai M, Kodama R, Takayama H. Involvement of glycoprotein VI in platelet thrombus formation on both collagen and von Willebrand factor surfaces under flow conditions. *Circulation*. 2002;106:266–272.

68. Reininger AJ, Heijnen HF, Schumann H, Specht HM, Schramm W, Ruggeri ZM. Mechanism of platelet adhesion to von Willebrand factor and microparticle formation under high shear stress. *Blood*. 2006;107:3537–3545.

69. Nesbitt WS, Giuliano S, Kulkarni S, Dopheide SM, Harper IS, Jackson SP. Intracellular calcium communication regulates platelet aggregation and thrombus growth. *J Cell Biol*. 2003;160:1151–1161.

70. García A, Prabhakar S, Brock CJ, et al. Extensive analysis of the human platelet proteome by two-dimensional gel electrophoresis and mass spectrometry. *Proteomics*. 2004;4:656–668.

71. Coppinger JA, O'Connor R, Wynne K, Flanagan M, Sullivan M, Maguire PB. Moderation of the platelet release response by aspirin. *Blood*. 2007;109:4786–4792.

72. Maguire PB, Wynne KJ, Harney DF, O'Donoghue NM, Stephen, SG, Fitzgerald DJ. Identification of the phosphotyrosine proteome from thrombin activated platelets. *Proteomics*. 2002;2:642–648.

73. Gnatenko DV, Dunn JJ, McCorkle SR, Weissmann D, Perrotta PL, Bahou WF. Transcript profiling of human platelets using microarray and serial analysis of gene expression. *Blood*. 2003;101:2285–2293.

74. Bugert P, Dugrillon A, Günaydin A, Eichler H, Klüter H. Messenger RNA profiling of human platelets by microarray hybridization. *Thromb Haemost*. 2003;90:738–748.

75. Sun L, Gorospe JR, Hoffman EP, Rao AK. Decreased platelet expression of myosin regulatory light chain polypeptide (MYL9) and other genes with platelet dysfunction and CBFA2/RUNX1 mutation: insights from platelet expression profiling. *J Thromb Haemost*. 2007;5:146–154.

76. Jones CI, Garner SF, Angenent W, et al. Mapping the platelet profile for functional genomic studies and demonstration of the effect size of the GP6 locus. *J Thromb Haemost*. 2007;5:1756–1765.

77. Nelson EJ, Nair SC, Peretz H, et al. Diversity of Glanzmann thrombasthenia in Southern India: 10 novel mutations identified among 15 unrelated patients. *J Thromb Haemost*. 2006;4:1730–1737.

78. Castro V, Kroll H, Origa AF, et al. A prospective study on the prevalence and risk factors for neonatal thrombocytopenia among 9332 unselected Brazilian newborns. *Transfusion*. 2007;47:59–66.

79. Freson K, Devriendt K, Matthijs G, et al. Platelet characteristics in patients with X-linked macrothrombocytopenia because of a novel GATA1 mutation. *Blood*. 2001;98:85–92.

16 Laboratory evaluation of heparin-induced thrombocytopenia

Theodore (Ted) E. Warkentin & Jane C. Moore

Departments of Pathology and Molecular Medicine, and Medicine
Michael G. DeGroote School of Medicine, McMaster University;
Hamilton Regional Laboratory Medicine Program
Hamilton, ON, Canada

Immune heparin-induced thrombocytopenia (HIT) is a "clinical-pathologic" syndrome, that is, the diagnosis is based upon the patient having clinical features consistent with HIT ("clinical") as well as the presence of pathogenic platelet-activating anti-platelet factor 4 (PF4)/heparin antibodies ("pathologic") [1, 2]. This concept underscores the importance of laboratory testing in supporting a diagnosis of HIT.

Assays for HIT antibodies can be broadly classified into: (a) platelet activation (or functional) assays; and (b) PF4-dependent antigen assays (immunoassays) [3, 4]. However, a key problem is that only a small minority of heparin-exposed patients who form anti-PF4/heparin antibodies detectable by immunoassay develop HIT. Thus, there is the potential for considerable HIT "overdiagnosis" [5].

In this chapter, we first provide an overview of the HIT syndrome, including key concepts relating to laboratory testing. We then discuss platelet activation assays, emphasizing washed platelet assays. We also review immunoassays, both enzyme-immunoassays (EIAs) as well as rapid particle-based immunoassays. We conclude by discussing the approach of the McMaster Platelet Immunology Laboratory to investigating HIT.

HIT syndrome

HIT can be defined as any clinical event (or events) best explained by the presence of platelet-activating anti-PF4/heparin antibodies ("HIT antibodies"); almost always, there is a history of concurrent or recent exposure to heparin [6]. Thrombocytopenia is the most common event, and is observed in at least 90–95% of patients, depending on how thrombocytopenia is defined. Table 16.1 summarizes the clinical and laboratory features of HIT. A key concept is that even when HIT is strongly suspected, if antibodies are not detectable, the patient does *not* have HIT. This statement particularly applies if negative results are obtained using two complementary—and both highly sensitive—assays, notably a washed platelet activation assay and an IgG-specific PF4-dependent EIA.

Central paradigm of HIT [5]

HIT is caused by antibodies of IgG class that produce strong activation of platelets via the platelet Fcγ IIa (IgG) receptors (FcγRIIa) [7]; these antibodies recognize large, multimolecular complexes of PF4 bound to heparin [8–11] and are already detectable in patient serum/plasma at the beginning of the HIT-associated platelet count decline [12]. There is usually (but not invariably) a proximate immunizing exposure to unfractionated heparin (UFH) or (less commonly) low-molecular-weight heparin (LMWH) or fondaparinux.

Quality in Laboratory Hemostasis and Thrombosis, Second Edition. Edited by Steve Kitchen, John D. Olson and F. Eric Preston.
© 2013 John Wiley & Sons, Ltd. Published 2013 by Blackwell Publishing Ltd.

Table 16.1 HIT as a clinical–pathological syndrome

Clinical	Pathological
At least one of: • **Thrombocytopenia**[a] • **Thrombosis** (e.g., *venous*: deep-vein thrombosis, pulmonary embolism, venous limb gangrene, adrenal hemorrhage,[c] cerebral vein thrombosis, splanchnic vein thrombosis; *arterial*: limb artery thrombosis, stroke, myocardial infarction, mesenteric artery thrombosis, miscellaneous artery; *microvascular*) • Necrotizing skin lesions at heparin injection sites[d] • Acute anaphylactoid reactions[e] • Disseminated intravascular coagulation (DIC)[f] Timing: above event(s) bear(s) temporal relation to a preceding immunizing heparin exposure[h] Absence of another more compelling explanation	Heparin-dependent, platelet-activating IgG[b] • Positive platelet activation assay (e.g., serotonin-release assay) • Positive anti-PF4/polyanion-IgG EIA (infers possible presence of platelet-activating IgG[g]

[a]>50% platelet count fall is seen in ~90% of patients; in 5–10%, the platelet fall is 30–50%.

[b]Heparin-dependent refers to inhibition of platelet activation or binding to PF4/heparin complexes in the presence of very high heparin concentrations. Acute serum or plasma should be used for testing, as HIT antibodies are transient.

[c]Adrenal hemorrhagic necrosis is a consequence of adrenal vein thrombosis.

[d] Non-necrotizing lesions (erythematous plaques) are less specific for HIT.

[e]Usually occur 5–30 minutes after intravenous heparin bolus; rarely, after subcutaneous heparin.

[f]10–15% of patients with HIT have overt (decompensated) DIC.

[g]In the appropriate context, a strong-positive EIA (either IgG-specific or polyspecific assay that detects IgG/A/M antibodies) can be used to infer presence of platelet-activating antibodies.

[h]Typical-onset (or delayed-onset) HIT begins 5–10 days after immunizing heparin exposure (usually, heparin given intra- or perioperatively); rapid-onset HIT can occur if heparin is given to a patient who already has circulating HIT antibodies, usually due to heparin given in the last 5–100 days.

Source: Modified from Warkentin [2], with permission from Elsevier.

Key concepts in HIT

Several concepts directly relate to issues of laboratory testing and the interpretation of test results.

Stoichiometric PF4: heparin ratios and high heparin inhibition

PF4 and heparin form immunogenic, multimolecular complexes only when both are present at stoichiometrically optimal concentrations (PF4: heparin molar ratio, approximately 1:1 to 2:1). Very high concentrations of heparin (10–100 U/mL) disrupt the complexes. This property is exploited in laboratory diagnostic testing: addition of high heparin inhibits platelet activation [13] and PF4-dependent immunoassays [10].

Iceberg model

The "iceberg model" of HIT illustrates that only a minority of anti-PF4/heparin antibodies identified by EIA are also detectable in a platelet activation assay (Figure 16.1) [14]. In this model, the portion of the iceberg that protrudes above the waterline corresponds to clinically evident HIT. The model infers that platelet activation assays and PF4-dependent EIAs both have high sensitivity for HIT diagnosis. However, the model also indicates that diagnostic specificity is much greater for platelet activation assays than for EIAs, particularly the "polyspecific" EIA that detects antibodies of any of the major immunoglobulin classes (IgG, IgA, IgM). This is because only a subset of IgG-class antibodies with platelet-activating properties has the potential to cause HIT. Figure 16.1 also shows that the greater the strength of the EIA test

175

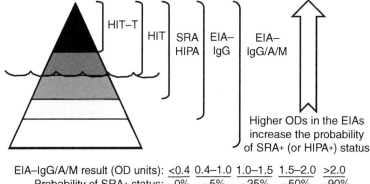

EIA–IgG/A/M result (OD units): <u>≤0.4</u> 0.4–1.0 1.0–1.5 1.5–2.0 >2.0
Probability of SRA+ status: ~0% ~5% ~25% ~50% ~90%

Figure 16.1 "Iceberg model" of HIT. Clinical HIT, comprising HIT with (HIT-T) or without thrombosis, is represented by the portion of the iceberg above the waterline; the portion below the waterline represents subclinical anti-PF4/heparin seroconversion. Three types of assays are highly sensitive for the diagnosis of HIT: the washed platelet activation assays (SRA and HIPA), the IgG-specific PF4-dependent EIAs (EIA-IgG), and the polyspecific EIAs that detects anti-PF4/heparin antibodies of the three major immunoglobulin classes (EIA-IgG/A/M). In contrast, diagnostic specificity varies greatly among these assays, being the highest for the platelet activation assays (SRA and HIPA) and lowest for the EIA-IgG/A/M. This is because the EIA-IgG/A/M is most likely to detect clinically irrelevant, non-platelet-activating anti-PF4/heparin antibodies. The approximate probability of SRA + status in relation to a given EIA result, expressed in OD units, was obtained from the literature [15]. EIA, enzyme-immunoassay; HIPA, heparin-induced platelet activation test; OD, optical density; SRA, serotonin-release assay. Reprinted from [14].

result—expressed in optical density (OD) units—the greater the likelihood that platelet-activating antibodies are present (*vide infra*) [15].

Timeline of HIT immune response

HIT antibodies are readily detectable in patient serum or plasma at the onset of the HIT-associated platelet count decline (Figure 16.2a) [12]. Moreover, when antibodies of two or three different immunoglobulin classes (IgG, IgA, IgM) are formed, they develop simultaneously, that is, there is no IgM precedence (Figure 16.2b) [12, 16]. This timeline infers that a negative test result should not be automatically repeated using a later blood sample, unless some change in the clinical situation occurs suggesting that a diagnosis of HIT should be newly considered [12, 14].

Serum versus plasma

In our laboratory, serum aliquots are heated at 56°C for 30 minutes, then centrifuged (10 minutes at 12,000 *g*) to remove fibrin(ogen) gel, before testing in the SRA [13]. The rationale using heat-inactivated serum is to reduce the risk of false-positive reactions due to thrombin. Although complement proteins are destroyed by heat inactivation, they are not required for IgG-dependent platelet activation in HIT. Plasma (treated as described above) can also be used for the SRA; however, substantially more fibrin(ogen) gel is formed during the heat-inactivation process.

For the EIA, either serum or plasma anticoagulated in sodium citrate or EDTA can be used [17]; however, plasma collected into sodium heparin will yield false-negative results due to high heparin inhibition effect, unless the heparin is first removed using a heparin-binding resin such as Ecteola cellulose (Sigma Aldrich, St Louis, MO) [18].

Positive control reagents

The most common positive HIT control reagents are stored sera (or plasmas) from patients with well-documented HIT. In our experience, such HIT sera obtained during clinical trials performed during the late 1980's and stored at −70°C continue to react well when used in the SRA or EIA more than two decades later [12, 19].

Most commercial assays also use (lyophilized) human serum or plasma controls. In the EIAs, the controls are also used to determine the stop time

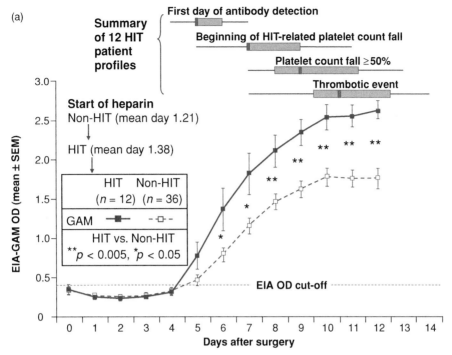

Figure 16.2 Characteristic timeline of HIT: anti-PF4/heparin antibodies (by EIA) per postoperative day in 12 patients with HIT and 36 seropositive non-HIT control patients. (a) Mean ($\pm$ SEM) optical density (OD) of anti-PF4/heparin antibodies detected using a commercial immunoassay (EIA–GAM) from Gen-Probe GTI Diagnostics Inc. that detects antibodies of all three immunoglobulin classes (IgG, IgA, IgM). HIT patients are indicated by solid squares, and seropositive non-HIT controls by open squares. On each day beginning on postoperative day 6, there is a significant difference in the mean of the OD levels between the patients with HIT and the seropositive non-HIT controls ($p < 0.05$ by non-paired t test). At the top of the figure, summary data for 12 HIT patient profiles are shown for four key events (first day of antibody detection, beginning of HIT-related platelet count fall, platelet count fall $\geq 50\%$, and thrombotic event), summarized as median (small squares within rectangles), IQR (rectangles), and range (ends of thin lines).

of the assay. Once the positive control reaches a designated level of reactivity, the assay is complete. For example, for the two EIAs provided by Gen-Probe GTI Diagnostics (Waukesha, WI), the reactivity is complete when the positive serum control reads $OD_{405} \geq 1.80$ U, and the negative serum control remains $OD_{405} \leq 0.30$ U [20, 21]. Corresponding cutoffs for the various Zymutest EIAs (Aniara, Mason, OH; manufactured by Hyphen-BioMed, Neuville-sur-Oise, France) are $OD_{450} \geq 1.0$ U (positive control) and ≤ 0.25 U (negative control), respectively [22, 23]. For the Asserachrom® EIAs manufactured by Diagnostica Stago (Asnières-sur-Seine, France), positive reagents (one strong, one weaker) are used to determine the cutoff in the particular assay run [24, 25].

Whereas the Gen-Probe GTI assays use human serum controls and the Stago assays lyophilized human plasma, the Zymutest assays employ an artificial positive control made by covalently linking polyclonal (rabbit) anti-PF4 affinity purified antibody with human IgG.

For the particle gel immunoassay (PaGIA), positive and negative serum controls are used that must react as expected in order to validate the assay [26]. Some investigators recommend using titrated commercial controls and (internal) HIT sera controls to identify faulty polymer lots [27].

Laboratories that perform the functional (platelet activation) assays usually employ well-characterized HIT sera. For assays such as the heparin-induced

177

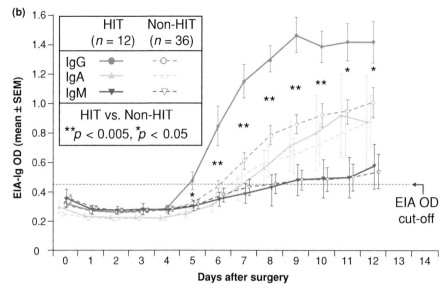

Figure 16.2 (b) Mean (± SEM) OD values of anti-PF4/heparin antibodies detected using an in-house immunoassay (EIA-Ig) that detects antibodies of the individual immunoglobulin classes, IgG (circles), IgA (triangles), and IgM (inverted triangles) for HIT (solid symbols) and non-HIT (open symbols). On each postoperative day beginning on day 5, there is a significant difference in the mean of the OD units for the IgG immunoassay between the patients with HIT and the seropositive non-HIT controls (**$p < 0.005$ for days 6–10; *$p < 0.05$ for days 5, 11, and 12). In addition, among the 34 non-HIT controls who tested positive for IgG antibodies, mean (± SEM) maximum OD values for the EIA-IgG were significantly greater in the eight patients who tested positive in the serotonin-release assay (SRA) compared with the 26 patients who tested negative in the SRA (1.30 ± 0.15 vs. 0.96 ± 0.07 units; $p = 0.025$). Among the 20 patients who tested positive in the SRA, mean (± SEM) maximum OD values for the EIA-IgG showed a trend to higher levels in the 12 patients with clinical HIT, compared with the eight seropositive non-HIT controls (1.63 ± 0.09 vs. 1.30 ± 0.15 units; $p = 0.059$). EIA, enzyme-immunoassay; HIT, heparin-induced thrombocytopenia. Reprinted, with permission [12].

platelet activation (HIPA) test (*vide infra*), it is recommended that the positive HIT control serum (diluted if necessary with normal serum) yield a positive result with a lag time of approximately 25 minutes (with buffer used as a negative control) [28]. This approach is chosen because the operator assesses platelet reactivities visually at 5 minute intervals, and the stop time is dependent on the optimal reactivity of the positive control.

In contrast, for the SRA, the reaction is allowed to proceed over a preset period of time (usually 1 hour). Here, the reactivities of a panel of positive sera (of graded reactivities), heat-aggregated IgG, and a negative serum are used for quality control (see "Approach of the McMaster Laboratory Immunology Laboratory").

A HIT-mimicking monoclonal antibody—known as KKO—has been developed [29]. In theory, this could be used as a positive control, but a disadvantage in functional assays is that human platelets differ in their responsiveness to murine monoclonal antibodies in a way that does not correlate well with reactivity to HIT antibodies [30].

The *External Quality Control of Diagnostic Assays* and *Tests Foundation* (ECAT) markets HIT controls but currently does not have controls for platelet activation assays. The *North American Specialized Coagulation Laboratory Association* (NASCOLA) runs proficiency testing programs and makes available samples of known HIT reactivity for laboratory validation.

Evaluation of pretest probability

Clinical scoring systems have been developed to help the clinician estimate the pretest probability of HIT

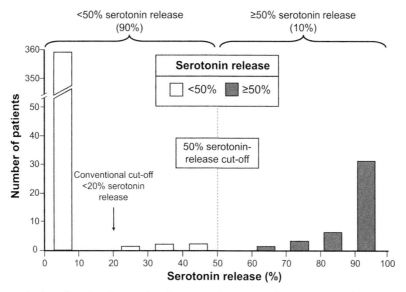

Figure 16.3 Dichotomization of results of serotonin-release assay (SRA) testing for HIT antibodies (n = 405 patients tested). The data are shown as deciles of mean percent serotonin-release (at 0.1 and 0.3 IU/mL) unfractionated heparin. The conventional cut-off defining a positive SRA test result is 20%; however, the author generally uses 50% as the cut-off (assuming all controls react as expected, including weak-positive control serum), as this better discriminates between HIT and non-HIT thrombocytopenia. Only ~10% of patients investigated for HIT achieved a positive test result at this cut-off. Overall, >97% of patients in this dataset tested either clearly negative (<20% serotonin-release) or strongly positive (≥80% serotonin-release). Reprinted from [15] with permission from John Wiley & Sons, Ltd.

[31, 32]. Since low scores are associated with low likelihood of HIT antibodies being present, it is reasonable to avoid testing in low pretest probability situations (to minimize risk of overdiagnosis). On the other hand, some patients who have never previously been exposed to heparin (and thus would have a low score) nevertheless test strongly positive for HIT antibodies, a syndrome known as "spontaneous HIT" [33]. It is believed that such patients may have been immunized by preceding bacterial infection (since bacteria bind PF4 in such a way to form the HIT antigens [34], and a chronic bacterial infection—periodontitis—has been linked with natural anti-PF4/heparin antibodies [35]) or other proinflammatory events such as surgery [36]. Thus, clinical judgment is required for deciding which individual patient should undergo testing for HIT.

Platelet activation assays

Platelet-activating properties of HIT antibodies correspond closely to the risk of developing thrombocytopenia; accordingly, platelet activation assays are the most useful for the laboratory diagnosis of HIT (Figure 16.1).

Platelet aggregation assays

The earliest platelet activation assays used aggregation of platelets (in citrate-anticoagulated platelet-rich plasma) [3, 4, 37]. However, suboptimal sensitivity [38] and specificity [39], and the inability to assess multiple test conditions (low throughput) have resulted in decreasing use of these assays.

Washed platelet activation assays: serotonin-release assay (SRA) and heparin-induced platelet activation (HIPA) test

Platelet activation assays that utilize "washed" platelets have superior operating characteristics for detecting HIT antibodies, that is, they have the highest sensitivity-specificity tradeoff [3, 4]. Figure 16.3

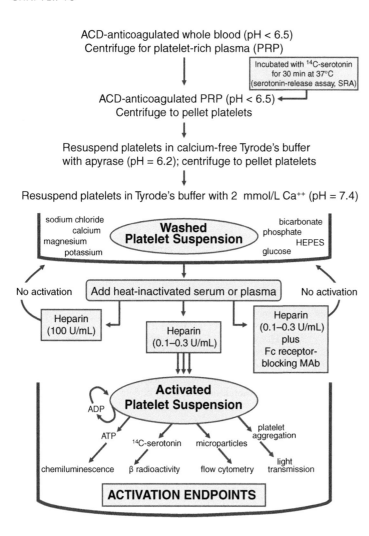

ACD-anticoagulated whole blood (pH < 6.5)
Centrifuge for platelet-rich plasma (PRP)

Incubated with ^{14}C-serotonin
for 30 min at 37°C
(serotonin-release assay, SRA)

ACD-anticoagulated PRP (pH < 6.5)
Centrifuge to pellet platelets

Resuspend platelets in calcium-free Tyrode's buffer
with apyrase (pH = 6.2); centrifuge to pellet platelets

Resuspend platelets in Tyrode's buffer with 2 mmol/L Ca^{++} (pH = 7.4)

sodium chloride
calcium
magnesium
potassium

**Washed
Platelet Suspension**

bicarbonate
phosphate
HEPES
glucose

No activation ← Add heat-inactivated serum or plasma → No activation

Heparin
(100 U/mL)

Heparin
(0.1–0.3 U/mL)

Heparin
(0.1–0.3 U/mL)
plus
Fc receptor-
blocking MAb

**Activated
Platelet Suspension**

ADP

ATP
^{14}C-serotonin   microparticles

platelet
aggregation

chemiluminescence   β radioactivity   flow cytometry   light
transmission

ACTIVATION ENDPOINTS

Figure 16.4 Schematic overview of washed platelet activation assays for HIT. HIT serum causes platelet activation at therapeutic (0.1–0.3 U/mL) heparin concentrations, but not in the presence of FcγRIIa-blocking monoclonal antibody or high (100 U/mL) heparin concentrations. Platelet activation by HIT serum is potentiated by ADP release from platelet dense granules. Various platelet activation endpoints can be used. False-positive results can be avoided if typical reaction profiles of non-HIT platelet activation triggers are recognized, for example, (1) residual thrombin (activation that progressively decreases from 0 to 0.1 to 0.3 to 100 U/mL heparin, and without inhibition in the presence of FcγRIIa-blocking monoclonal antibody); (2) immune complexes (activation at no, low, and high heparin concentrations, with inhibition by FcγRIIa-blocking monoclonal antibody); and (3) thrombotic thrombocytopenic purpura serum (variable activation in the presence of heparin that is not inhibited by FcγRIIa-blocking monoclonal antibody). ACD, acid-citrate-dextrose; ADP, adenosine diphosphate; ATP, adenosine triphosphate; PRP, platelet-rich plasma. Reprinted from [4].

shows the "dichotomizing" nature of the SRA; in general, samples test either negative or strongly positive, with relatively few samples yielding weak or moderate serotonin release [15].

Platelets are washed in apyrase-containing buffer (to maintain sensitivity to adenosine diphosphate (ADP)—an important potentiator of HIT antibody-induced platelet activation [40])—and are resuspended in divalent cation-containing buffer (Figure 16.4) [3, 4]. The McMaster Platelet Immunology Laboratory measures release of [^{14}C]-serotonin to quantitate platelet activation [4, 13, 41], although other platelet activation endpoints can be used. Indeed, in central Europe, the HIPA test—which assesses platelet aggregation visually in microtiter wells with rotating

steel balls used to agitate the platelets—is commonly used [28, 42]. Platelet activation can also be quantitated using flow cytometric endpoints, for example, platelet-derived microparticles [43].

It is important to use platelets obtained from blood donors ("pedigree" donors) whose platelets are pretested and known to react well to HIT antibodies [41]. Table 16.2 shows the results of an early experiment performed in our laboratory: platelet donors used in the SRA can be ranked hierarchically from the strongest to weakest. HIT sera can also be ranked hierarchically; in this way, "weak positive" HIT sera can be identified, which serve an important quality control function (see "Approach of the McMaster Platelet Immunology Laboratory").

Table 16.2 Hierarchically ordered reactions of ten HIT sera tested against ten normal platelet donors: 100 serum-platelet pairs[a]

HIT sera (S1–S10)	Normal platelet donors: strongest (P1) to weakest (P10)									
	P1 84%	P2 71%	P3 68%	P4 54%	P5 53%	P6 41%	P7 40%	P8 39%	P9 37%	P10 30%
S1 85%	+ + + +	+ + + +	+ + + +	+ + + +	+ + + +	+ + + +	+ + +	+ + + +	+ +	+ + +
S2 84%	+ + + +	+ + + +	+ + + +	+ + + +	+ + + +	+ + +	+ + +	| + + +	+ + +	+ + +
S3 69%	+ + + +	+ + + +	+ + + +	+ + +	+ + +	+ +	+ + +	+ +	+ +	+ +
S4 61%	+ + + +	+ + + +	+ + +	+ + +	+ + +	+ +	+ +	+ +	+ +	+
S5 56%	+ + + +	+ + +	+ + +	+ +	+ + +	+ +	+ +	+	+	+
S6 51%	+ + +	+ + +	+ + +	+ + +	+ +	+ +	+ +	+ +	+	+
S7 44%	+ + + +	+ + +	+ + +	+	+ +	+	+	+	+ +	–
S8 30%	+ + + +	+ +	+ + +	+	+	+	–	–	–	–
S9 24%	+ + +	+ +	+	+ +	+	–	–	–	–	–
S10 11%	+ +	+	+	–	–	–	–	–	–	–

[a]Ten HIT sera and ten platelet donors are ranked from strongest to weakest (S1–S10 and P1–P10, respectively), according to the mean percentage of [14C]serotonin release when considering all 100 serum-platelet donor pairs (10 pairs corresponding to each HIT serum and each normal platelet donor). For each serum-platelet donor pair, the individual amount of serotonin release is summarized as follows: 80–100% release, + + + +; 60–79% release, + + +; 40–59% release, + +; 20–39% release, +; <20% release, –. Overall, there is a graded pattern of reactivity among the individual reaction pairs that is hierarchical (i.e., there are no unexpected weak or strong reactions among the pairs). All negative reactions (<20% release) were found in the lower right portion of the table. Conversely, the strongest reactions (>80% release) were found in the upper left portion of the table. Modified from [4].

Although the use of pedigree blood donors is common in North America, in Europe random donor platelets (obtained through blood donation centers) are used to perform the HIPA test. To compensate for the issue of variable donor reactivity, the HIPA is usually performed using four random donors, with only two or three positive tests (depending on the laboratory) required for a positive test.

Sometimes test sera yield an "indeterminate" test result, that is, the results cannot be used to classify a serum as either positive or negative [44]. One common "indeterminate" reaction profile is when the serum induces platelet activation at all heparin concentrations, including at 100 U/mL heparin, but with inhibition by $Fc\gamma RIIa$-blocking monoclonal antibody. When this occurs, it is recommended that the assay be repeated using different platelet donors, and using a different heat-inactivated serum aliquot; approximately half the time, the subsequent test yields a clear negative or positive result [44]. However, if a patient serum yields a repeated indeterminate result, then the SRA cannot be used to determine whether the patient has platelet-activating HIT antibodies or not, and an immunoassay must be used.

In prospective studies, approximately 50% of heparin-treated patients who had a positive SRA developed a platelet count fall suggestive of HIT (Table 16.3) [45–49]. This implies that there are patient-dependent factors that influence risk of HIT, for example, platelet-associated PF4 levels [50].

Whole blood impedance aggregometry

A multiple electrode platelet aggregometer, known as Multiplate® (Dynabyte Medical, Munich, Germany), can be used to test patient serum or platelet-poor plasma (in citrate anticoagulant) against citrate-anticoagulated whole blood obtained from a normal platelet donor, thus avoiding platelet handling and preparation as required for other platelet activation assays. Two sets of electrodes (impedance sensors) detect platelet aggregation. Two studies [51, 52] reported the use of this technology for detecting HIT antibodies through heparin-dependent platelet aggregation; one study [51] noted the sensitivity to be lower than that of a washed platelet SRA, but similar to that of standard platelet aggregometry.

PF4-dependent enzyme-immunoassays

Three commercial EIAs are marketed in the United States; in addition, some research laboratories employ "in-house" EIAs (Table 16.4). We refer to these as

Table 16.3 SRA versus EIAs. Frequency of thrombocytopenia (>50% platelet count fall) among anti-PF4/heparin EIA + patients (polyspecific or IgG-specific assay) who received heparin (UFH or LMWH): a comparison of SRA + versus SRA– status

SRA status	Positive in polyspecific EIA (IgG/A/M)	Positive in IgG-specific EIA
A. Postorthopedic surgery patients[a]		
SRA +	12/24	12/24
SRA–	0/58	0/16
p	<0.0001	0.0009
B. Venous thromboembolism patients[b]		
SRA +	4/4	4/4
SRA–	0/15	0/6
p	0.0003	0.0048
C. Postcardiac surgery patients		
SRA +	4/11	NA
SRA–	0/152	NA
p	<0.0001	NA

EIA, enzyme-immunoassay; NA, not available; SRA +, positive in the serotonin-release assay; SRA–, negative in the serotonin-release assay.

[a]For the data shown, the cut-off for a positive SRA was 20% serotonin-release. For study A (postorthopedic surgery), if instead a 50% serotonin-release cut-off is used, the comparisons (polyspecific EIA) yield similar results: 11/20 vs. 1/62 (p < 0.0001), and unchanged data for study B (venous thromboembolism patients).

[b]For the venous thromboembolism study, all positive EIA results shown were ≥1.0 units of optical density (OD).

Source: [45–49]

"PF4-dependent" EIAs, since PF4 is always used, whereas the PF4-binding polyanion can differ. Both IgG-specific and polyspecific (i.e., detecting IgG, IgA, and/or IgM) assays are marketed; in general, IgG-specific assays have much greater diagnostic specificity without significant loss of diagnostic sensitivity [19, 46, 53–55].

The major problem with PF4-dependent EIAs is their relatively low diagnostic specificity for HIT, compared with washed platelet activation assays: EIAs are much more likely to detect clinically insignificant antibodies (Table 16.3). However, their sensitivity for detecting clinically relevant HIT antibodies approaches 100% [15, 56].

Some investigators—and one manufacturer (Gen-Probe GTI Diagnostics) recommend performing a high heparin maneuver to increase diagnostic specificity [20, 21, 57, 58]. In this "confirmatory procedure," the EIA is repeated with 100 U/mL heparin. High heparin concentrations disrupt the antigenic PF4/heparin complexes, and thus reactivity is usually inhibited by >50%. However, this maneuver only increases diagnostic specificity to a minor degree, since both pathogenic and non-pathogenic anti-PF4/heparin antibodies are usually inhibited by high heparin. Also, in practice, relatively few positive samples are not inhibited by high heparin. Of concern, occasionally a true-positive HIT serum/plasma will fail to be inhibited by the high heparin procedure (perhaps because of very high antibody titers), thus risking sample misclassification [59, 60]. For this reason, some workers recommend using the high heparin procedure only when the OD is only weakly positive (<1.0 OD units) [61]: In this situation, the failure of high heparin

Table 16.4 PF4-dependent EIAs

Manufacturer	PF4 (source)	Polyanion	Assay	Ab classes
Diagnostica Stago	Recombinant	Heparin	Asserachrom HPIA	IgG/A/M
Gen-Probe GTI Diagnostics[a]	Platelets (outdated)	Polyvinyl sulfonate (PVS)	PF4 Enhanced PF4 IgG	IgG/A/M IgG
HYPHEN Biomed	Platelet lysate	Heparin bound to protamine	Zymutest HIA	IgG/A/M IgG, IgA, IgM
McMaster Platelet Immunology Laboratory	Platelets (outdated)	Heparin	'In-house'	IgG, IgA, IgM

[a]Gen-Probe GTI Diagnostics was acquired by Hologic in 2012, and is now renamed as 'Hologic Gen-Probe'.

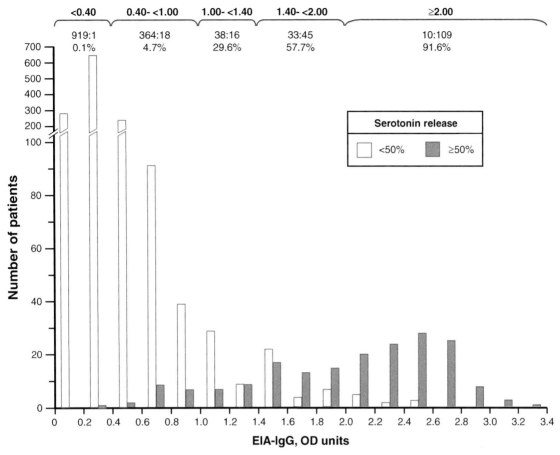

Figure 16.5 Predictivity of the EIA–IgG for a positive SRA. For each of five groups of quantitative EIA–IgG data (<0.40, 0.40 to <1.00, 1.00 to <1.40, 1.40 to <2.00, and ≥2.00 OD U), the percent of samples yielding a positive SRA result (≥50% serotonin-release) is shown. The probability of a positive SRA result varied considerably, in relation to the magnitude of the EIA result, expressed in OD units. For the EIA–IgG ("in-house" assay of the McMaster Platelet Immunology Laboratory), the probability of a positive SRA result did not reach ≥50% until the OD value was approximately 1.20–1.40 U or greater. Reprinted from [15] with permission from John Wiley & Sons, Ltd.

to inhibit binding indicates that platelet-activating antibodies are unlikely to be present, without the risk of sample misclassification that can result when the high heparin step is used for samples yielding higher reactivity in the EIA.

The probability that a positive EIA indicates the presence of (pathologic) platelet-activating antibodies is directly related to the strength of the EIA result, expressed in OD units (Figure 16.5) [15]. In one study, for every 1.0 U increase in OD, the probability of a positive SRA increased by 40 (odds ratio), or, expressed another way, from ∼5% to ∼25% to ∼95%

for OD values of 0.5, 1.5, and 2.5, respectively (cutoff defining a negative result, 0.40 OD units) [15]. This strong relationship between OD values and a positive platelet activation assay can be seen with different EIAs and different washed platelet activation assays [62]. Although IgG-specific assays have greater diagnostic specificity than do polyspecific EIAs, a strong positive polyspecific EIA is far more predictive of HIT than is a weakly positive IgG-specific assay [54]. Higher OD levels have also been shown to correlate with greater risk of HIT on clinical grounds [57], and with increased frequency of thrombosis [63–65].

Particle Gel Immunoassay
(DiaMed ID-PaGIA Heparin/PF4 antibody test)

- Test serum containing positive or negative HIT IgG
  is mixed with red polystyrene beads (shown as
  small blue circles in the figure) coated with PF4-heparin

- The test mixture is then added to the particle gel
  immunoassay tube containing anti-human IgG

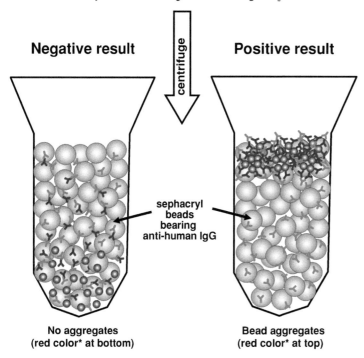

Negative result

centrifuge

Positive result

sephacryl
beads
bearing
anti-human IgG

**No aggregates
(red color* at bottom)**

**Bead aggregates
(red color* at top)**

*Represented by small blue circles.

Figure 16.6 Schematic drawing showing
the particle gel immunoassay assay
(PaGIA) using gel centrifugation
technology. Note the use of a secondary
anti-antibody to facilitate particle
agglutination. Reprinted from [3] with
permission from Elsevier.

PF4-dependent particle-based immunoassays (rapid assays)

Particle gel immunoassay

The particle gel immunoassay (PaGIA) utilizes a gel centrifugation technology system that is commonly available in blood banks. The manufacturer (DiaMed, a subsidiary of Bio-Rad Laboratories) has manufactured red, high-density polystyrene beads to which PF4/heparin complexes have been bound; after patient serum or plasma is added, anti-PF4/heparin antibodies (if present) bind to the antigen-coated beads [66, 67].

However, since IgG-class antibodies do not agglutinate polystyrene beads well, a secondary anti-human immunoglobulin antibody has been added into the sephacryl gel. The rationale behind this (and other gel centrifugation assays) is that upon centrifugation, agglutinated beads (indicating the presence of anti-PF4/heparin antibodies) do not migrate through the sephacryl gel, whereas non-agglutinated beads (indicating the absence of antibodies) will pass through the gel, thus forming a red band at the bottom (Figure 16.6). The PaGIA has been used for several years in Europe, Asia, and Canada (but is not available in the United States).

The assay will occasionally "miss" a true positive HIT result, and thus its sensitivity (~95%) is not as high as that of the EIA (~99%) [54, 55]. In some cases, faulty lots may have accounted for suboptimal sensitivity [27]. The diagnostic specificity of the PaGIA appears to be intermediate between that of the (washed) platelet activation assay and EIA [54, 55, 67].

Several investigators have combined the PaGIA with a pretest probability score [68, 69]; here, a low score plus a negative PaGIA rules out HIT. Other investigators have pointed out that performing the test at higher dilutions of patient serum improves its diagnostic utility. Here, a titer of 1:4 or higher is much more indicative of HIT than a positive using neat or 1:2 diluted serum/plasma [70]. These investigators also found that a titer of 32 or greater essentially indicated 100% probability for the presence of platelet-activating antibodies [71]. This mirrors the observations in PF4-dependent EIAs, where very strong positive results (OD >2.0) have at least 90% predictivity for the presence of platelet-activating antibodies.

Particle immunofiltration assay

An assay from Akers Biosciences (Thorofare, NJ), known as the PIFA® Heparin/PF4 Rapid Assay, is currently marketed in the United States. It utilizes a "Particle ImmunoFiltration Assay" (PIFA) system, wherein patient serum is added to a reaction well containing dyed particles coated with PF4 (not PF4/heparin); the lack of requirement for heparin presumably reflects formation of HIT antigens through close approximation of PF4 tetramers achieved under the conditions of PF4 binding to the particles. Subsequently, non-agglutinated—but not agglutinated particles—will migrate through the membrane filter. Thus, a negative test is shown by a blue color in the result well, whereas no color indicates a positive test. The assay, however, performed poorly in two reference laboratories [72], and no published studies attesting to its validity are available; therefore, its use is not recommended.

Instrumentation-based immunoassays

Two automated assays that utilize proprietary instruments, one based on agglutination of latex particles and the other on chemiluminescence, have recently

been developed by Instrumentation Laboratory (Bedford, MA) [73, 74]. The HemosIL HIT-Ab(PF4-H), which is performed using an ACL TOP® Family analyzer, is a latex particle enhanced immunoturbidimetric assay that detects anti-PF4/heparin antibodies of all immunoglobulin classes [73]. In this assay, a suspension of polystyrene latex particles coated with mouse monoclonal anti-PF4/heparin reacts with a solution containing PF4/polyvinyl sulfonate (PVS) (the reaction buffer also contains a blocking agent against human anti-mouse antibodies to minimize this interference on the assay results). To this is added patient sample (citrated plasma); if patient anti-PF4/heparin antibodies are not present, the HIT-mimicking monoclonal antibody coated onto the latex particles will bind with the PF4/PVS reagent, and agglutination will occur. However, if the patient plasma contains anti-PF4/heparin antibodies, then agglutination will be inhibited. In this competitive agglutination system, the degree of agglutination is inversely proportional to the level of antibodies in the patient sample, as assessed by decrease in light transmittance. (The assay is calibrated using a buffer containing monoclonal anti-PF4/heparin.) Thus, a positive sample will result in a *lower* OD than negative control samples. The software automatically reports the results in U/mL as the inverse proportion. If a strong positive result causes the OD to measure outside the test range (0–5.7 U/mL), the instrument automatically reruns the test after making an on-board dilution and correcting the final result for the dilution factor; thus, the effective measuring range is up to 16 U/mL. A positive test is a result ≥1.0 U/mL. The technology allows for on-demand single-patient testing, so that a result can be provided within 15 minutes of sample preparation.

In a study of 414 patient samples that compared the HemosIL HIT-Ab (PF4-H) with the Stago EIA, overall agreement was seen in 88% of samples (co-negativity, 95%; co-positivity 60%) [73]. However, patient information was not available, and no platelet activation assay was used, so implications of discrepant results could not be ascertained.

The HemosIL HIT-Ab(PF4-H) assay is not currently available in the United States, China, or Japan, but is available elsewhere.

The chemiluminescence assays (HemosIL AcuStar HIT-IgG (PF4-H), HemosIL AcuStar HIT-Ab (PF4-H)) which are performed using an ACL AcuStar® system instrument, are also based on binding of anti-PF4/

heparin antibodies to PF4/PVS [74]. Here, magnetic particles coated with PF4/PVS capture anti-PF4/heparin antibodies present within a patient sample. After incubation, magnetic separation, and a wash step, a tracer consisting of an isoluminol-labeled anti-human IgG antibody (or a mixture of three isoluminol-labeled monoclonal antibodies (anti-IgG, -IgA, and -IgM)) is added, which binds to the captured anti-PF4/H antibodies on the particles. After a second incubation, magnetic separation, and a wash step, reagents that trigger the luminescent reaction are added, and the emitted light is measured as relative light units (RLUs) by the instrument's optical system. The RLUs are directly proportional to the concentration of anti-PF4/heparin antibodies in the sample. This assay can be performed with serum or plasma and can distinguish between different immunoglobulin classes. It shows a wide range of reactivity, and thus stronger results may indicate a higher likelihood of HIT [74].

In a study of 102 patients with suspected HIT (including 17 patients with a diagnosis of HIT confirmed by intermediate or high 4Ts score, positive PaGIA, and positive platelet aggregation assay), both the IgG-specific and the polyspecific assays detected all 17 patients (i.e., no false negatives) [74]. As expected, diagnostic specificity was greater for the HemosIL AcuStar HIT-IgG $_{(PF4-H)}$ assay compared with the polyspecific test (96% vs. 81%).

The HemosIL AcuStar HIT panel assays are available in all countries except the United States, Canada, China, and Japan.

Fluid-phase immunoassays

All of the PF4-dependent EIAs and particle-based immunoassays described above involve the binding of HIT antibodies to PF4/(polyanion) bound to a solid phase. However, surface-adsorbed proteins can undergo denaturation, potentially compromising test sensitivity and specificity [75]. Two fluid-phase immunoassays have been developed to overcome these problems.

Sepharose G fluid-phase EIA

Newman, Swanson, and Chong [76] developed a fluid-phase EIA in which anti-PF4/heparin IgG antibodies bind to PF4/heparin antigens (PF4, 5% biotinylated)

in the fluid phase, with subsequent capture of the antigen–antibody complexes by protein G sepharose. After washing, the amount of biotin-PF4/heparin–antibody complexes immobilized to the beads is measured using peroxidase substrate after initial incubation with streptavidin-conjugated peroxidase.

This assay improves test specificity for at least two reasons. First, the fluid-phase EIA minimizes nonspecific binding of antibody as can occur with cryptic antigens formed on PF4 when it binds to a solid phase. Second, Sepharose G only binds antibodies of IgG class, thus avoiding detection of (non-pathogenic) IgA and IgM.

In our laboratory, we have used this fluid-phase EIA primarily in performing studies of cross-reactivity of HIT antibodies against LMWH and heparinoids, such as danaparoid sodium [77]. The reason is that cross-reactivity, especially with danaparoid, is usually weak, and we wanted to be certain that any cross-reactivity detected against PF4/danaparoid represented "true" cross-reactivity rather than spurious reactivity related to binding against denatured antigens.

Gold nanoparticle-based fluid-phase EIA (lateral-flow immunoassay)

A rapid nanoparticle-based fluid-phase EIA is marketed in Europe by Milenia Biotec (Giessen, Germany) [78]. In this "lateral-flow immunoassay" (LFI), capillary action causes the test sample to flow laterally along a solid phase (test strip). Flow commences after 5 μL of patient serum and two drops of reagent (ligand-labeled PF4/polyanion complexes) are added to the sample pad. During their migration through the test strip, the ligand-labeled PF4/polyanion complexes come into contact with (red-colored) gold nanoparticles, which are coated with anti-ligand. At the same time, anti-PF4/polyanion antibodies (if present) bind to the PF4/polyanion complexes. These complexes continue to migrate to the test line, where immobilized goat anti-human IgG captures the IgG/PF4/polyanion complexes to which the gold nanoparticles are also bound (through the ligand–anti-ligand interaction) [78]. A positive reaction is a bold-colored line. A control antibody (anti-ligand antibody) is included on each test strip and should result in a bold line at the end of the test strip, irrespective of test sample positivity or negativity; this ensures that proper reagent application and sample migration has occurred. The turnaround time for the LFI (after preparation of patient serum) is only 15 minutes; further, the single-assay design facilitates on-demand testing [79]. Results can be read visually or quantitatively with a reader.

In an evaluation of this assay by the Platelet Immunology Laboratory in Giessen, Germany, the investigators found that the HIT–LFI to have high sensitivity for detecting platelet-activating HIT antibodies, but with the additional advantage of fewer false-positive results compared with the PaGIA and two other commercial IgG-specific EIAs [78].

Approach of the McMaster platelet immunology laboratory

The McMaster Platelet Immunology Laboratory emphasizes the SRA for laboratory diagnosis of HIT. The "in-house" IgG anti-PF4/heparin EIA is used primarily for quality assurance [14]. However, if a patient sample yields an indeterminate pattern of reactivity by SRA in repeat assays performed using two platelet pools prepared from different pedigree donors, then the EIA assay is used to provide a result.

The SRA is a complicated assay and depends on technical expertise, use of a radioactive isotope (^{14}C), and both intra- and inter-assay validation. Each assay is set up using a mixture of platelets obtained from two well-characterized (pedigree) donors, free from all platelet-inhibiting medications for >72 hours. The donors are selected from a pool of 20 pre-screened donors known to react well in the HIT assay. The platelets are isolated, washed, and labeled with ^{14}C-serotonin and used within 4 hours of collection to ensure optimal reactivity. Each patient sample is tested in duplicate with pharmacologic (0.1 and 0.3 U/mL) and high (100 U/mL) concentrations of UFH, and a pharmacologic concentration (0.1 U/mL) of the LMWH, enoxaparin. In addition, platelets pre-incubated with the FcγRIIa-blocking monoclonal antibody (IV.3) are added to samples with 0.1 U/mL UFH. In the final reaction, heat-inactivated patient serum (20 μL) is diluted 1:4, as the other reaction constituents total 80 μL in volume [13].

Historically, the SRA result is considered positive if the test sample causes ≥20% serotonin release at pharmacologic UFH concentrations, and <20% serotonin release (inhibition) at 100 U/mL of UFH and in the presence of IV.3; a negative test is defined as <20% serotonin release at all heparin concentrations [13].

However, in our experience, "true" HIT is associated with much stronger serotonin release, usually >80% peak serotonin release ("strong" positive), but sometimes 50–79% serotonin release ("moderate" positive).

A total of eight serum controls are run in each assay—two negative and six positive controls obtained from clinical samples, as follows: two strong-positive sera; two weak/moderate-positive sera (20–79% serotonin-release), and two "standardized" controls (i.e., very strong HIT sera that have been diluted to 1/64 and 1/128 to assess variability in assay performance over time). The panel of controls affirms that the labeled platelets are reactive and that the dilutions of heparin are appropriate. An immune complex control (heat-aggregated human IgG) is added, with and without IV.3, to ensure that the platelets respond to an "IgG agonist" and also to validate the FcγRIIa inhibition step.

A 100% release (total) and blank control are included in each assay and these results are used to perform the calculations of percent release. The percent reactivity of the blank is typically only 2–6% of the total, and is an important indication that the platelets are not releasing serotonin spontaneously.

Prospective platelet donors confirm that they have not recently taken any medication that may affect platelet function. Of primary concern is acetylsalicylic acid (ASA), including external ASA-containing rubs or ointments. The next most common impeding drug is ibuprofen (present in many over-the-counter cold and flu preparations). Also, allergy medication is important to ask about, since antihistamines can impact platelet function. Naturopathic medications are also ruled out.

As noted, the in-house IgG-specific anti-PF4/heparin EIA is used primarily for quality-control purposes, since serum (or plasma) yielding a positive SRA is also expected to test positive in the EIA; if not, the validity of the SRA result should be reassessed. The EIA is also used to resolve the anti-PF4/heparin antibody status of samples that consistently yield "indeterminate" results in the SRA. Here, although we consider an OD ≥0.45 as a positive result in the IgG anti-PF4/heparin EIA, we rate samples that yield an OD result of >1.0 U as indicating a possible diagnosis of HIT, and samples with OD >1.5 U as indicating a probable diagnosis of HIT (Figure 16.5).

In summary, laboratory quality control maneuvers used at the McMaster lab include [3]: (a) selection of suitable platelet donors (because of hierarchical variability in platelet donor reactivity to IgG agonists); (b) use of "weak" and "strong" positive control HIT serum (to be sure the platelets have acceptable reactivity); (c) demonstration that reactivity of immune complexes (as well as any putative positive HIT serum) can be inhibited by an FcγRIIa-blocking monoclonal antibody; (d) demonstrating that high heparin concentrations inhibit the reactivity of HIT serum; (e) corroborating the presence of anti-PF4/heparin antibodies by the IgG-specific PF4/heparin-EIA. Through all of these maneuvers, the combination of the SRA and EIA–IgG methods yields very high sensitivity for clinically relevant HIT antibodies, while maintaining high diagnostic specificity. Nevertheless, the clinical picture is important to take into account, because patients do not necessarily develop HIT even if platelet-activating antibodies are detectable.

References

1. Warkentin TE, Greinacher A, Gruel Y, Aster RH, Chong BH, On behalf of the Scientific and Standardization Committee of the International Society on Thrombosis and Haemostasis. Laboratory testing for heparin-induced thrombocytopenia: a conceptual framework and implications for diagnosis. *J Thromb Haemost.* 2011;9:2498–2500.
2. Warkentin TE. Agents for the treatment of heparin-induced thrombocytopenia. *Hematol/Oncol Clin N Am.* 2010;24:755–775.
3. Warkentin TE, Sheppard JA. Testing for heparin-induced thrombocytopenia antibodies. *Transfus Med Rev.* 2006;20:259–272.
4. Warkentin TE, Greinacher A. Laboratory testing for heparin-induced thrombocytopenia. In: Warkentin TE, Greinacher A, eds. *Heparin-Induced Thrombocytopenia.* 5th ed. Boca Raton, FL: CRC Press; 2013:272–314.
5. Warkentin TE. HIT paradigms and paradoxes. *J Thromb Haemost.* 2011;9(suppl 1):105–117.
6. Warkentin TE. Heparin-induced thrombocytopenia: pathogenesis and management. *Br J Haematol.* 2003;121:535–555.
7. Kelton JG, Sheridan D, Santos A, Steeves K, Smith C, Brown C. Heparin-induced thrombocytopenia: laboratory studies. *Blood.* 1988;72:925–930.
8. Amiral J, Bridey F, Dreyfus M, Vissac AM, Fressinaud E, Wolf M. Platelet factor 4 complexed to heparin is

the target for antibodies generated in heparin-induced thrombocytopenia. *Thromb Haemost.* 1992;68:95–96.
9. Kelton JG, Smith JW, Warkentin TE, Hayward CPM, Denomme GA, Horsewood P. Immunoglobulin G from patients with heparin-induced thrombocytopenia binds to a complex of heparin and platelet factor 4. *Blood.* 1994;83:3232–3239.
10. Greinacher A, Pötzsch B, Amiral J, Dummel V, Eichner A, Mueller-Eckhardt C. Heparin-associated thrombocytopenia: isolation of the antibody and characterization of a multimolecular PF4-heparin complex as the major antigen. *Thromb Haemost.* 1994;71:247–251.
11. Visentin GP, Ford SE, Scott JP, Aster RH. Antibodies from patients with heparin-induced thrombocytopenia/thrombosis are specific for platelet factor 4 complexed with heparin or bound to endothelial cells. *J Clin Invest.* 1994;93:81–88.
12. Warkentin TE, Sheppard JA, Moore JC, Cook RJ, Kelton JG. Studies of the immune response in heparin-induced thrombocytopenia. *Blood.* 2009;113:4963–4969.
13. Sheridan D, Carter C, Kelton JG. A diagnostic test for heparin-induced thrombocytopenia. *Blood.* 1986;67:27–30.
14. Warkentin TE. How I diagnose and manage HIT. *Hematology Am Soc Hematol Educ Program.* 2011;2011:143–149.
15. Warkentin TE, Sheppard JI, Moore JC, Sigouin CS, Kelton JG. Quantitative interpretation of optical density measurements using PF4-dependent enzyme-immunoassays. *J Thromb Haemost.* 2008;6:1304–1312.
16. Greinacher A, Kohlmann T, Strobel U, Sheppard JA, Warkentin TE. The temporal profile of the anti-PF4/heparin immune response. *Blood.* 2009;113:4970–4976.
17. Krakow EF, Goudar R, Petzold E, Suvarna S, Last M, Welsby IJ. Influence of sample collection and storage on the detection of platelet factor 4-heparin antibodies. *Am J Clin Pathol.* 2007;128:150–155.
18. Warkentin TE, Sheppard JI. Clinical sample investigation (CSI) hematology: pinpointing the precise onset of heparin-induced thrombocytopenia (HIT). *J Thromb Haemost.* 2007;5:636–637.
19. Warkentin TE, Sheppard JI, Moore JC, Kelton JG. The use of well-characterized sera for the assessment of new diagnostic enzyme-immunoassays for the diagnosis of heparin-induced thrombocytopenia. *J Thromb Haemost.* 2010;8:216–218.
20. PF4 Enhanced® [package insert]. Waukesha, WI: Gen-Probe GTI Diagnostics; revised 8 Jun 2011.
21. PF4 IgG™ [package insert]. Waukesha, WI: Gen-Probe GTI Diagnostics; revised 8 Jun 2011.

22. Zymutest HIA IgGAM [package insert]. Mason, OH: Aniara; revised 26 Oct 2007.

23. Zymutest HIA IgG [package insert]. Mason, OH: Aniara; revised 23 Oct 2007.

24. Asserachrom® HPIA – IgG [package insert]. Asnière-sur-Seine, France: Diagnostica Stago, January 2011.

25. Asserachrom® HPIA [package insert]. Asnière-sur-Seine, France: Diagnostica Stago, January 2011.

26. ID-PaGIA Heparin/PF4 Antibody Test [package insert]. Cressier, France: DiaMed GmbH, May 2010.

27. Schneiter S, Colucci G, Sulzer I, Barizzi G, Lämmle B, Alberio L. Variability of anti-PF4/heparin antibody results obtained by the rapid testing system ID-H/PF4-PaGIA. *J Thromb Haemost*. 2009;7:1649–1655.

28. Eichler P, Budde U, Haas S, Kroll H, Loreth RM, Meyer O. First workshop for detection of heparin-induced antibodies: validation of the heparin-induced platelet activation test (HIPA) in comparison with a PF4/heparin ELISA. *Thromb Haemost*. 1999;81:625–629.

29. Arepally GM, Kamei S, Park KS, Kamei K, Li ZQ, Liu W, et al. Characterization of a murine monoclonal antibody that mimics heparin-induced thrombocytopenia antibodies. *Blood* 2000;95:1533–1540.

30. Denomme GA, Warkentin TE, Horsewood P, Sheppard JA, Warner MN, Kelton JG. Activation of platelets by sera containing IgG1 heparin-dependent antibodies: an explanation for the predominance of the FcγRIIa "low responder" (his$_{131}$) gene in patients with heparin-induced thrombocytopenia. *J Lab Clin Med*. 1997;130:278–284.

31. Lo GK, Juhl D, Warkentin TE, Sigouin CS, Eichler P, Greinacher A. Evaluation of pretest clinical score (4 T's) for the diagnosis of heparin-induced thrombocytopenia in two clinical settings. *J Thromb Haemost*. 2006;4:759–765.

32. Cuker A, Arepally G, Crowther MA, Rice L, Datko F, Hook K. The HIT Expert Probability (HEP) Score: a novel pre-test probability model for heparin-induced thrombocytopenia based on broad expert opinion. *J Thromb Haemost*. 2010;8:2642–2650.

33. Warkentin TE, Makris M, Jay RM, Kelton JG. A spontaneous prothrombotic disorder resembling heparin-induced thrombocytopenia. *Am J Med*. 2008;121:632–636.

34. Krauel K, Pötschke C, Weber C, Kessler W, Fürll B, Ittermann T. Platelet factor 4 binds to bacteria, inducing antibodies cross-reacting with the major antigen in heparin-induced thrombocytopenia. *Blood*. 2011;117:1370–1378.

35. Greinacher A, Holtfreter B, Krauel K, Gätke D, Weber C, Ittermann T. Association of natural anti-platelet factor 4/heparin antibodies with periodontal disease. *Blood*. 2011;118:1395–1401.

36. Jay RM, Warkentin TE. Fatal heparin-induced thrombocytopenia (HIT) during warfarin thromboprophylaxis following orthopedic surgery: another example of 'spontaneous' HIT? *J Thromb Haemost*. 2008;6:1598–1600.

37. Chong BH, Burgess J, Ismail F. The clinical usefulness of the platelet aggregation test for the diagnosis of heparin-induced thrombocytopenia. *Thromb Haemost*. 1993;69:344–350.

38. Greinacher A, Amiral J, Dummel V, et al. Laboratory diagnosis of heparin-associated thrombocytopenia and comparison of platelet aggregation test, heparin-induced platelet activation test, and platelet factor 4/heparin enzyme-linked immunosorbent assay. *Transfusion*. 1994;34:381–385.

39. Goodfellow KJ, Brown P, Malia RG, Hampton KK. A comparison of laboratory tests for the diagnosis of heparin-induced thrombocytopenia (HIT) [Abstr]. *Br J Haematol*. 1998;101:89.

40. Polgár J, Eichler P, Greinacher A, Clemetson KJ. Adenosine diphosphate (ADP) and ADP receptor play a major role in platelet activation/aggregation induced by sera from heparin-induced thrombocytopenia patients. *Blood*. 1998;91:549–554.

41. Warkentin TE, Hayward CPM, Smith CA, Kelly PM, Kelton JG. Determinants of donor platelet variability when testing for heparin-induced thrombocytopenia. *J Lab Clin Med*. 1992;120:371–379.

42. Greinacher A, Michels I, Kiefel V, Mueller-Eckhardt C. A rapid and sensitive test for diagnosing heparin-associated thrombocytopenia. *Thromb Haemost*. 1991;66:734–736.

43. Lee DH, Warkentin TE, Denomme GA, Hayward CPM, Kelton JG. A diagnostic test for heparin-induced thrombocytopenia: detection of platelet microparticles using flow cytometry. *Br J Haematol*. 1996;95:724–731.

44. Moore JC, Arnold DM, Warkentin TE, Warkentin AE, Kelton JG. An algorithm for resolving 'indeterminate' test results in the platelet serotonin release assay for investigation of heparin-induced thrombocytopenia. *J Thromb Haemost*. 2008;6:1595–1597.

45. Warkentin TE, Levine MN, Hirsh J, Horsewood P, Roberts RS, Gent M. Heparin-induced thrombocytopenia in patients treated with low-molecular-weight heparin or unfractionated heparin. *N Engl J Med*. 1995;332:1330–1335.

46. Warkentin TE, Sheppard JI, Moore JC, Moore KM, Sigouin CS, Kelton JG. Laboratory testing for the antibodies that cause heparin-induced thrombocytopenia: how much class do we need? *J Lab Clin Med*. 2005;146:341–346.

47. Linkins LA, Lee DH. Frequency of heparin-induced thrombocytopenia. In: Heparin-Induced Thrombocytopenia. 5th ed. Warkentin TE, Greinacher A, eds. Boca Raton, FL: CRC Press; 2013:110–150.

48. Warkentin TE, Davidson BL, Büller HR, Gallus A, Gent M, Lensing AWA. Prevalence and risk of pre-existing heparin-induced thrombocytopenia antibodies in patients with acute VTE. *Chest*. 2011;140:366–373.

49. Poupard C, May MA, Regina S, Marchand M, Fusciardi J, Gruel Y. Changes in platelet count after cardiac surgery can effectively predict the development of pathogenic heparin-dependent antibodies. *Br J Haematol*. 2005;128:837–841.

50. Rauova L, Zhai L, Kowalska MA, Arepally GM, Cines DB, Poncz M. Role of platelet surface PF4 antigenic complexes in heparin-induced thrombocytopenia pathogenesis: diagnostic and therapeutic implications. *Blood*. 2006;107:2346–2353.

51. Elalamy I, Galea V, Hatmi M, Gerotziafas GT. Heparin-induced multiple electrode aggregometry: a potential tool for improvement of heparin-induced thrombocytopenia diagnosis. *J Thromb Haemost*. 2009;7:1932–1934.

52. Morel-Kopp MC, Aboud M, Tan CW, Kulathilake C, Ward C. Whole blood impedance aggregometry detects heparin-induced thrombocytopenia antibodies. *Thromb Res*. 2010;125:e234–e239.

53. Lindhoff-Last E, Gerdsen F, Ackermann H, Bauersachs R. Determination of heparin-platelet factor 4-IgG antibodies improves diagnosis of heparin-induced thrombocytopenia. *Br J Haematol*. 2001;113:886–890.

54. Bakchoul T, Giptner A, Bein G, Santoso S, Sachs UJH. Prospective evaluation of immunoassays for the diagnosis of heparin-induced thrombocytopenia. *J Thromb Haemost*. 2009;7:1260–1265.

55. Warkentin TE, Linkins LA. Immunoassays are not created equal. *J Thromb Haemost*. 2009;7:1256–1259.

56. Greinacher A, Juhl D, Strobel U, Wessel A, Lubenow N, Selleng K. Heparin-induced thrombocytopenia: a prospective study on the incidence, platelet-activating capacity and clinical significance of anti-PF4/heparin antibodies of the IgG, IgM, and IgA classes. *J Thromb Haemost*. 2007;5(8):1666–1673.

57. Whitlatch NL, Perry SL, Ortel TL. Anti-heparin/platelet factor 4 antibody optical density values and the confirmatory procedure in the diagnosis of heparin-induced thrombocytopenia. *Thromb Haemost*. 2008;100:678–684.

58. Whitlatch NL, Kong DF, Metjian AD, Arepally GM, Ortel TL. Validation of the high-dose heparin confirmatory step for the diagnosis of heparin-induced thrombocytopenia. *Blood*. 2010;116:1761–1766.

59. Warkentin TE, Sheppard JI. No significant improvement in diagnostic specificity of an anti-PF4/polyanion immunoassay with use of high heparin confirmatory procedure. *J Thromb Haemost*. 2006;4:281–282.

60. Selleng S, Schreier N, Wollert HG, Greinacher A. The diagnostic value of the anti-PF4/heparin immunoassay high-dose heparin confirmatory test in cardiac surgery patients. *Anesth Analg*. 2011;112:774–776.

61. Althaus K, Strobel U, Warkentin TE, Greinacher A. Combined use of the high heparin step and optical density to optimize diagnostic sensitivity and specificity of an anti-PF4/heparin enzyme-immunoassay. *Thromb Res*. 2011;128:256–260.

62. Greinacher A, Ittermann T, Bagemühl J, et al. Heparin-induced thrombocytopenia: towards standardization of platelet factor 4/heparin antigen tests. *J Thromb Haemost*. 2010;8:2025–2031.

63. Zwicker JI, Uhl L, Huang WY, Shaz BH, Bauer KA. Thrombosis and ELISA optical density values in hospitalized patients with heparin-induced thrombocytopenia. *J Thromb Haemost*. 2004;2:2133–2137.

64. Altuntas F, Metavosyan K, Burner J, Shen YM, Sarode R. Higher optical density of an antigen assay predicts thrombosis in patients with heparin-induced thrombocytopenia. *Eur J Haematol*. 2008;80:429–435.

65. Baroletti S, Hurwitz S, Conti NA, Fanikos J, Piazza G, Goldhaber SZ. Thrombosis in suspected heparin-induced thrombocytopenia occurs more often with high antibody levels. *Am J Med*. 2012;125:44–49.

66. Meyer O, Salama A, Pittet N, Schwind P. Rapid detection of heparin-induced platelet antibodies with particle gel immunoassay (ID-HPF4). *Lancet*. 1999;354:1525–1526.

67. Eichler P, Raschke R, Lubenow N, Meyer O, Schwind P, Greinacher A. The new ID-heparin/PF4 antibody test for rapid detection of heparin-induced antibodies in comparison with functional and antigenic assays. *Br J Haematol*. 2002;116:887–891.

68. Poupard C, Gueret P, Fouassier M, Ternisien C, Trossaert M, Régina S. Prospective evaluation of the '4Ts' score and particle gel immunoassay specific to heparin/PF4 for the diagnosis of heparin-induced thrombocytopenia. *J Thromb Haemost*. 2007;5:1373–1379.

69. Bryant A, Low J, Austin S, Joseph JE. Timely diagnosis and management of heparin-induced thrombocytopenia in a frequent request, low incidence single centre using clinical 4T's score and particle gel immunoassay. *Br J Haematol*. 2008;143:721–726.

70. Alberio L, Kimmerle S, Baumann A, Taleghani BM, Demarmels Biasiutti FD, Lämmle B. Rapid determination of anti-heparin/platelet factor 4 antibody titers in the diagnosis of heparin-induced thrombocytopenia. *Am J Med*. 2003;114:528–536.

71. Nellen V, Sulzer I, Barizzi G, Lämmle B, Alberio L. Rapid exclusion or confirmation of heparin-induced thrombocytopenia; a single-centre experience with 1,291 patients. *Haematologica*. 2012;97:89–97.

72. Warkentin TE, Sheppard JI, Raschke R, Greinacher A. Performance characteristics of a rapid assay for anti-PF4/heparin antibodies, the Particle ImmunoFiltration Assay. *J Thromb Haemost*. 2007;5:2308–2310.

73. Davidson SJ, Ortel TL, Smith LJ. Performance of a new, rapid, automated immunoassay for the detection of anti-platelet factor 4/heparin complex antibodies. *Blood Coagul Fibrinolysis*. 2011;22:340–344.

74. Legnani C, Cini M, Pili C, Boggian O, Frascaro M, Palareti G. Evaluation of a new automated panel of assays for the detection of anti-PF4/heparin antibodies in patients suspected of having heparin-induced thrombocytopenia. *Thromb Haemost*. 2010;104:402–409.

75. Nagi PK, Ackermann F, Wendt H, Savoca R, Bosshard HR. Protein A antibody-capture ELISA (PACE): an ELISA method to avoid denaturation of surface-adsorbed antigens. *J Immunol Methods*. 1993;158:267–276.

76. Newman PM, Swanson RL, Chong BH. Heparin-induced thrombocytopenia: IgG binding to PF4-heparin complexes in the fluid phase and cross-reactivity with low molecular weight heparin and heparinoid. *Thromb Haemost*. 1998;80:292–297.

77. Warkentin TE, Cook RJ, Marder VJ, Sheppard JA, Moore JC, Eriksson BI, et al. Anti-platelet factor 4/heparin antibodies in orthopedic surgery patients receiving antithrombotic prophylaxis with fondaparinux or enoxaparin. *Blood*. 2005;106:3791–3796.

78. Sachs UJ, von Hesberg J, Santoso S, Bein G, Bakchoul T. Evaluation of a new nanoparticle-based lateral-flow immunoassay for the exclusion of heparin-induced thrombocytopenia (HIT). *Thromb Haemost*. 2011;106:1197–1202.

79. Cuker A. Heparin-induced thrombocytopenia (HIT) in 2011: an epidemic of overdiagnosis. *Thromb Haemost*. 2011;106:993–994.

17 Laboratory evaluation of von Willebrand disease: phenotypic analysis

Emmanuel J. Favaloro

Department of Hematology, ICPMR, Westmead Hospital, Westmead, NSW, Australia

Introduction and background

von Willebrand disease (vWD) and von Willebrand factor (vWF): von Willebrand disease (vWD) is now recognized to be the most common inherited bleeding disorder [1]. Individuals with vWD have defects in, or reduced levels of, von Willebrand factor (vWF), an adhesive plasma protein essential for primary hemostasis [1–4]. In plasma, vWF exists in a multimeric dimer configuration, ranging in size from small ("low molecular weight"; LMW) to "intermediate molecular weight" (IMW) to very large "high molecular weight" (HMW) forms. The larger the vWF molecule, the greater the overall number of individual adhesion sites, and thus the greater the overall adhesive capacity. vWD is very heterogeneous and may be characterized by quantitative or qualitative defects in vWF. Comprehensive laboratory testing is therefore required to define specific defects. The current vWD classification scheme is detailed elsewhere [2], and summarized below. Although genetic testing is available in some geographic localities and useful for some selective clinical investigations, it is not indicated for most. Genetic testing for vWD is the subject of another chapter in this book (Chapter 18). For practical purposes, a diagnosis of vWD, consistent with clinical findings, and confirmed by phenotypic hemostasis testing, is accepted as sufficient evidence for vWD.

Type 1 vWD is caused by partial deficiency in vWF, whereas Type 3 vWD occurs when vWF is essentially absent (i.e., both are "quantitative" defects) [1–4]. In contrast, individuals suffering from qualitative defects are classified as Type 2, of which there are four subtypes 2A, 2B, 2M, and 2N [1–4]. Type 2A individuals suffer decreased vWF-dependent adhesion that is associated with a loss of HMW vWF multimers. Type 2B variants show an increased affinity of vWF for platelet glycoprotein Ib α (GPIBA), and sometimes also a loss of HMW vWF and mild thrombocytopenia. Type 2M variants have decreased platelet-dependent adhesion associated with evidence of a dysfunctional vWF molecule (activity decreased relative to antigen) that is not caused by a loss of HMW vWF. Type 2N variants have normal vWF platelet function; however, they demonstrate a markedly decreased affinity of vWF for factor VIII (FVIII) usually causing a reduced circulating FVIII. The correct classification of an individual's vWD is important not only because the presenting biological activity of vWF determines the hemorrhagic risk, but also because the subsequent clinical management may differ accordingly.

A number of other disorders can mimic vWD, because of similarities in clinical presentation and/or laboratory results. These disorders include "platelet-type" (PT-, or "pseudo-") vWD (a hereditary platelet GPIBA disorder caused by mutations in the *GPIBA* gene), and acquired vWD-like disorders associated with myeloproliferative disease or presenting as auto-anti-vWF antibody syndromes [5–7].

Quality in Laboratory Hemostasis and Thrombosis, Second Edition. Edited by Steve Kitchen, John D. Olson and F. Eric Preston.
© 2013 John Wiley & Sons, Ltd. Published 2013 by Blackwell Publishing Ltd.

Fundamental problems with the phenotypic evaluation of vWD

vWD heterogeneity and assay limitations: Because of individual assay limitations and evident vWD heterogeneity, no single laboratory procedure is able to detect all forms of vWD. For example, a normal level of plasma vWF protein ("antigen"; measured by the vWF:Ag assay) does not discount vWD, as many Type 2 vWD individuals will have levels that fall within the normal reference range; these cases will, therefore, only be identified by the performance of additional *functional* vWF assays [1–4, 8]. Secondly, a low plasma level of vWF:Ag will suggest vWD, but cannot, in isolation, identify the underlying subtype. Accordingly, overall laboratory investigation for vWD requires a panel of tests. The classically used "vWD-screening" panel normally comprises FVIII coagulant (FVIII:C), vWF:Ag, *and* vWF function, typically using the ristocetin cofactor (vWF:RCo) assay, and, in some laboratories, the collagen binding (vWF:CB) assay and/or other vWF "activity" assays [1–4, 8].

The test panel of FVIII:C, vWF:Ag, vWF:RCo, and vWF:CB will *identify* the majority of vWD cases, and supplementary tests can then be used to further *classify* the identified vWD. These include ristocetin-induced platelet aggregation (RIPA), vWF:Multimer analysis, and vWF:FVIII binding (vWF:FVIIIB) assays. Other more recent diagnostic developments are also influencing vWD diagnostics.

Preanalytical variables: It is important to be aware of preanalytical variables (as summarized in Chapter 5 and elsewhere) [9, 10], as these cause substantial problems for the identification of vWD. In brief, collection of blood into inappropriate tubes, delayed transport of blood or of separated plasma, inappropriate transport of refrigerated whole blood or of nonfrozen plasma, and inappropriate processing of whole blood or separated plasma (e.g., by filtration) can potentially lead to false identification of vWD in non-vWD individuals, or to false identification of Type 2 vWD in Type 1 vWD individuals. Poor collection techniques or difficult collections may also lead to partial sample clotting, and loss of HMW vWF because of entrapment or platelet activation.

vWF is an acute phase reactant causing levels to vary considerably in the same patient when studied on different occasions. Plasma levels of vWF may be related to exercise, inflammation, stress, diurnal variation (higher levels later in the day), and hormonal influences (e.g., fluctuations within menstrual cycles and higher levels in pregnancy). ABO blood groups also influence vWF levels, with lower levels in O blood group individuals compared to non-O blood group. vWF levels also increase with age. A diagnosis of vWD must take all these potential factors into account. At the very least, all tests should be repeated for confirmation using a freshly collected sample, taken some weeks apart, before making or excluding a definitive diagnosis of vWD. The investigations should also be repeated when normal results are obtained in individuals with a convincing clinical history of bleeding (e.g., the stress of a hospital visit may temporarily correct the abnormality).

Clinical evaluation, personal, and family histories: A diagnosis of vWD should also not be made without a full and comprehensive clinical and family history and physical evaluation. Although important in the workup of vWD, this aspect of diagnosis is not covered by this report, and the reader is referred elsewhere for details [3].

Phenotypic assays used in the diagnosis of vWD

Routine coagulation tests: The prothrombin time (PT) and activated partial thromboplastin time (APTT) are the two most widely used clot-based assays. The PT is not sensitive to deficiencies or defects in either FVIII:C or vWF. The APTT is sensitive to deficiencies or defects in FVIII:C and since FVIII:C levels might be low in individuals with vWD, the APTT has some limited value as a screening test for vWD. However, a normal APTT will not exclude vWD. If vWD is suspected, appropriate specific and sensitive assays should always be performed.

[Skin] bleeding times (SBT) and PFA-100®: SBT procedures are neither specific for, nor highly sensitive to the presence of, vWD, and are thus not recommended for this purpose. If the laboratory has a PFA-100®, this might be a better option for use as a vWD-screening tool in selected test cases as highlighted elsewhere [11, 12].

Platelet counts and platelet morphology: This is often worthwhile, especially when the individual initially presents and the clinical history is unclear. Both platelet count and platelet size should be evaluated.

193

Individuals with Type 2B vWD and PT-vWD will sometimes present with mild thrombocytopenia [7]. Alternatively, platelet counts and platelet morphology may differentially define an alternate platelet-related disorder or deficiency to explain a bleeding propensity [13].

Platelet function analysis: RIPA is a useful diagnostic test for vWD (see below), otherwise standard platelet function testing per se is of no value in the diagnosis of vWD. Nevertheless, comprehensive platelet function would be indicated to define potential platelet abnormalities in the event that vWD investigations prove to be negative in individuals with strong clinical histories. Similarly, the possibility of a combined disorder needs to be considered when vWF levels are only mildly reduced in an individual with a clinically significant bleeding disorder [13, 14].

Sensitive and specific laboratory assays for vWD

FVIII:C: Testing for FVIII:C should always be included in a phenotypic workup for possible vWD. Although a number of methodologies are available, the "one-stage" clot-based assay is generally employed by most laboratories for technical simplicity. Generally, the lower the FVIII:C, the more severe the vWD and the hemorrhagic risk. FVIII:C testing alone is, however, insufficient to identify, diagnose, or exclude vWD (i.e., a normal level of FVIII:C will not always exclude vWD, and an abnormal level will not necessarily define vWD, nor give information on the vWD subtype). Details regarding assays for coagulation factors are found elsewhere in this book (Chapter 10).

vWF:Ag: Many methods are available, although most laboratories now perform an enzyme-linked immunosorbent assay (ELISA) procedure or newer automated technologies such as immunoturbidimetric or latex immunoassays (LIA) [4]. Although LIA-based methodologies will continue to gain popularity due to automation, one drawback is the potential interference of rheumatoid factor. Interestingly, LIA assays also tend to provide higher values for vWF:Ag than do ELISA assays [15], and may also show slightly inferior sensitivity to low vWF levels [16]. Used alone, determination of vWF:Ag will help *detect* all Type 3 vWD and *identify* most Type 1 vWD, but will *miss* many Type 2 vWD individuals. Also, whilst a low level may suggest vWD, it will provide no information on the disease subtype.

Functional vWF assays I: vWF:RCo and vWF:Act assays—vWF:RCo is the original functional vWF assay, and is classically performed using a platelet agglutination procedure, but has also now been automated on many instruments [4]. vWF:RCo assesses the ability of plasma vWF to bind to normal platelets in the presence of ristocetin, and has some capacity to preferentially recognize HMW forms. Thus, plasma from individuals with Types 2A, 2B, and usually 2M vWD will tend to give lower vWF:RCo results than vWF:Ag (i.e., show functional vWF discordance), due to the absence of HMW vWF (Type 2B vWD), IMW and HMW vWF (Type 2A vWD), or the presence of functionally defective vWF (Type 2M vWD). However, there are notable assay problems that diminish the overall effectiveness of vWF:RCo, including assay reproducibility (i.e., high variability; intra-assay, interassay, and interlaboratory) and low-level vWF sensitivity issues [4, 16].What this means in practice is that the test needs to be repeated several times for confirmation, and levels under 20 U/dL cannot be accurately determined by many methods. This is a serious assay limitation, given that most severe cases of vWD present with levels of vWF:RCo below 20 U/dL. More recent modifications to automated vWF:RCo testing may have overcome some of these limitations [17, 18].

Because of the above, and because of the labor intensiveness of the classical vWF:RCo assay, several functional vWF alternatives continue to evolve [4, 8]. Some methodologies include the incorporation of monoclonal antibodies (MAB) to functional epitopes in vWF, binding of vWF to collagen, and the use of recombinant platelet receptor binding (e.g., using glycocalicin, which is a plasma analogue of GPIBA) or MAB to these receptors. Only some of these assays use ristocetin. One method, now commercially marketed as a vWF "activity" ("vWF:Act") assay, utilizes a MAB against vWF in an ELISA. Several versions have been developed, none of which incorporate ristocetin, but these are not considered suitable as alternatives to classical vWF:RCo [4, 8, 19].

Although two different versions of a "genuine" vWF:RCo ELISA have been described [20–22], with each correlating well to classical vWF:RCo assays by agglutination, neither has been generally adopted by laboratories nor otherwise independently validated. Cross-laboratory studies for both these assays are also lacking at this time.

The most recent entry into the vWF "Activity" assay group comprises automated LIA-based assays [4]. Currently, there are limited high-quality data on the utility of these assays for the diagnosis of vWD. Although studies to date are encouraging, these tests do not entirely correlate with vWF:RCo, particularly for type 2A and 2M vWD; hence they cannot be considered a replacement for vWF:RCo [4, 23, 24]. Also encouraging are attempts to develop better ristocetin-based assays using flow cytometry [25, 26].

Functional vWF Assays II: vWF:CB Assays—The vWF:CB is typically performed by ELISA, although a flow cytometry-based method has been described [4, 8]. A number of different commercial ELISA-based kits are available [27]. vWF:CB gives some estimate of the level of vWF present, but its greatest strength, when appropriately optimized, is its ability to selectively detect primarily HMW vWF (i.e., most functional, adhesive, and hemostatically potent forms of vWF) [4, 8]. The vWF:CB is generally more sensitive to HMW forms of vWF than vWF:RCo, although efficacy depends on various factors, and not all vWF:CB assays behave identically [4, 8, 27]. This standardization issue has delayed their more general incorporation into laboratory practice, and has been extensively discussed in previous reviews [4, 8].

In brief, the following can be emphasized:
(i) Type I/III collagen-mixture preparations (from equine or bovine tendon) are, in general, better able to preferentially detect HMW vWF than either purified human-derived Type III collagen or purified animal-derived Type I collagen, although those based on "purified" Type I or Type III collagen can be made to be effective [8, 27].
(ii) Some purified, human-derived Type III collagen systems (in-house and commercial) appear to bind vWF too well, and thus may not show selective discrimination of HMW vWF, and some purified Type I collagen systems may bind vWF too poorly, leading to poor reproducibility issues, particularly at low levels of vWF [8, 27].
(iii) The observation that collagen binding assays bind HMW vWF more readily has been demonstrated in studies of factor concentrates as well as in plasma systems [8].

Technically, vWF:CB ELISA assays use similar procedural steps to vWF:Ag ELISA assays, but rely on the ability of vWF to adhere to collagen. The potential significance of this as an *in vivo* correlate has yet to be fully evaluated. However, vWF binding to tissue matrix proteins including collagen is a primary hemostatic mechanism following injury, and it needs to be recognized that this adhesive activity is distinct to that identified by vWF:RCo assays. The potential importance of this is explored in more detail elsewhere [4].

RIPA procedure—The RIPA assay assesses an individual's platelet rich plasma (PRP) for sensitivity to ristocetin at various concentrations (typically, using at least two to three distinct concentrations over the range 0.5–1.5 mg/mL for light transmittance aggregometry (LTA) systems) [3, 13, 28]. Ristocetin sensitivity in RIPA is dependent on both the level and functional activity of vWF. Normal individuals show platelet agglutination at (and above) 1.0–1.5 mg/mL ristocetin, but typically not at or below 0.5 mg/mL (in LTA systems). Patients with Type 3 vWD will typically not show any platelet agglutination even using high concentrations because they essentially lack vWF. The level of platelet agglutination using PRP from individuals with Type 1 vWD will depend on the presenting plasma level of vWF. However, RIPA is somewhat insensitive to mild quantitative deficiencies, and individuals with moderate loss of vWF (e.g., presenting with levels above 30 U/dL vWF) may show normal RIPA. Alternatively, individuals with severe Type 1 vWD (i.e., <15 U/dL vWF) or severe Type 2A vWD will tend to show no aggregation (or only mild aggregation) with ≤1.5 mg/mL ristocetin. In contrast, individuals with Type 2B vWD (and those with PT-vWD) show an enhanced agglutination response, and PRP will typically agglutinate with ≤0.5 mg/mL ristocetin [3, 7]. However, the platelets of some individuals with 2B vWD will only agglutinate at slightly higher concentrations (0.7 mg/mL) [29], providing difficulties in the detection of 2B vWD given the proximity of this concentration to the standard normal cut-off value (0.8–1.0 mg/mL for LTA) [30]. Nevertheless, RIPA is recommended for use to confirm or subtype vWD in all patients showing a consistent discordance in functional vWF versus vWF:Ag (i.e., low vWF:RCo/vWF:Ag and/or vWF:CB/vWF:Ag) and also to differentially diagnose Type 2B and PT-vWD (see later) [3, 7].

vWF:Multimer assay—This gel-electrophoresis procedure identifies vWF of differing molecular weight, as well as identifying certain vWF-structural abnormalities [31, 32]. Because of test complexity, time, and cost, it is now only performed by a limited

195

number of expert laboratories (e.g., only a single laboratory in Australia). Although this procedure still has a place in vWD testing and diagnosis, its use is diminishing as alternative (easier to perform and faster) tests are improving. Although this analysis is difficult to perform well, it remains a major part of determining the type of vWD in those patients who have an apparent dysfunction of vWF [2]. Newer testing that is more easily performed may replace multimeric analysis in the future; however, the multimeric data are currently required to meet international recommendations for determining the type of vWD [2, 3]. Frozen plasma samples can be shipped effectively to laboratories specializing in this testing.

Because multimer analysis is difficult to perform well, there is a high diagnostic error rate [32–34]. Thus, it can be more misleading to include poor multimer data within the diagnosis of vWD than to exclude it from the investigation [32–34]. Also, it is not generally appropriate to assess vWF:multimers during the initial vWD investigation process unless there are compelling clinical reasons. vWF:multimers are not generally indicated when previous vWF testing using FVIII:C, vWF:Ag and functional vWF assays are consistently normal, and platelet function testing has excluded a platelet dysfunction, unless there is compelling evidence of muco-cutaneous bleeding (in this case, a vWF structural abnormality is still feasible, although unlikely). vWF:multimers are also not generally indicated when previous vWF testing is suggestive of a quantitative vWF defect (i.e., Type 1 or Type 3 vWD), since this will merely act to confirm the loss of vWF already identified by previous testing.

In contrast, vWF:multimer testing may be useful when functional discordance has been identified (i.e., low vWF:RCo/vWF:Ag and/or low vWF:CB/vWF:Ag). Nevertheless, the initial recommended approach would be to perform the RIPA analysis first (see below). vWF:multimers may then be useful to help identify, distinguish, or confirm Type 2A vWD (loss of HMW and IMW vWF), Type 2B vWD (loss of HMW and occasionally IMW vWF), and Type 2M vWD (no significant loss of HMW or IMW vWF). Other qualitative defects (abnormal triplet patterns or smearing) may also be visible in multimer gel patterns and potentially useful to identify unusual subtypes of vWD.

vWF:FVIII binding assay—This assay assesses the ability of an individual's vWF to bind FVIII and is used to differentially diagnose Type 2N vWD. In the normal individual, FVIII circulates bound to vWF and has a half-life of 8–12 hours. When vWF is structurally abnormal (e.g., Type 2N vWD) or absent (i.e., Type 3 vWD), the half-life of FVIII is reduced to minutes and since the synthetic rate does not adequately compensate, this results in a lower plasma concentration. Clinical manifestations of Type 2N vWD are those of hemophilia A. The vWF:FVIIIB assay is most frequently used for the differential diagnosis of hemophilia A and Type 2N vWD, rather than for the usual clinical presentations of vWD. This assay is typically performed as an ELISA-like procedure, and may also involve a chromogenic assay step [35, 36]. A disproportion of bound vWF and bound FVIII identified in this assay (i.e., FVIII to vWF ratio <0.6) is suggestive of a Type 2N vWD defect. This diagnosis can also be addressed with molecular methods, discussed in Chapter 18.

vWF:FVIIIB should always be performed for newly identified individuals that give a clinical presentation of hemophilia A, particularly where the genetic inheritance does not fit the classical hemophilia pattern (which is sex-linked, whereas Type 2N vWD is not). The penetrance of Type 2N vWD may also be geographically based; for example, the disorder appears to be more common in north Europe (particularly in France, where it was originally identified), but is less common in more distant localities (e.g., relatively rare in Australia) [36].

A diagnostic laboratory process for vWD

If vWD is suggested by clinical review, then the performance of routine coagulation tests such as PT and APTT is optional, as is the performance of the PFA-100® (Figure 17.1) [3, 4, 8]. However, the performance of a platelet count is indicated together with FVIII:C plus vWF:Ag plus at least one (but preferably multiple) vWF functional assay(s). If only a single functional vWF assay is able to be supported by laboratories, the vWF:CB may be favored over the vWF:RCo for the reasons extensively outlined elsewhere [4, 8, 27, 33, 37]. In brief, the vWF:CB (i) more consistently and correctly identifies Types 2A and 2B vWD, (ii) is generally less variable in terms of intra-assay, interlaboratory, and interassay results, (iii) is

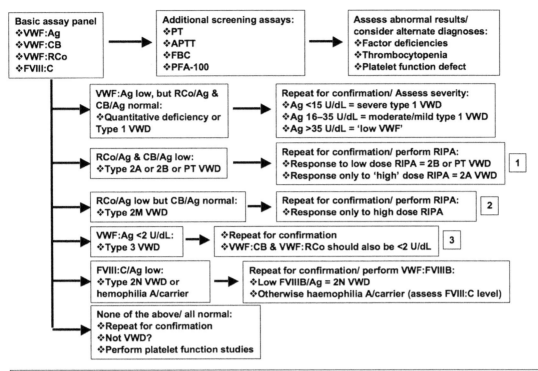

Figure 17.1 One recommended approach to the investigation of vWD, as essentially utilized in our laboratory. Where abnormal test results are obtained that suggest vWD using the basic assay panel, further specific testing can then be employed on a case-by-case basis to aid in vWD type discrimination. Ag, von Willebrand factor antigen result; APTT, activated partial thromboplastin time; CB/Ag, ratio of vWF:CB to vWF:Ag; FBC, full blood count; FVIIIB, level of factor VIII bound in a von Willebrand factor–FVIII binding assay; FVIII:C, factor VIII coagulant; PFA-100, platelet function analyzer-100; gp1BA, glycoprotein 1b alpha gene; LIA, Latex immunoassay; PT, prothrombin time; PT vWD, platelet type vWD; RCo/Ag, ratio of vWF:RCo to vWF:Ag; RIPA, ristocetin-induced platelet agglutination assay; vWD, von Willebrand disease/disorder; vWF, von Willebrand factor; vWF:Ag, von Willebrand factor antigen (assay); vWF:CB, von Willebrand factor collagen binding (assay); vWF:FVIIIB, von Willebrand factor–FVIII binding assay; vWF:RCo, von Willebrand factor ristocetin cofactor (assay).

usually more sensitive to low levels of vWF (important for proper identification of severe Type 1, Type 2, and Type 3 vWD), and (iv) uses similar methodology to vWF:Ag and thus is "easier" to perform. Nevertheless, a diagnostic test panel that excludes the vWF:RCo may miss some patients with platelet function discordant Type 2M vWD [1, 4, 8, 19, 23, 38]. However, my view also maintains that it is no longer appropriate for laboratories to deploy the vWF:RCo as the sole vWF functional assay, since this approach will lead to the misdiagnosis of up to a quarter of vWD cases being investigated, as well as potentially missing some (matrix-binding-function-discordant) Type 2M vWD cases [1, 4, 8, 32, 33, 37, 38]. Within this context, it is also important to consider the type of collagen used in the vWF:CB assay, or the commercial kit's sensitivity or otherwise to these 2M vWD cases. Thus, not only will this sub-type of type 2M vWD be

197

missed if vWF:CB assays are not performed, but different vWF:CB assays may also differ in their relative sensitivities [38].

Based on the initial test findings, plus the degree of clinical evidence, further evaluation may or may not be required (Figure 17.1). Although the recommended steps outlined in this chapter will cover most situations appropriately, vWD does not always present in "textbook" fashion. Clinicians should at all times be guided by their patient's clinical history and their local expert hemostasis laboratory's advice.

Exclusion of vWD: If all initial phenotypic test results are normal, and if the clinical suspicion is low, then further investigation may not be warranted, as vWD is highly unlikely. Alternatively, if results are normal, but the clinical suspicion is high, then the test processes should be repeated for confirmation to discount a potential laboratory testing or collection artifact. Repeat testing is also required if the initial sampling occurred at an inappropriate time (e.g., during pregnancy or during acute stress when vWF levels might be falsely elevated). The supplementary tests of vWF:multimers and RIPA might be indicated if there is a strong clinical history of mucocutaneous bleeding even if the standard phenotypic tests (FVIII:C, vWF:Ag, vWF:RCo, vWF:CB) are all consistently normal, because an unusual or rare presentation of vWD is still feasible. vWF is a complex molecule, with multiple functional domains. We simply do not have all the required laboratory tools to identify all possible types of vWD. Although current testing should identify all currently known forms of vWD, there is no doubt that some forms of vWD are yet to be discovered, and potentially represented by abnormalities in vWF structure that current tests cannot identify.

Similarly, vWF:FVIIIB testing might also be indicated where there is a strong clinical history of hemophilia-like bleeding, even if the standard phenotypic tests (FVIII:C, vWF:Ag, vWF:RCo, vWF:CB) are all consistently normal, because the standard testing will occasionally miss some forms of Type 2N vWD [36]. Finally, should all currently available vWF tests be normal, platelet function testing would then be indicated to identify a potential platelet dysfunction [13, 14].

Making a diagnosis of vWD: If any or all phenotypic test results are abnormal, then follow-up testing is indicated and is dependent on the initial pattern of results. Repeat testing for confirmation is usually indicated to exclude potential testing/collection artifacts, and because of assay variability and sampling issues. Repeat confirmation is particularly important when vWF:RCo is being employed as the sole functional vWF assay. It is important to repeat *all* the assays (i.e., vWF:Ag, vWF:RCo, vWF:CB, FVIII:C) on the second sample.

Identification of Type 1 vWD: If all initial phenotypic tests (i.e., vWF:Ag, vWF:RCo, vWF:CB, FVIII:C) show low levels, but are proportionally similar (i.e., concordant test patterns obtained on initial *and* repeat testing), then Type 1 vWD is most likely (Table 17.1 and Figure 17.1). vWF:multimers are generally unnecessary (as the vWF distribution pattern will typically be normal and the overall relative intensity of multimer bands will simply correlate with the level of vWF). Further confirmation of severity using RIPA may be useful in some cases. In some cases, a desmopressin challenge (or DDAVP trial), as typically performed for therapy assessment, may also have additional diagnostic utility, given that post DDAVP laboratory findings can be used to firm up a diagnosis [39]. Thus, in Type 1 vWD, post DDAVP laboratory findings should also show a Type 1 vWD laboratory test pattern. The PFA-100® may also have a role in this post DDAVP evaluation setting [40].

Identification of Type 2 vWD—A discordant pattern is obtained if functional test results (i.e., FVIII:C, vWF:CB, and/or vWF:RCo) are substantially lower than vWF:Ag (Table 17.1 and Figure 17.1). In these cases, Type 2A, 2B, 2N, or 2M vWD is likely. It should be noted that discordance using a vWF:Ag and vWF:RCo test combination is not always apparent upon single testing; again, it is important to repeat the assays to confirm or discount previous findings. If discordance between vWF:Ag and "vWF:function" (i.e., vWF:RCo and/or vWF:CB) is confirmed upon repeat testing, then there is an indication to perform RIPA analysis. If RIPA is reduced, then Type 2A or Type 2M vWD is suggested. If RIPA is enhanced, then Type 2B vWD or PT-vWD is suggested.

In Type 2A vWD and in Type 2B vWD, vWF:CB/vWF:Ag ratios generally tend to be lower than vWF:RCo/vWF:Ag, because the vWF:CB is generally more sensitive to the loss of HMW vWF than vWF:RCo. In Type 2M vWD, vWF:RCo/vWF:Ag ratios generally tend to be lower than vWF:CB/vWF:Ag because most cases of Type 2M

Table 17.1 Typical laboratory patterns in vWD[a]

vWD type:	1	2A	2B[b]	2N	2M	3
Laboratory assay:						
(i) Screening tests:						
PT	Normal	Normal	Normal	Normal	Normal	Normal
APTT	Elevated (/normal)	Elevated (/normal)	Normal (/elevated)	Elevated (/normal)	Normal (/elevated)	Elevated
Platelet count	Normal	Normal	Low (/normal)	Normal	Normal	Normal
PFA-100® (closure time; CT)	Elevated/ (normal)	Elevated/no closure	Elevated/no closure	Normal	Elevated/no closure	Elevated/no closure
(ii) Diagnostic assays: [c, d, e]						
FVIII:C	Low (/normal)	Low (/normal)	Low/normal	Proportionally low	Normal/low	Low ("<20 U/dL")
vWF:Ag	Low ("<50 U/dL")	Low (/normal)	Low/normal	Normal (/low)	Normal/low	Very low ("<5 U/dL")
vWF:RCo	Low/ (occasionally normal)	Low ("<30 U/dL")	Low (occasionally normal)	Normal (/low)	Low (/normal)	Very low ("<5 U/dL")
vWF:CB	Low/ (occasionally normal)	Very low ("<15 U/dL")	Low ("<40 U/dL")	Normal (/low)	Low (/normal)	Very low ("<5 U/dL")
vWF:RCo to vWF:Ag ratio[f, g]	Normal (">0.6")	Low ("<0.6")	Low ("<0.6")	Normal (">0.6")	Low/normal	variable— don't use
vWF:CB to vWF:Ag ratio[f, g]	Normal (">0.6")	Low ("<0.6")	Low ("<0.6")	Normal (">0.6")	Low/normal	variable— don't use
(iii) Confirmative/ vWD subtyping assays:						
vWF:FVIII binding assay:						
bound FVIII/ bound vWF ratio:	Normal (">0.6")	Normal (">0.6")	Normal (">0.6")	Low ("<0.6")	Normal (">0.6")	variable— don't use
RIPA—ristocetin:						
Low dose (0.5 mg/mL):	Absent	Absent	Present	Absent	Absent	Absent
1.0 mg/mL:	Reduced (/normal)	Reduced	Normal	Normal	Reduced (/normal)	Absent
1.5 mg/mL:	Reduced (/normal)	Reduced (/normal)	Normal	Normal	Reduced (/normal)	Absent

(*Continued*)

Table 17.1 (*Continued*)

vWD type:	1	2A	2B[b]	2N	2M	3
vWF:Multimer pattern	Normal pattern, vWF reduced	Large to intermediate multimers missing	Large multimers missing	Normal	Normal vWF multimer distribution (but with possible abnormal bands)	multimers "absent"

[a]Values within the table are approximate guide values only; different laboratories may derive different reference ranges.

[b]Pseudo- or 'platelet-type' (PT) vWD patterns are similar to those for Type 2B vWD.

[c]For vWF and FVIII: values >50 U/dL usually considered normal; however, single or individual 'normal' assay results cannot discount vWD.

[d]For vWF and FVIII: values <50 U/dL usually considered abnormal; however, single or individual 'abnormal' assay results do not diagnose vWD.

[e]Normal reference ranges vary between laboratories, tests and methods; lower vWF values expected in blood group O individuals.

[f]For 2A vWD, CB/Ag ratio generally lower than RCo/Ag because vWF:CB generally more sensitive to loss of HMW vWF than vWF:RCo.

[g]For 2M vWD, discordance in RCo/Ag or CB/Ag depends on the specific defect defined by the 2M vWD (i.e., platelet adhesion or matrix adhesion).

However, most Type 2M vWD so far defined show inherent vWF-platelet-adhesion defect (not inherent vWF-collagen adhesion defect), so, in these cases of Type 2M, RCo/Ag ratio is lower than CB/Ag ratio.

vWD so far described show an inherent vWF-platelet-adhesion defect rather than a vWF-collagen-adhesion defect. If required, Types 2A and 2M vWD can be differentiated using vWF:multimer analysis. Types 2A and 2M vWD can often also be differentiated by differential test patterns with vWF:CB and vWF:RCo, whereby vWF:RCo/vWF:Ag ratios are typically low, but vWF:CB/vWF:Ag ratios are often normal [1, 4, 19, 38]. It might also be useful to perform RIPA testing, or a DDAVP trial, as these will also facilitate differentiation between these two disorders [4, 39, 40].

If RIPA analysis shows enhanced responsiveness (i.e., at ≤0.5 mg/mL), then Type 2B or a PT-vWD is indicated [4, 7]. Mixtures of platelets and plasma from patients and normal subjects can help to identify if the defect is plasma- or platelet-related [7]. Thus, Type 2B vWD will show enhanced ristocetin responsiveness in mixed samples comprising normal platelets and patient plasma, but generally not with patient platelets and normal plasma. PT-vWD will show the opposite pattern, and give enhanced ristocetin responsiveness in mixed samples comprising patient platelets and normal plasma, but not with normal platelets and

patient plasma. Differentiation between Type 2B and PT-vWD is important since individuals with these disorders are managed differently.

Phenotypic discordance between vWF:Ag and FVIII:C (i.e., FVIII/vWF ratio <0.7), confirmed by repeat testing, usually indicates hemophilia A, but Type 2N vWD is possible. Some guidance will be offered by family history studies (i.e., sex-linked or not). If Type 2N vWD is suspected, then specific vWF:FVIIIB testing should be performed. If the FVIII bound to vWF is reduced in this assay (ratio of FVIII/vWF <0.6), then Type 2N vWD is likely [35, 36]. Alternatively, if the FVIII bound to vWF in the vWF:FVIIIB assay is not reduced (ratio of bound FVIII/vWF >0.6), then Type 2N vWD is unlikely, and hemophilia A is probable. Discrimination of Type 2N vWD from hemophilia A is clinically important, both from the viewpoint of treatment modalities and also genetic counseling. It is important to note, however, that a lack of discordance between vWF and FVIII:C screening assays will not always exclude Type 2N vWD [35, 36], so direct analysis using the specific vWF:FVIIIB assay should always be performed if there is a clinical suspicion of Type 2N vWD, even if initial vWF and FVIII:C discordance is not observed. Type 2N vWD can also be defined by molecular methods (see Chapter 18).

Identification of Type 3 vWD: If the initial test results reveal that vWF was not detectable using any vWF assay (i.e., vWF:Ag, vWF:CB, and vWF:RCo), then Type 3 vWD is suggested. Repeat testing should be performed to confirm the severity of the disease. Remember that low-level sensitivity issues may be a problem, particularly with vWF:RCo [16]. Molecular manifestations of Type 3 vWD are addressed in Chapter 18.

Desmopressin challenge, factor concentrate pharmacokinetic (PK) studies and vWF propeptide testing: Although therapeutic management of vWD is not a focus of this review, it is also important to consider the potential value of a desmopressin challenge or factor concentrate PKs to the diagnosis of vWD. Assessment of vWF propeptide levels may also be useful in the context of vWD studies and may permit more clinically relevant diagnosis and better discrimination of Types 1, 2A, 2M, and 3 vWD, as well as identifying vWF "secretory" vWD defects versus "clearance" defects [2, 39–41]. vWF propeptide levels are often evaluated within the context of a DDAVP trial, but can also be assessed without such a trial [41].

Recommendations and conclusions

1 Assessment of vWD requires both a thorough clinical evaluation and appropriate laboratory testing.
2 All relevant clinical criteria should be considered, especially bleeding and family history, but also age, gender, recent drug history, ABO blood group, pregnancy, and estrogen replacement therapy.
3 As a screening process, and to exclude the presence of other hypocoagulopathic disorders, it would be reasonable to perform PT, APTT, fibrinogen, thrombin time, platelet count, FVIII:C, and vWF:Ag plus at least one (but preferably two) functional vWF assays (i.e., vWF:CB and vWF:RCo). If time is critical, a more pragmatic approach (e.g., inclusion of PFA-100® and specific coagulation factors) might be indicated.
4 Alternatively, if vWD is strongly suggested by clinical history, family studies, or previous testing, then a more direct comprehensive laboratory assessment is indicated. This may include retesting of the initial test panel for confirmation, plus RIPA and/or vWF:multimers and/or vWF:FVIIIB studies as specifically indicated.
5 All abnormal laboratory results should be repeated at least once, in order to confirm previous findings and to exclude potential specimen collection, laboratory testing, or artifacts. Similarly, when there is a moderate or strong clinical index of suspicion, all borderline or normal laboratory findings should also be repeated for confirmation (because of assay variation and individual fluctuations). Tests should also be repeated if the original sampling period might have resulted in spurious findings (e.g., samples taken during pregnancy, or from anxious patients (especially pediatric samples), or subsequent to strenuous exercise, as elevated vWD and FVIII:C may arise and mask a possible vWD).
6 The possibility of a platelet defect, or some specific factor deficiency should also be considered if clinically indicated (e.g., abnormal bleeding but normal vWF studies, or severe abnormal bleeding but only moderately low vWF).

Acknowledgments

The author would like to thank all personnel from his laboratory for the ongoing technical support over the past many years.

References

1. Favaloro EJ. Von Willebrand disease: local diagnosis and management of a globally distributed bleeding disorder. *Semin Thromb Hemost.* 2011;37:440–455.
2. Sadler JE, Budde U, Eikenboom JCJ, et al. Update on the pathophysiology and classification of von Willebrand disease: a report of the Subcommittee on von Willebrand Factor. *J Thromb Haemost.* 2006;4:2103–2114.
3. Laffan M, Brown SA, Collins PW, et al. The diagnosis of von Willebrand disease: a guideline from the UK Haemophilia Centre Doctors' Organization. *Haemophilia.* 2004;10:199–217.
4. Favaloro EJ. Diagnosis and classification of von Willebrand disease: a review of the differential utility of various functional von Willebrand factor assays. *Blood Coag Fibrinolysis.* 2011;22:553–564.
5. Ball J, Malia RG, Greaves M, Preston FE. Demonstration of abnormal factor VIII multimers in acquired von

Willebrand's disease associated with a circulating inhibitor. *Br J Haematol.* 1987;65:95–100

6. Franchini M, Lippi G, Favaloro EJ. Etiology and diagnosis of acquired von Willebrand syndrome. *Clin Adv Hematol Oncol.* 2010;8:20–24.

7. Favaloro EJ. Phenotypic identification of platelet-type von Willebrand disease and its discrimination from type 2B von Willebrand disease: a question of 2B or not 2B? A story of nonidentical twins? Or two sides of a multidenominational or multifaceted primary-hemostasis coin? *Semin Thromb Hemost.* 2008;34:113–127.

8. Favaloro EJ. An update on the von Willebrand factor collagen binding assay: 21 years of age and beyond adolescence, but not yet a mature adult. *Semin Thromb Hemost.* 2007;33:727–744.

9. Favaloro EJ, Lippi G, Adcock DM. Preanalytical and postanalytical variables: the leading causes of diagnostic error in hemostasis? *Semin Thromb Hemost.* 2008;34:612–634.

10. Favaloro EJ, Funk (Adcock) D, Lippi G. Preanalytical variables in coagulation testing associated to diagnostic errors in hemostasis. *Lab Med.* 2012;43:54-60.

11. Favaloro EJ. The utility of the PFA-100® in the identification of von Willebrand disease: A concise review. *Semin Thromb Hemost.* 2006;32:537–545.

12. Favaloro EJ. Clinical Utility of the PFA-100. *Semin Thromb Hemost.* 2008;34:709–733.

13. Favaloro EJ, Lippi G, Franchini M. Contemporary platelet function testing. *Clin Chem Lab Med.* 2010;48:579–598.

14. Mezzano D, Quiroga T, Pereira J. The level of laboratory testing required for diagnosis or exclusion of a platelet function disorder using platelet aggregation and secretion assays. *Semin Thromb Hemost.* 2009;35:242–254.

15. Favaloro EJ, Bonar R, Meiring M, Street A, Marsden K; RCPA QAP in Haematology. 2B or not 2B? Disparate discrimination of functional VWF discordance using different assay panels or methodologies may lead to success or failure in the early identification of type 2B VWD. *Thromb Haemost.* 2007;98:346–358.

16. Favaloro EJ, Bonar R, Marsden K (on behalf of the RCPA QAP Haemostasis Committee). Lower limit of assay sensitivity: an under-recognised and significant problem in von Willebrand disease identification and classification. *Clin Lab Sci.* 2008;21:178–185.

17. Hillarp A, Stadler M, Haderer C, Weinberger J, Kessler CM, Romisch J. Improved performance characteristics of the von Willebrand factor ristocetin cofactor activity assay using a novel automated assay protocol. *J Thromb Haemost.* 2010;8:2216–2223.

18. Favaloro EJ, Mohammed S, McDonald J. Validation of improved performance characteristics for the automated von Willebrand factor ristocetin cofactor activity assay. *J Thromb Haemost.* 2010;8:2842–2844.

19. Favaloro EJ. Diagnosis of type 1 versus 2A and 2M von Willebrand disease. *Haemophilia.* 2012;18:e9–e11.

20. Vanhoorelbeke K, Cauwenberghs N, Vauterin S, Schlammadinger A, Mazurier C, Deckmyn H. A reliable and reproducible ELISA method to measure ristocetin cofactor activity of von Willebrand factor. *Thromb Haemost.* 2000;83:107–113.

21. Federici AB, Canciani MT, Forza I, et al. A sensitive ristocetin co-factor activity assay with recombinant glycoprotein Ibα for the diagnosis of patients with low von Willebrand factor levels. *Haematologica.* 2004;89:77–85.

22. Vanhoorelbeke K, Pareyn I, Schlammadinger A, et al. Plasma glycocalicin as a source of GPIb alpha in the von Willebrand factor in the ristocetin cofactor ELISA. *Thromb Haemost.* 2005;93:165–171.

23. Rodgers SE, Lloyd JV, Mangos HM, Duncan EM, McRae SJ. Diagnosis and management of adult patients with von Willebrand disease in South Australia. *Semin Thromb Hemost.* 2011;37:535–541.

24. Chen D, Tange JI, Meyers BJ, Pruthi RK, Nichols WL, Heit JA. Validation of an automated latex particle-enhanced immunoturbidimetric von Willebrand factor activity assay. *J Thromb Haemost.* 2011;9:1993–2002.

25. Chen D, Daigh CA, Hendricksen JI, Pruthi RK, Nichols WL, Heit JA, Owen WG. A highly-sensitive plasma von Willebrand factor ristocetin cofactor (VWF:RCo) activity assay by flow cytometry. *J Thromb Haemost.* 2008;6:323–330.

26. Giannini S, Mezzasoma AM, Leone M, Gresele P. Laboratory diagnosis and monitoring of desmopressin treatment of von Willebrand's disease by flow cytometry. *Haematologica.* 2007;92:1647–1654.

27. Favaloro EJ. Evaluation of commercial von Willebrand factor collagen binding assays to assist the discrimination of types 1 and 2 von Willebrand disease. *Thromb Haemost.* 2010;104:1009–1021.

28. Favaloro EJ. Internal Quality Control and External Quality Assurance of Platelet Function Tests. *Semin Thromb Hemost.* 2009;35:139–149.

29. Federici AB, Mannucci PM, Castaman G, et al. Clinical and molecular predictors of thrombocytopenia and risk of bleeding in patients with von Willebrand disease type 2B: a cohort study of 67 patients. *Blood.* 2009;113:526–534.

30. Favaloro EJ, Koutts J. 2B or not 2B? Masquerading as von Willebrand disease? *J Thromb Haemost.* 2012;10:317–319.

31. Adcock DM, Bethel M, Valcour A. Diagnosing von Willebrand disease: a large reference laboratory's perspective. *Semin Thromb Hemost.* 2006;32:472–479.

32. Meijer P, Haverkate F. An external quality assessment program for von Willebrand factor laboratory analysis: an overview from the European concerted action on thrombosis and disabilities foundation. *Semin Thromb Hemost*. 2006;32:485–491.

33. Chandler WL, Peerschke EI, Castellone DD, Meijer P, on behalf of the NASCOLA Proficiency Testing Committee. von Willebrand factor assay proficiency testing: the North American Specialized Coagulation Laboratory Association experience. *Am J Clin Pathol*. 2011;135:862–869.

34. Favaloro EJ. Detailed von Willebrand factor multimer analysis in patients with von Willebrand disease in the European study, molecular and clinical markers for the diagnosis and management of type 1 von Willebrand disease (MCMDM-1VWD): a rebuttal. *J Thromb Haemost*. 2008;6:1999–2001.

35. Rodgers SE, Lerda NV, Favaloro EJ, et al. Identification of von Willebrand's disorder type 2N (Normandy) in Australia: A cross-laboratory investigation using different methodologies. *Am J Clin Pathol*. 2002;118:269–276.

36. Favaloro EJ, Mohammed S, Koutts J. Identification and prevalence of von Willebrand Disease type 2N (Normandy) in Australia. *Blood Coag Fibrinolysis*. 2009;20:706–714.

37. Favaloro EJ, Bonar R, Kershaw G, et al. Reducing errors in identification of von Willebrand disease: The experience of the Royal college of Pathologists of Australasia Quality Assurance Program. *Semin Thromb Hemost*. 2006;32:505–513.

38. Keeling D, Beavis J, Marr R, Sukhu K, Bignell P. A family with type 2M VWD with normal VWF:RCo but reduced VWF:CB and a M1761K mutation in the A3 domain. *Haemophilia*. 2012;18:e33.

39. Favaloro EJ, Thom J, Patterson D, et al. Desmopressin therapy to assist the functional identification and characterisation of von Willebrand disease: differential utility from combining two (VWF:CB and VWF:RCo) von Willebrand factor activity assays? *Thromb Res*. 2009;123:862–868.

40. Favaloro EJ, Thom J, Patterson D, et al. Potential supplementary utility of combined PFA-100 and functional VWF testing for the laboratory assessment of desmopressin and factor concentrate therapy in von Willebrand disease. *Blood Coag Fibrinolysis*. 2009;20:475–483.

41. Casonato A, Daidone V, Roberto Padrini R. Assessment of von Willebrand Factor Propeptide Improves the Diagnosis of von Willebrand Disease. *Semin Thromb Hemost*. 2011;37:456–463.

42. Budde U, Pieconka A, Will K, Schneppenheim R. Laboratory testing for von Willebrand disease: contribution of multimer analysis to diagnosis and classification. *Semin Thromb Hemost*. 2006;32:514–521.

18 Laboratory analysis of von Willebrand disease: molecular analysis

Anne C. Goodeve[1,2] *& Ian R. Peake*[1]

[1] Sheffield Haemostasis Research Group, Department of Cardiovascular Science, University of Sheffield, Sheffield, UK
[2] Sheffield Diagnostic Genetic Service, Sheffield Children's NHS Foundation Trust, Sheffield, UK

Introduction

The common inherited bleeding disorder, von Willebrand disease (VWD), results from deficient or defective plasma von Willebrand factor (VWF). Two important hemostatic roles are played by VWF: binding to and thus protecting factor VIII (FVIII) from premature proteolytic degradation, whilst delivering it to the sites of vascular damage plus binding platelets to subendothelium at these same sites. The disorder is divided into three types: types 1 and 3 are partial and virtually complete quantitative deficiencies whereas type 2 represents qualitative defects and is further divided into four subtypes: 2A, 2B, 2M, and 2N dependent upon the function perturbed [1]. The VWF gene (*VWF*), located on chromosome 12 encodes the large 2813-amino acid VWF protein. Its repeated domain structure is illustrated in Figure 18.1.

VWF comprises 52 exons that span 178 kb of genomic DNA. *VWFP*, an incomplete pseudogene on chromosome 22, has 97% sequence similarity to the gene [2], and may complicate molecular analysis. PCR primer design must therefore be biased toward amplification of the gene and not the pseudogene. *VWF* mutation analysis has been undertaken since the gene was first cloned in the 1980s [3]. The International Society on Thrombosis and Haemostasis Scientific and Standardisation Committee on VWF (ISTH SSC on VWF) database (VWFdb) [4] lists information on previously identified *VWF* mutations and currently has 560 entries, giving an indication of the extent of analysis undertaken by many laboratories worldwide.

Mutation analysis was initially undertaken to understand the molecular basis of VWD. Subsequently, some mutation analysis has moved into diagnostic laboratories and analysis is currently undertaken in both research and diagnostic situations. This article considers particularly quality control issues in molecular genetic analysis of VWD and so has relevance especially for diagnostic laboratories. However, many of the issues discussed also apply to obtaining correct mutation results in the research setting. Only a brief description of VWD types and mutations responsible is presented, as this information is abundantly available elsewhere [1, 5, 6].

Type 3 VWD

This is the severest form of VWD where plasma VWF levels are generally undetectable. It is autosomal recessively inherited and has a prevalence between 0.5 and 6 per million population [7–9]. Type 3 VWD is most common in populations where consanguineous relationships are common. Carriers are often asymptomatic but homozygous or compound heterozygous affected individuals can have severe bleeding problems that may require the infusion of blood products containing VWF.

A number of population-based studies have sought mutations in patients with type 3 VWD [10–13], many

Quality in Laboratory Hemostasis and Thrombosis, Second Edition. Edited by Steve Kitchen, John D. Olson and F. Eric Preston.
© 2013 John Wiley & Sons, Ltd. Published 2013 by Blackwell Publishing Ltd.

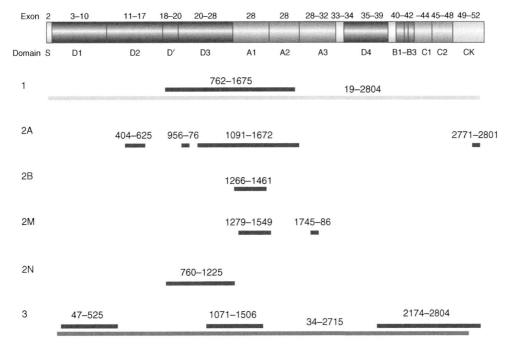

Figure 18.1 Location of VWF point mutations in patients with von Willebrand disease (VWD). The top panel shows VWF domain structure with the exons encoding each domain indicated. The panels below show the main location of mutations identified in each VWD type. The dark blue line in type 1 VWD denotes the most common mutation locations while the pale blue line denotes the less commonly occurring mutations. In type 3 VWD, the dark blue line denotes missense mutation locations while the mid blue line denotes null allele locations.

of which are reported on VWFdb [4, 14]. Only a small number of large deletions have been reported, but this may partly result from the difficulty, until recently, in identifying large heterozygous deletions (see below). Point mutations are located throughout *VWF* (Figure 18.1) and largely result in the lack of VWF expression (null alleles).

An increasing number of diagnostic laboratories offer full analysis of *VWF* for mutations. This comprises dosage analysis to determine presence of large deletions or duplications, plus DNA sequence analysis of exons 1–52 covering the entire protein-coding region, including intron–exon boundaries. Prenatal diagnosis in VWD is infrequently requested and is generally carried out only in cases of type 3 disease.

Type 2 VWD

Type 2 VWD patients have plasma VWF that has abnormal function in relation to the binding of VWF to platelets via the GpIbα receptor, to subendothelium or to circulating factor VIII.

Type 2A VWD

Classic type 2A VWD is dominantly inherited and results from missense mutations within the A2, or less frequently A1 domains of VWF encoded by exon 28 [15]. These mutations can result in VWF that shows increased susceptibility to proteolysis by ADAMTS13, the plasma metalloprotease which moderates VWF function by cleavage, thus reducing the number of the largest, most hemostatically active multimeric forms of VWF in plasma [16]. Mutations in the D3 domain, encoded by sequence variants in exons 22 and 25–27 have been reported recently [17], with a distinct type 2A(IIE) multimer profile on high-resolution gels that reflect reduced ADAMTS13 proteolysis through reduced satellite ("triplet") bands. Missense mutations frequently result in the loss or gain of cysteine

205

residues. Rarer missense mutations that can be either dominantly or recessively inherited affect dimerization (CK domain, exon 52), demonstrated through odd-sized multimer bands (2A (IID)) or multimerization (D2 domain, exons 11–17, 2A (IIC)), which is recessively inherited. Second mutations may be non-expressed in recessively inherited cases.

In practice, sequence analysis of exon 28 often reveals a causative mutation that is highly penetrant and dominantly inherited. Type 2A VWD is a moderately severe bleeding condition and knowledge of the causative mutation within a family can be of value in genetic counseling and in confirming an individual's diagnosis when phenotypic tests are uninformative or unavailable. If an exon 28 mutation is not identified or recessive inheritance is suspected, other regions of *VWF* may be analyzed (exons 22, 25–27, 11–17, and 52) (Figure 18.1).

Type 2B VWD

Type 2B VWD is characterized by plasma VWF that has increased ability to bind to platelets through the GpIbα receptor, demonstrated in the laboratory by enhanced ristocetin-induced platelet agglutination (RIPA). This can result in platelet microthrombi and a reduced platelet count (thrombocytopenia) for the majority of type 2B mutations, particularly when patients are exposed to stress [18]. As a result, and also due to enhanced ADAMTS13 cleavage resulting from the altered VWF conformation [19], the plasma multimeric profile in type 2B VWD may show reduced levels of HMW VWF multimers. Missense mutations in type 2B VWD are found in the A1 domain that affect confirmation of the GpIbα binding site and analysis of *VWF* exon 28 will reveal mutations in most cases [15]. However, the possibility of platelet-type-pseudo VWD (PT-VWD) should also be contemplated if analysis of exon 28 does not identify a mutation. Missense mutations affecting two *GPIBA* codons have been identified; p.Gly249 and p.Met255 (legacy numbering Gly233, Met239) along with a single report of a 27 bp in-frame deletion p.Pro449_Ser457del (c.1345_1371del27) [20, 21]. These can readily be sought using one or two PCR amplifications and DNA sequence analysis. Mutations are listed on the Human Gene Mutation Database (HGMD) [22] and on the PT-VWD Registry and Database [23]. The relative frequency of 2B VWD and PT-VWD has been

investigated and PT-VWD may account for up to 15% of apparent 2B cases [21].

Type 2B VWD is dominantly inherited often with high penetrance, so knowledge of the causative mutation within a family can be of value in genetic counseling. Knowledge of the mutation could also guide treatment decisions; treatment with desmopressin increases the level of the patient's plasma VWF and can result in increased platelet–platelet binding through VWF and an increased risk of thrombocytopenia. However, this appears not to occur for all type 2B mutations; in patients with p.P1266L and p.R1308L mutations, no thrombocytopenia was reported [18]. It can also be important in differential diagnosis between type 2B VWD and PT-VWD, as treatment of the latter may also include platelet concentrates [24].

Type 2M VWD

Type 2M VWD is currently defined as occurring in individuals whose plasma VWF shows reduced ability to bind to platelets via GpIbα, or reduced ability to bind subendothelium and where HMW multimers are present [1]. This type can be difficult to distinguish from type 2A or type 1 without high-resolution multimer analysis. Missense mutations have been reported within the carboxyl terminal of the A1 domain [4] and in the A3 domain [25–27], with case reports in the D4–CK domains [4, 28] and in the D3 domain [28]. The condition is dominantly inherited often with high penetrance. Patients with A1 domain mutations may respond poorly to desmopressin and for this reason a precise diagnosis based on causative mutation detection would seem appropriate. Analysis of at least exon 28 should be undertaken.

Type 2N VWD

Type 2N VWD is characterized by reduced levels of plasma FVIII, often lower than the VWF levels, which can be within the normal range. Mutations affect the ability of VWF to bind FVIII (VWF:FVIIIB). Recessive inheritance of the disorder results from one of the three different scenarios: (1) homozygous missense mutation affecting VWF:FVIIIB; (2) compound heterozygous inheritance of two different missense mutations, both of which affect VWF:FVIIIB; and (3) one missense mutation affecting VWF:FVIIIB plus a nonexpressed (null) second allele. The latter situation occurs frequently [14], with p.R854Q occurring on at least one allele in up to 90% of European patients with type 2N VWD [15]. Missense mutations largely lie in the D′ domain encoded by exons 18–20, but case reports of mutations from exons 17–27 have been published [4]. As in type 3 VWD, mutations resulting in a null allele can be anywhere in *VWF*. Heterozygotes for a single missense mutation occasionally present with mildly reduced FVIII levels and a bleeding history [29], but they are frequently asymptomatic.

Phenotypically, the disorder often appears very similar to mild hemophilia A and bleeding is largely due to the reduced FVIII level, apart from in those patients who also have abnormal multimers [6]. A phenotypic VWF:FVIIIB assay can determine whether VWF has a reduced ability to bind FVIII and a commercial version of the assay has just become available [30–32]. Unless there is a reasonably extensive family history of bleeding, the two disorders cannot readily be discriminated by inheritance pattern and this may be further complicated as some female hemophilia carriers have low FVIII levels and experience bleeding symptoms. *VWF* or *F8* mutation analysis is frequently requested in order to discriminate mild hemophilia A (in males), symptomatic hemophilia A carriership (in females), and 2N VWD.

Type 2 VWD summary

Mutations in type 2 VWD have been reasonably well characterized and there is correlation between mutation location and VWF function affected, enabling targeted mutation analysis in many cases. Knowledge of the causative mutation(s) within a family can add to the ability to predict bleeding risk within individuals and can help to guide therapeutic decisions.

Type 1 VWD

Type 1 VWD is the commonest form of the disorder with up to 70% of cases being so classified. Originally, it was defined as affecting those VWD patients with reduced plasma levels of normal VWF as assessed by a normal ratio of protein to function (VWF:RCo/VWF:Ag as a specific activity) and a normal multimeric profile [33]. More recently [1], it has been accepted that subtle changes in the multimeric profile can be seen in the plasma VWF of some cases of type 1, notably in those most severely affected with the lowest levels of plasma VWF. The VWF:RCo/VWF:Ag ratio (which has been used to discriminate between type 1 and 2A, 2B, or 2M VWD), may also be below 0.7 [34], but the reliability of this assessment at low levels of VWF is poor [15].

Recently published multicenter studies on type 1 VWD from the United Kingdom, Europe, and Canada [35–38] have revealed extensive information on the mutations that can be found in type 1 VWD. The EU study [36, 38] used a nonselective recruitment strategy and consequently, 38% of the recruited index cases (IC) showed some evidence of abnormal multimer structure but not typical of types 2A or 2B VWD [36, 39]. In all but one of these 57 cases, a potentially causative mutation was identified and levels of plasma VWF:Ag were low (median 19 IU/dL) [36]. Of the remaining index cases with normal multimers, 54% had a detected change in *VWF*. In the Canadian study [35], which was more selective in its recruitment strategy, 63% had detectable *VWF* alterations. In the UK study [37], with recruitment criteria intermediate between the above two studies, candidate mutations were identified in 53% of cases. 65% of identified mutations from the three studies were missense, about 25% were predicted to result in in-frame deletions/insertions, exon skipping, or were promoter region changes, whilst the remaining 15% were predicted to result in null alleles [40]. Between 10% and 15% of patients had more than one candidate mutation identified, which included both allelic (including gene conversions) [35] and compound heterozygous changes [36].

The value of *VWF* analysis in type 1 VWD has been a matter of some debate particularly as it appears that mutations in this type of VWD, especially in the milder forms are less frequent and when present may demonstrate incomplete penetrance [5]. Within the complete EU cohort [36] of index cases with ≤20 IU/dL VWF:Ag, 97% had a detectable *VWF* mutation with 62% of these being fully penetrant and dominantly inherited. As such, knowledge of the mutation has potential benefit in genetic counseling as for type 2 VWD. IC with >40 IU/dL had only 46% chance of having a *VWF* change whilst 27% of their families demonstrated fully penetrant VWD. Several candidate mutations appeared to be incompletely penetrant and in many cases could be described as risk factors for bleeding. Determining sequence variants in such families has limited value in genetic counseling. For those patients with VWF:Ag between 21 and 40 IU/dL, 86% had a detectable *VWF* change, with 44% being fully penetrant and dominantly inherited. The penetrance and diagnostic significance of these "mutations" was very variable. Other factors, notably ABO blood group also influence VWF level and thus VWD penetrance, as demonstrated by the common variant p.Y1584C [41].

Mutation analysis

Point mutations

Two different approaches have been applied to *VWF* point mutation analysis using a mutation screening technique to seek amplicons with sequence alterations followed by DNA sequencing of those that indicate a sequence change, for example, confirmation-sensitive gel electrophoresis (CSGE) or single-strand confirmation polymorphism analysis [11, 36, 42] and direct DNA sequencing of all exons and intron–exon boundaries [43]. The latter approach has become more common as DNA sequencing has become cheaper and easier to undertake.

Screening techniques, for example, CSGE are poor for many regions of *VWF* due to the high number of single-nucleotide polymorphisms (SNP). The VWFdb [4] and the single nucleotide polymorphism database (dbSNP) [44] can be used to identify SNP locations within the gene and highlight those where, due to the presence of several SNP or particularly common SNP, sequencing alone should be used. Heterozygous SNP(s) result in a migration change indicating the presence of sequence alteration(s) and the amplicon bearing them requires sequencing to characterize the variant, so such SNP-containing regions should be sequenced from the outset. Regions of *VWF* known to lack SNP can be screened. However, no screening technique has 100% sensitivity for the detection of all sequence variants and the use of such techniques will result in some sequence variants remaining undetected.

The use of a single set of thermocycling conditions for PCR amplification [43] plus common-tailed PCR primers (e.g., using M13 sequences) to simplify DNA sequencing reaction set up can greatly enhance the speed of molecular analysis. Practice guidelines for DNA sequencing and analysis using software tools to identify mutations are available [5, 45].

Large deletions and duplications

Homozygous deletions of an exon up to the entire *VWF* gene resulting in type 3 VWD have been recognized for several years [4]. However, heterozygous large deletions along with homozygous or heterozygous large duplications have not been readily detectable until the recent advent of dosage analysis techniques. Multiplex ligation-dependent probe amplification (MLPA) is the most commonly used of these and has identified large heterozygous deletions in type 3 VWD [46, 47] and heterozygous deletions have also been described in types 1 and 2 VWD [47–49]. In type 3 VWD, screening for large deletions/duplications prior to analysis of the gene for point mutations may save time and resources, as they appear to be most common in this VWD type.

Mutation analysis in VWD

When is it necessary?
For a condition like VWD where patients may have differing levels of severity and where the disease may show autosomal dominant or recessive inheritance, decisions on whether *VWF* gene analysis is necessary for the benefit of the patient and their family are complex. The variable penetrance of clinical VWD within a family adds to this complexity.

The following points should be considered when, in a diagnostic setting, *VWF* analysis is contemplated. The same considerations could also be addressed in the research environment when assessing the value of gene analysis in understanding the etiology of VWD.
1 The clinical severity of the condition that is present in the index case and affected family members. It is clear that *VWF* mutations are highly prevalent in the severest forms of VWD and that these mutations are highly penetrant. In milder cases of type 1 VWD, any candidate mutations identified are likely to display incomplete penetrance, in that not all the individuals inheriting the change will have symptoms. Such sequence alterations should be treated as risk factors for bleeding.
2 The value of *VWF* analysis in relation to the desirability of early neonatal diagnosis or, in the severest forms, prenatal diagnosis.

3 The possible association between a particular mutation and treatment.

4 The value of *VWF* analysis as a complement to phenotypic analysis where the latter results are unclear.

5 The cost benefit of *VWF* analysis.

What to analyze?

Table 18.1 suggests regions of *VWF* that should be analyzed in each VWD type.

Missing mutations and too many mutations

Mutations are not found in all VWD patients, even in phenotypically well-characterized VWD, and there are many possible explanations for this. Dosage analysis has only recently been introduced and the extent of contribution of large deletions and duplications to VWD pathogenesis is not yet established. In type 3 VWD, between 83% and 100% of predicted mutations were identified in large cohort studies [50]

whereas in type 2 VWD, more than 80% of expected mutations are identified (Enayat S, personal communication, October 2007). In type 1 VWD, a candidate mutation may be identified in up to 70% of cases [35–37, 51, 52]. Mutations may be missed by the analysis or lie outside the regions of the gene analyzed. *VWF* has an unusually large number of SNP; PCR primers should be checked whenever there is a new build of the human genome to determine whether there are SNPs within the primer sequences used for PCR amplification. An online tool, SNPCheck, is available to facilitate this analysis [53]. If only one allele has amplified due to allele dropout, an undetected candidate mutation on the nonamplified allele may be missed. Occasionally, the converse is seen; an apparently homozygous mutation may seemingly pass from one generation to the next due to allele dropout of the normal allele.

Intronic sequence alterations leading to changes in splicing may occur. Although not yet reported in VWD, examples of point mutations deep in introns

Table 18.1 Suggested extent of *VWF* analysis in patients with VWD

VWD type	Initial screen of exon no.	Additional screen of exon no./gene	Comments
1	18–28	Promoter-17 and 29–52, 1–52 dosage analysis	55% mutations located in central *VWF* region but significant proportion elsewhere. Heterozygous large deletions/duplications can be identified by dosage analysis
2A	28	11–17, 22, 25–27, 52, 1–52 dosage analysis	Screen additional exons if exon 28 mutation not identified or recessive inheritance is suspected. In the latter case, the second mutation may be a null allele, which can be located throughout *VWF*. Heterozygous large deletions/duplications can be identified by dosage analysis
2B	28	*GP1BA*	Screen *GP1BA* for mutations resulting in PT-VWD if exon 28 mutation is not identified. Plasma mixing studies may also clarify phenotype
2M	28	29–32, 52	Mutations 3′ of exon 28 have occasionally been identified [6]
2N	18–20	17, 21–27 *F8*	Screen additional exons if no missense mutations identified in exons 18–20. Phenotype analysis may indicate whether two VWF-FVIIIB missense mutations or a missense plus a null mutation are expected. Mutations resulting in null alleles can be located throughout *VWF*. If no mutations are identified, (mild) hemophilia A, or hemophilia A carriership may be responsible for the phenotype and the *F8* gene can be analyzed.
3	1–52 dosage analysis	1–52 point mutation analysis	Mutations are located throughout *VWF*, with no particular hotspot. Heterozygous large deletions/duplications can be identified by dosage analysis. Linkage analysis is possible for PND.

creating novel splice sites that lead to aberrant mRNA species have been described in hemophilia A and disrupt normal FVIII production [54, 55]. The mutations were detected using mRNA analysis and this may be helpful where *VWF* mutations cannot be identified in genomic DNA. Alterations in splicing may also result from changes to splice enhancers and repressors [56], whose role has not yet been explored in VWD.

The recent studies on type 1 VWD [35–37] analyzed the *VWF* promoter region and identified a number of sequence alterations. The majority were absent from normal individuals but the pathogenic significance of only one mutation; a 13 bp deletion, has so far been demonstrated [57]. It is possible that other promoter sequence variants could result in reduced VWF expression from one allele. Promoter analysis may be justified in the future if such variants are shown to contribute significantly to reduced VWF levels.

In a small number of patients, more mutations than expected are detected; these may result from gene conversion [58] mediated by *VWFP* [59]. Up to five different single-nucleotide substitutions have been reported to occur on a single allele as a result of gene conversion [35]. All of the above possibilities should be borne in mind and mentioned where relevant when reporting mutations identified.

Some sequence variants, previously reported as candidate mutations, may have only a minor or no effect on VWF expression, for example, pR924Q and p.P2063S, and so are erroneously thought to contribute significantly to disease pathogenesis [60–62].

Prenatal diagnosis

Prenatal diagnosis is rarely requested in VWD, but type 3 VWD families who already have one affected child may wish to know the VWD status of further pregnancies. In these instances, where the familial mutation(s) has already been identified, the mutation(s) can be sought by targeted PCR and DNA sequencing or by dosage analysis. Where familial mutations have not been identified prior to pregnancy and time for mutation analysis is short, linkage analysis can be used. *VWF* has a number of short tandem repeat (STR) polymorphisms located in intron 40

[63, 64] and the promoter [65]. These can be analyzed singly using PCR amplification and gel electrophoresis or can be fluorescently labeled, amplified as a multiplex, and genotyped using a DNA sequencer [66].

Maternal and chorionic villus sample (CVS) DNA should be analyzed to confirm that maternal cell contamination of fetal material is absent; practice guidelines are available [67]. This can be achieved using, for example, the Powerplex 16 system (Promega) where a number of STR loci from around the genome are analysed. At least two separate CVS fronds should be independently analyzed [68].

Internal quality control

Guidelines on internal quality control in molecular genetics describe procedures to achieve reliable results [68].

A water blank should be included with every PCR amplification to ensure that there is no contamination of PCR reagents by exogenous DNA. No amplified product should be visible in the amplification from this tube. Whenever any product is seen, all simultaneously amplified PCR products should be discarded.

Ensure that only *VWF*, and not *VWFP*, has been amplified. PCR primers should be designed with both gene and pseudogene sequences available and mismatches with *VWFP* incorporated at the 3′ end. One should suspect that *VWFP* has also been amplified if a number of apparently heterozygous changes are seen within one amplicon. Gene–pseudogene mismatch positions may be responsible.

Always repeat the sequence of an amplicon in which a candidate mutation has been identified, preferably on a separately extracted DNA sample (from a blood sample taken on a different day if possible), or at least from a separate PCR amplification.

A second scientist should independently check sequences, nucleotide number, and base change, and its predicted effect on the protein.

When analyzing family members for a previously identified mutation, include a familial positive control where possible. If the mutation in the index case was not originally determined by the laboratory undertaking the analysis of a subsequent family member and the DNA sample from the index case is not available, the report should highlight the identity of the laboratory undertaking the original analysis and their report date. This is particularly important where the familial mutation is absent.

When a sequence alteration is identified, the use of VWFdb [4], dbSNP [44] and a review of the literature using both legacy and HGVS VWF numbering (legacy cDNA numbering was from the transcription start site, 250 bp 5′ to the currently used A of the initiation codon. Legacy amino acid numbering was from Ser764 of mature VWF, rather than from the initiator methionine) should identify reports of the variant. If it has been previously reported as a mutation, determine whether the phenotype of the current patient is similar to that in previous patients. If it is not, review the patient phenotype and be cautious.

For previously unreported missense mutations, a number of online predictions of pathogenicity based on amino acid evolutionary conservation can be used [69]; these include SIFT, PolyPhen2, and Align GVGD. The combined use of such predictions can be undertaken to try and achieve a consensus and to help predict the possible deleterious nature of any change. Practice guidelines are available [69].

Similarly, if a sequence alteration is suspected to have an effect on mRNA splicing, a number of prediction tools are available. In a comparative analysis of their performance, the four best performing algorithms were NNSplice, MaxEntScan, Gene-Splicer, and SSFL [70]. At the consensus donor and acceptor splice site dinucleotides, GT and AG, the algorithms always predict a large change in splice site signal. Variations in the sequence further away than −10 or +7 from the splice junction do not predict any reduction in the signal, but are useful within that interval. The prediction tools can also be used to identify new splice sites that may be created further into the introns. Where an effect on splicing is likely, follow-up by platelet mRNA analysis can confirm the prediction [71].

External quality control

No materials are currently available for external quality control. Immortalized cell line DNA containing known *VWF* mutations may become available in the future through the UK National Institute for Biological Standards and Control (NIBSC).

External quality assessment

An external quality assessment (EQA) scheme is available through UK NEQAS for Blood Coagulation on the molecular genetics of hemophilia [72]. This scheme runs twice-yearly exercises that assess proficiency in the genetic analysis of hemophilia A, hemophilia B, and VWD [73]; other hemostasis genetic analysis EQA schemes may also be available. As with other molecular genetic EQA schemes, the three areas of clerical accuracy, genotyping, and interpretation are examined. Marks are lost for errors in each of these three areas. Essential content for genetic analysis reports is given below.

Reporting

The development of standard templates for commonly used report types can help to avoid missing essential information. Reports should be written so that they can follow the patient and be interpreted by different health care professionals. A practice guideline describes essential components [74].

Nomenclature

Standard abbreviations for VWF and its activities should follow ISTH SSC on VWF recommendations [75]. Nucleotide and amino acid numbering and nomenclature for sequence alterations should follow current Human Genome Variation Society (HGVS) recommendations [76, 77] with nucleotide numbering from the "A" of the initiator ATG and amino acid numbering from the first methionine. GenBank reference sequences with version numbers should be stated for both cDNA and protein (currently NM_000552.3 and NP_000543.2).

Report inclusions

The following information is required by UK NEQAS to be present in genetic analysis reports, as it is necessary for complete understanding of patient mutation data and its interpretation.

1 The laboratory name, address, and contact details for the individual(s) undertaking VWD genetic analysis.

2 The identity of the patient by first name, family name, date of birth plus at least one further unique identifier, such as the hospital number.

3 Referring clinician's name and address and those for recipients of any copies.

4 Clinical question being investigated.

5 Patient's levels for VWF:Ag, VWF:RCo, and FVIII:C. Where relevant, also the results of other phenotypic assays such as VWF:FVIIIB, RIPA, platelet count, and multimer analysis.

6 Disease and gene being examined, with gene name (VWF) following HUGO Gene Nomenclature Committee (HGNC) recommendations [78].

7 Overall results or conclusion clearly visible, for example, in bold text.

8 The extent of molecular analysis undertaken and if relevant, reference to the method. This can be added as a footnote.

9 The relationship between the patient and the index case where there is a family history of VWD.

10 Where a mutation(s) was identified, whether the individual was homozygous, heterozygous, or compound heterozygous (if known).

11 The nucleotide change and predicted effect on the protein as a single block of text, following HGVS guidelines, for example, c.3614G>A, predicted to result in p.Arg1205His. This enables others transcribing the mutation data from the text, the best chance of correctly copying the mutation.

12 The numbering scheme used should also be stated. VWF follows HGVS conventions where nucleotide and amino acid numbering are from the "A" of the methionine start codon.

13 The reference cDNA and protein sequences used for comparison with the patient sequence should be stated. These can be added as footnotes.

14 Conclusion regarding whether a mutation(s) identified is commensurate with the phenotype. Be cautious with novel sequence alterations (exclude SNP, use relevant prediction software).

15 For previously reported mutations, reference to the publication with sufficient information for the reader to obtain the reference themselves.

16 Where a mutation(s) was identified, implications for family members.

17 If no mutation was identified, possible reasons why (it could lie in unanalyzed regions of the gene, etc.) and suggestions of any further analysis that could

be undertaken, including additional phenotype analysis.

18 Reports should be clear, succinct, and accurate.

19 Two suitably qualified health care professionals should check and then sign reports for accuracy of all information.

20 Where appropriate, the possibility of errors due to factors beyond the control of the laboratory (e.g., the need for family relationships stated on the referral being correct) should be mentioned.

Implementation of the above recommendations into both clinical reports and other descriptions of mutations, where relevant, should help to enhance the accuracy of the information transmitted.

References

1. Sadler JE, Budde U, Eikenboom JC, et al. Update on the pathophysiology and classification of von Willebrand disease: a report of the Subcommittee on von Willebrand Factor. *J Thromb Haemost*. 2006;4:2103–2114.

2. Mancuso DJ, Tuley EA, Westfield LA, et al. Human von Willebrand factor gene and pseudogene: structural analysis and differentiation by polymerase chain reaction. *Biochemistry*. 1991;30:253–269.

3. Mancuso DJ, Tuley EA, Westfield LA, et al. Structure of the gene for human von Willebrand factor. *J Biol Chem*. 1989;264:19514–19527.

4. VWFdb. International Society on Thrombosis and Haemostasis Scientific and Standardization Committee VWF Information Homepage. http://www.vwf.group .shef.ac.uk. Accessed 18 Nov 2011.

5. Keeney S, Bowen D, Cumming A, Enayat S, Goodeve A, Hill M. The molecular analysis of von Willebrand disease: a guideline from the UK Haemophilia Centre Doctors' Organisation Haemophilia Genetics Laboratory Network. *Haemophilia*. 2008;14:1099–1111.

6. Goodeve AC. The genetic basis of von Willebrand disease. *Blood Rev*. 2010;24:123–134.

7. Mannucci PM, Bloom AL, Larrieu MJ, Nilsson IM, West RR. Atherosclerosis and von Willebrand factor. I. Prevalence of severe von Willebrand's disease in western Europe and Israel. *Br J Haematol*. 1984;57:163–169.

8. Lak M, Peyvandi F, Mannucci PM. Clinical manifestations and complications of childbirth and replacement therapy in 385 Iranian patients with type 3 von Willebrand disease. *Br J Haematol*. 2000;111:1236–1239.

9. Berliner SA, Seligsohn U, Zivelin A, Zwang E, Sofferman G. A relatively high frequency of severe (type III) von Willebrand's disease in Israel. *Br J Haematol*. 1986;62:535–543.

10. Schneppenheim R, Krey S, Bergmann F, et al. Genetic heterogeneity of severe von Willebrand disease type III in the German population. *Hum Genet*. 1994;94:640–652.

11. Baronciani L, Cozzi G, Canciani MT, et al. Molecular defects in type 3 von Willebrand disease: updated results from 40 multiethnic patients. *Blood Cells Mol Dis*. 2003;30:264–270.

12. Gupta PK, Saxena R, Adamtziki E, et al. Genetic defects in von Willebrand disease type 3 in Indian and Greek patients. *Blood Cells Mol Dis*. 2008;41:219–222.

13. Sutherland MS, Keeney S, Bolton-Maggs PH, Hay CR, Will A, Cumming AM. The mutation spectrum associated with type 3 von Willebrand disease in a cohort of patients from the north west of England. *Haemophilia*. 2009;15:1048–1057.

14. Hampshire DJ, Goodeve AC. The International Society on Thrombosis and Haemostasis von Willebrand disease database: an update. *Sem Thromb Hemost*. 2011;37:470–479.

15. Meyer D, Fressinaud E, Mazurier C. Clinical, laboratory, and molecular markers of type 2 von Willebrand disease. In: Federici AB, Lee CA, Berntorp E, Lillicrap D, Montgomery RR, eds. *von Willebrand Disease: Basic And Clinical Aspects*. 1st ed. Chichester, West Sussex: Blackwell Publishing Ltd; 2011.

16. Hassenpflug WA, Budde U, Obser T, et al. Impact of mutations in the von Willebrand factor A2 domain on ADAMTS13-dependent proteolysis. *Blood*. 2006;107:2339–2345.

17. Schneppenheim R, Michiels JJ, Obser T, et al. A cluster of mutations in the D3 domain of von Willebrand factor correlates with a distinct subgroup of von Willebrand disease: type 2A/IIE. *Blood*. 2010;115:4894–4901.

18. Federici AB, Mannucci PM, Castaman G, et al. Clinical and molecular predictors of thrombocytopenia and risk of bleeding in patients with von Willebrand disease type 2B: a cohort study of 67 patients. *Blood*. 2009;113:526–534.

19. Rayes J, Hommais A, Legendre P, et al. Effect of von Willebrand disease type 2B and type 2M mutations on the susceptibility of von Willebrand factor to ADAMTS-13. *J Thromb Haemost*. 2007;5:321–328.

20. Othman M, Notley C, Lavender FL, et al. Identification and functional characterization of a novel 27-bp deletion in the macroglycopeptide-coding region of the GPIBA gene resulting in platelet-type von Willebrand disease. *Blood*. 2005;105:4330–4336.

21. Hamilton A, Ozelo M, Leggo J, et al. Frequency of platelet type versus type 2B von Willebrand disease. an international registry-based study. *Thromb Haemost*. 2011;105:501–508.

22. HGMD. The Human Gene Mutation Database at the Institute of Medical Genetics in Cardiff. http://www.hgmd.cf.ac.uk/ac/index.php. Accessed 16 Oct 2011.

23. Othman M. Platelet type von Willebrand disease registry and database; PT-VWD.org. http://www.pt-vwd.org/. Accessed 16 Oct 2011.

24. Miller JL. Platelet-type von Willebrand disease. *Thromb Haemost*. 1996;75:865–869.

25. Ribba AS, Loisel I, Lavergne JM, et al. Ser968Thr mutation within the A3 domain of von Willebrand factor (VWF) in two related patients leads to a defective binding of VWF to collagen. *Thromb Haemost*. 2001;86:848–854.

26. Riddell AF, Gomez K, Millar CM, et al. Characterization of W1745C and S1783A: 2 novel mutations causing defective collagen binding in the A3 domain of von Willebrand factor. *Blood*. 2009;114:3489–3496.

27. Flood VH, Lederman CA, Wren JS, et al. Absent collagen binding in a VWF A3 domain mutant: utility of the VWF:CB in diagnosis of VWD. *J Thromb Haemost*. 2010;8:1431–1433.

28. James PD, Notley C, Hegadorn C, et al. Challenges in defining type 2M von Willebrand disease: results from a Canadian cohort study. *J Thromb Haemost*. 2007;5:1914–1922.

29. Hilbert L, Jorieux S, Proulle V, et al. Two novel mutations, Q1053H and C1060R, located in the D3 domain of von Willebrand factor, are responsible for decreased FVIII-binding capacity. *Br J Haematol*. 2003;120:627–632.

30. Nesbitt IM, Goodeve AC, Guilliatt AM, Makris M, Preston FE, Peake IR. Characterisation of type 2N von Willebrand disease using phenotypic and molecular techniques. *Thromb Haemost*. 1996;75:959–964.

31. Zhukov O, Popov J, Ramos R, et al. Measurement of von Willebrand factor-FVIII binding activity in patients with suspected von Willebrand disease type 2N: application of an ELISA-based assay in a reference laboratory. *Haemophilia*. 2009;15:788–796.

32. Veyradier A, Caron C, Ternisien C, et al. Validation of the first commercial ELISA for type 2N von Willebrand's disease diagnosis. *Haemophilia*. 2011;17:944–951.

33. Sadler JE. A revised classification of von Willebrand disease. For the Subcommittee on von Willebrand Factor of the Scientific and Standardization Committee of the International Society on Thrombosis and Haemostasis. *Thromb Haemost*. 1994;71:520–525.

34. Federici AB, Castaman G, Mannucci PM. Guidelines for the diagnosis and management of von Willebrand disease in Italy. *Haemophilia*. 2002;8:607–621.

35. James PD, Notley C, Hegadorn C, et al. The mutational spectrum of type 1 von Willebrand disease: results from a Canadian cohort study. *Blood*. 2007;109:145–154.

213

36. Goodeve A, Eikenboom J, Castaman G, et al. Phenotype and genotype of a cohort of families historically diagnosed with type 1 von Willebrand disease in the European study, Molecular and Clinical Markers for the Diagnosis and Management of Type 1 von Willebrand Disease (MCMDM-1VWD). *Blood.* 2007;109:112–121.

37. Cumming A, Grundy P, Keeney S, et al. An investigation of the von Willebrand factor genotype in UK patients diagnosed to have type 1 von Willebrand disease. *Thromb Haemost.* 2006;96:630–641.

38. Hampshire DJ, Burghel GJ, Goudemand J, et al. Polymorphic variation within the VWF gene contributes to the failure to detect mutations in patients historically diagnosed with type 1 von Willebrand disease from the MCMDM-1VWD cohort. *Haematologica.* 2010;95:2163–2165.

39. Budde U, Schneppenheim R, Eikenboom J, et al. Detailed von Willebrand factor multimer analysis in patients with von Willebrand disease in the European study, molecular and clinical markers for the diagnosis and management of type 1 von Willebrand disease (MCMDM-1VWD). *J Thromb Haemost.* 2008;6:762–771.

40. Collins PW, Cumming AM, Goodeve AC, Lillicrap D. Type 1 von Willebrand disease: application of emerging data to clinical practice. *Haemophilia.* 2008;14:685–696.

41. Davies JA, Collins PW, Hathaway LS, Bowen DJ. Effect of von Willebrand factor Y/C1584 on in vivo protein level and function and interaction with ABO blood group. *Blood.* 2007;109:2840–2846.

42. Hashemi Soteh M, Peake IR, Marsden L, et al. Mutational analysis of the von Willebrand factor gene in type 1 von Willebrand disease using conformation sensitive gel electrophoresis: a comparison of fluorescent and manual techniques. *Haematologica.* 2007;92:550–553.

43. Corrales I, Ramirez L, Altisent C, Parra R, Vidal F. Rapid molecular diagnosis of von Willebrand disease by direct sequencing. Detection of 12 novel putative mutations in VWF gene. *Thromb Haemost.* 2009;101:570–576.

44. NCBI. db SNP. http://www.ncbi.nlm.nih.gov/projects/SNP./ Accessed 08 Nov 2011.

45. Ellard S, Charlton R, Yau M, et al. Practice guidelines for Sanger sequencing analysis and interpretation. http://www.cmgs.org/BPGs/best_practice_guidelines.htm. Accessed 15 Nov 2011.

46. Cabrera N, Casana P, Cid AR, et al. First application of MLPA method in severe von Willebrand disease. Confirmation of a new large VWF gene deletion and identification of heterozygous carriers. *Br J Haematol.* 2011;152:240–242.

47. Yadegari H, Driesen J, Hass M, Budde U, Pavlova A, Oldenburg J. Large deletions identified in patients with von Willebrand disease using multiple ligation-dependent probe amplification. *J Thromb Haemost.* 2011;9:1083–1086.

48. Sutherland MS, Cumming AM, Bowman M, et al. A novel deletion mutation is recurrent in von Willebrand disease types 1 and 3. *Blood.* 2009;114:1091–1098.

49. Casari C, Pinotti M, Lancellotti S, et al. The dominant-negative von Willebrand factor gene deletion p.P1105_C1926delinsR: molecular mechanism and modulation. *Blood.* 2010;116(24):5371–5376.

50. Goodeve AC, Schneppenheim R. Molecular diagnosis of von Willebrand disease: the genotype. In: Federici AB, Berntorp E, Lee C, Lillicrap D, Montgomery R.R, eds. *von Willebrand's Disease: Basic and Clinical Aspects.* Chichester, UK: Wiley-Blackwell; 2011.

51. Robertson JD, Yenson PR, Rand ML, et al. Expanded phenotype–genotype correlations in a pediatric population with type 1 von Willebrand disease. *J Thromb Haemost.* 2011;9:1752–1760.

52. Johansson AM, Hallden C, Sall T, Lethagen S. Variation in the VWF gene in Swedish patients with type 1 von Willebrand disease. *Ann Hum Genet.* 2011.

53. NGRL. SNPCheck. ngrl.manchester.ac.uk/SNPCheckV2/snpcheck.htm. Accessed 08 Nov 2011.

54. Bagnall RD, Waseem NH, Green PM, Colvin B, Lee C, Giannelli F. Creation of a novel donor splice site in intron 1 of the factor VIII gene leads to activation of a 191 bp cryptic exon in two haemophilia A patients. *Br J Haematol.* 1999;107:766–771.

55. Castaman G, Giacomelli SH, Mancuso ME, et al. Deep intronic variations may cause mild hemophilia A. *J Thromb Haemost.* 2011;9:1541–1548.

56. Wang GS, Cooper TA. Splicing in disease: disruption of the splicing code and the decoding machinery. *Nat Rev Genet.* 2007;8:749–761.

57. Othman M, Chirinian Y, Brown C, et al. Functional characterization of a 13-bp deletion (c.-1522_-1510del13) in the promoter of the von Willebrand factor gene in type 1 von Willebrand disease. *Blood.* 2010;116:3645–3652.

58. Chen JM, Cooper DN, Chuzhanova N, Ferec C, Patrinos GP. Gene conversion: mechanisms, evolution, and human disease. *Nat Rev Genet.* 2007;8:762–775.

59. Gupta PK, Adamtziki E, Budde U, et al. Gene conversions are a common cause of von Willebrand disease. *Br J Haematol.* 2005;130:752–758.

60. Berber E, James PD, Hough C, Lillicrap D. An assessment of the pathogenic significance of the R924Q von Willebrand factor substitution. *J Thromb Haemost.* 2009;7:1672–1679.

61. Hickson N, Hampshire D, Winship P, et al. von Willebrand factor variant p.Arg924Gln marks an allele associated with reduced von Willebrand factor and factor VIII levels. *J Thromb Haemost*. 2010;8:1986–1993.

62. Eikenboom J, Hilbert L, Ribba AS, et al. Expression of 14 von Willebrand factor mutations identified in patients with type 1 von Willebrand disease from the MCMDM-1VWD study. *J Thromb Haemost*. 2009;7:1304–1312.

63. Peake IR, Bowen D, Bignell P, et al. Family studies and prenatal diagnosis in severe von Willebrand disease by polymerase chain reaction amplification of a variable number tandem repeat region of the von Willebrand factor gene. *Blood*. 1990;76:555–561.

64. van Amstel HK, Reitsma PH. Tetranucleotide repeat polymorphism in the *VWF* gene. *Nucleic Acids Res*. 1990;18:4957.

65. Zhang ZP, Deng LP, Blomback M, Anvret M. Dinucleotide repeat polymorphism in the promoter region of the human von Willebrand factor gene (*VWF gene*). *Hum Mol Genet*. 1992;1:780.

66. Vidal F, Julia A, Altisent C, Puig L, Gallardo D. Von Willebrand gene tracking by single-tube automated fluorescent analysis of four short tandem repeat polymorphisms. *Thromb Haemost*. 2005;93:976–981.

67. Allen S, Mountford R, Butler A, Mann K, Treacy B. Practice guidelines for the testing for maternal cell contamination (MCC) in prenatal samples for molecular studies. http://www.cmgs.org/BPGs/best_practice_guidelines.htm. Accessed 14 Nov 2011.

68. Patton S, Stenhouse S. Practice guidelines for internal quality control within the molecular genetics laboratory. http://www.cmgs.org/BPGs/best_practice_guidelines.htm. Accessed 16 Nov 2011.

69. Bell J, Bodmer D, Sistermans E, Ramsden S. Practice guidelines for the interpretation and reporting of unclassified variants (UVs) in clinical molecular genetics.

http://cmgsweb.shared.hosting.zen.co.uk/BPGs/Best_Practice_Guidelines.htm. Accessed 16 November 2011.

70. Hellen B. Splice site tools: a comparative analysis report http://www.ngrl.org.uk/Manchester/sites/default/files/publications/Informatics/NGRL_Splice_Site_Tools_Analysis_2009.pdf. Accessed 13 Nov 2011.

71. Corrales I, Ramirez L, Altisent C, Parra R, Vidal F. The study of the effect of splicing mutations in von Willebrand factor using RNA isolated from patients' platelets and leukocytes. *J Thromb Haemost*. 2011;9(4):679–688.

72. UKNEQAS. UK NEQAS for blood coagulation. http://www.ukneqasbc.org/content/Pageserver.asp. Accessed 16 Nov 2011.

73. Perry DJ, Goodeve A, Hill M, Jennings I, Kitchen S, Walker I. The UK National External Quality Assessment Scheme (UK NEQAS) for molecular genetic testing in haemophilia. *Thromb Haemost*. 2006;96:597–601.

74. Treacy RJL, Robinson DO. Best practice guidelines for reporting molecular genetics results. http://www.cmgs.org/BPGs/best_practice_guidelines.htm. Accessed 08 Nov 2011.

75. Mazurier C, Rodeghiero F. Recommended abbreviations for von Willebrand factor and its activities. *Thromb Haemost*. 2001;86:712.

76. HGVS. Nomenclature for the description of sequence variations homepage. http://www.hgvs.org/mutnomen/. Accessed 08 November 2011.

77. Goodeve AC, Reitsma PH, McVey JH, Working Group on Nomenclature of the Scientific and Standardisation Committee of the International Society on Thrombosis and Haemostasis. Nomenclature of genetic variants in hemostasis. *J Thromb Haemost*. 2011;9:852–855.

78. HGNC. HUGO Gene Nomenclature Committee information homepage. http://www.genenames.org/. Accessed 13 Nov 2011.

PART 4

Quality in Thrombophilia Testing and Monitoring Anticoagulation

19 Quality issues in heritable thrombophilia testing

Isobel D. Walker[1,2] & Ian Jennings[2]
[1]University of Glasgow, Scotland, UK
[2]UK NEQAS for Blood Coagulation, Sheffield, UK

Introduction

There is convincing evidence that deficiencies of the natural anticoagulants antithrombin, protein C, and protein S are associated with an increased risk of venous thrombosis. Retrospective cohort analyses of family studies indicate a roughly tenfold increase in risk compared to nondeficient subjects. It has been suggested that the risk of venous thrombosis increases with a dose–response effect with decreasing plasma levels of antithrombin, protein C, and protein S. Single point mutations in the genes encoding coagulation factors V and II, Factor V Leiden, and the prothrombin G20210A mutation, increase the risk of venous thrombosis three- to sevenfold. Until recently, the number of requests for thrombophilia tests was rising year after year challenging resource allocation in already overstretched health budgets. This led to serious discussions about who should be tested and why, what components and parameters should be measured, and what methods should be used and how should the results be interpreted?

The thrombophilia screen: what to include?

The term thrombophilia "screen" is unfortunate since it implies testing or "screening" unselected subjects. Nonetheless, it is in widespread use and is a useful shorthand for describing the list of tests a laboratory would usually perform in response to a request for thrombophilia testing. Investigations for heritable thrombophilia usually include antithrombin, protein C, and protein S assays; tests for factor V Leiden; and the prothrombin G20210A mutation.

It has also been suggested that a thrombin clotting time and a prothrombin time be incorporated in the initial testing. The thrombin clotting time will detect heparin contamination of the sample and fibrinogen abnormalities. The prothrombin time is useful in the interpretation of low protein C or protein S results. An activated partial thromboplastin time (aPTT) is also often included in the initial testing as, depending on the sensitivity of the reagent used, it may identify some patients with acquired antiphospholipid antibodies. A prolonged aPTT will also serve as an indicator of heparin contamination of the sample and there is evidence suggesting that a shortened aPTT may indicate increased venous thrombosis risk [1].

Familial thrombosis due to dysfibrinogenemia is rare, but may be considered in individuals with a strong family history of venous thrombosis if no other defect has been found. Activated protein C (APC) resistance in the absence of factor V Leiden and elevated plasma factor VIII have been associated with an increased risk of venous thrombosis but the risk is only of the order two- to threefold based on case control studies. Some authors have however recommended including an assay of clotting factor VIII in the thrombophilia screen and some also suggest including a test which will detect APC resistance not due to

Table 19.1 Suggested first line investigations. Discussion of the suggested methods is included in the text

	Test type	Method (see text for discussion)
Coagulation screen	Functional	Activated partial thromboplastin time, prothrombin time, and thrombin clotting time
Antithrombin	Functional	Heparin cofactor activity with bovine thrombin or factor Xa substrate
Protein C	Functional	Chromogenic activity
Protein S	Immunologic	Free protein S antigen
Activated protein C resistance	Functional	Predilution of test plasma in factor V depleted plasma
or factor V Leiden	DNA based	
Prothrombin G20210A	DNA based	
In addition, tests for acquired antiphospholipids are usually included		
Lupus anticoagulant	Functional	Clotting-based tests
Anticardiolipins	Immunologic	

factor V Leiden. Elevated homocysteine levels have been associated with an increased risk of venous thrombosis but there is no evidence that reducing plasma homocysteine levels reduces recurrent venous thrombosis risk. Assaying homocysteine or testing for the presence of the C677T methylene tetrahydrofolate reductase (MTHFR) mutation that is associated with a mild elevation in plasma homocysteine levels is not clinically useful in preventing venous thrombotic disease. Tests for fibrinolytic activity, widely used in early thrombophilia investigations, are considered too difficult to standardize and interpret to include in thrombophilia screening profiles. Furthermore, their clinical utility in thrombophilia testing is accepted as very limited. The tests that may be included in a thrombophilia screen are shown in Table 19.1. Possible additional tests are listed in Table 19.2. Diagnostic laboratories performing thrombophilia testing for heritable defects would usually extend to testing for acquired antiphospholipid antibodies and include functional testing for lupus anticoagulant activity and immunological testing for anticardiolipins and/or $\beta_2$glycoprotein1.

Which methods?

Given the general requirement to contain costs, routine diagnostic laboratories need to ensure that their testing profile includes methods that are as sensitive and specific as possible.

Table 19.2 Possible additional investigations

Parameter	Method
Activated protein C resistance	Original (unmodified) test
Antithrombin antigen	Immunologic assay
Protein C antigen	Immunologic assay
Protein C activity	Clotting-based functional assay
Total Protein S antigen	Immunologic assay
Protein S activity	Clotting-based functional assay
Fibrinogen	Clotting-based functional assay
Fibrinogen	Immunologic assay
FVIII, FIX, FXI	Clotting-based functional assays
Homocysteine	Functional or immunologic assay

Antithrombin

Antithrombin is the most important inhibitor of thrombin and also inhibits other coagulation serine proteases including activated factor X (factor Xa), factors IXa, XIa, XIIa, and tissue factor-bound factor VIIa. Antithrombin has two important functional regions: a thrombin-binding domain at Arg393-Ser394 (at the carboxy-terminal end of the molecule) and a heparin-binding site at its amino terminus. In the absence of heparin, antithrombin inactivates thrombin slowly—progressive antithrombin activity. Heparin binding to antithrombin produces a conformational change in antithrombin that accelerates by

4000-fold, the rate of complex formation between antithrombin and serine proteases. This rapid inactivation of thrombin and factor Xa in the presence of heparin is referred to as the heparin cofactor activity of antithrombin.

Two major types of heritable antithrombin deficiency are recognized. Type I deficiency is characterized by a quantitative reduction of qualitatively (functionally) normal antithrombin; antithrombin antigen and activity levels are concordantly reduced. Type II deficiency is due to the production of a qualitatively abnormal protein. Antithrombin activity is significantly reduced but antithrombin antigen levels are normal or near normal. Type II antithrombin deficiency is subclassified according to the site of the molecular defect. Reactive site variants have mutations near the thrombin-binding site and have decreased activity in both progressive antithrombin activity and heparin cofactor activity assays. Heparin-binding site variants are due to mutations at the amino terminus. Affected individuals generally have reduced heparin cofactor activity (approximately 50% of normal) but normal progressive antithrombin activity. Pleiotropic effect variants are the result of mutations at the carboxy-terminal end of the antithrombin molecule. Affected individuals may exhibit reductions in both the heparin binding and progressive antithrombin activity.

Distinction between the types and subtypes of antithrombin deficiency is of clinical relevance since the incidence of thrombosis is higher in association with type I deficiency and type II reactive site defects than in type II heparin-binding site defects. An initial classification into type I or type II can be made by comparing the result of an immunological assay with the result of an antithrombin heparin cofactor assay.

Antithrombin assays—problems and dilemmas
Only functional assays of heparin cofactor activity will detect both the type I and type II antithrombin deficiencies. Type II defects, present in approximately 40% of subjects with antithrombin deficiency and a thrombotic history, may remain undetected if only an immunologic assay is used. Furthermore, immunologic assays of antithrombin have been shown to have a greater interlaboratory coefficient of variation than functional assays.

The incubation time of plasma with heparin and thrombin is critical. Maximal sensitivity of thrombin-based antithrombin assays to some heparin-binding defects occurs when the incubation time is reduced to 20 seconds, although incubation times up to 50 seconds will still detect other defects [2]. Since the majority of currently used antithrombin heparin cofactor activity assays utilize a long incubation, the methods used in most routine diagnostic laboratories do not detect heparin-binding defects. This may be of no clinical significance, given the low prevalence of thrombotic events in subject with these defects. Crossed immunoelectrophoresis with heparin is a simple tool that may be used to detect type II heparin-binding site variants.

Heparin cofactor II is a confounding factor in antithrombin heparin cofactor activity assays. Antithrombin heparin cofactor assays using human thrombin may overestimate antithrombin activity since 20–30% of the total activity measured may be due to heparin cofactor II activity. Bovine thrombin is minimally inhibited by heparin cofactor II. Heparin cofactor II does not inhibit factor Xa and requires concentrations of heparin of at least 1 unit/mL in the reaction mixture to function as an efficient inhibitor of thrombin [3]. Antithrombin heparin cofactor assay methods measuring plasma anti-factor Xa activity or that measuring anti-IIa activity in the presence of 0.22 M NaCl exclude the influence of heparin cofactor II activity. A UK National External Quality Assessment Scheme (NEQAS) exercise demonstrated good sensitivity of bovine thrombin and Xa-based assays to a rare but clinically important antithrombin variant (antithrombin Wobble) but 40% of centers employing human thrombin-based assays failed to report reduced antithrombin activity in this plasma (unpublished data).

The missense substitution Ala384Ser (Cambridge II) is a relatively prevalent variant in Caucasian populations [4, 5]. It is not detectable by assay of antithrombin antigen or by the anti-Xa heparin cofactor activity [6]. Endogenous thrombin generation is increased but less so than in subjects with quantitative deficiencies of antithrombin [7]. In a study of 20 patients with antithrombin Cambridge II, antithrombin antigen and activity levels as measured by anti-Xa assay were within the normal ranges but, compared with controls, antithrombin activity measured in a chromogenic assay using bovine thrombin was mildly (but significantly) reduced [4]. This study also demonstrated an adjusted odds ratio of 9.75 of developing venous thrombosis associated with the Cambridge II variant—placing the thrombotic risk somewhere between that associated with a mild prothrombotic polymorphism (such as factor V Leiden) and that associated with severe thrombophilic mutations (such as type 1 antithrombin deficiency). Other studies have failed to find an increased prevalence of the Cambridge II mutation in patients with venous thrombosis [8]. The clinical relevance of antithrombin Cambridge II is unclear [8], but it may be reasonable to speculate that, in populations where both itself and the factor V Leiden mutation are prevalent, compound heterozygosity (antithrombin Cambridge II/factor V Leiden) may be clinically important.

In an exercise in which the UK National External Quality Assessment Scheme for Blood Coagulation (NEQAS BC) circulated a sample from a patient with antithrombin Cambridge II (Figure 19.1), almost half of the centers using human thrombin-based assays and 80% of those using factor Xa-based assays reported antithrombin activity levels of 80 IU/dL or greater.

If it is considered necessary for a routine diagnostic laboratory to be able to detect antithrombin

Cambridge II, an assay employing bovine thrombin would be preferable to an anti-Xa-based assay, but antithrombin Cambridge II heterozygotes have only mildly impaired anti-IIa activity and even an assay using bovine thrombin may miss affected subjects [9]. Plasma methods for detection of antithrombin deficiency may have to be complemented with a genetic test for the point mutation to avoid underdiagnosing the Cambridge II variant.

Protein C

APC with its cofactor protein S inactivates the coagulation cascade cofactors, Va and VIIIa, reducing the thrombin-generating capacity of blood. Protein C, the vitamin K-dependent zymogen of APC, is synthesized in the liver.

As with antithrombin deficiency, familial protein C deficiency can be classified on the basis of phenotypic analysis employing functional and immunologic assays. Type I, accounting for 75% of heritable protein C deficiency, is characterized by concordant reductions of functional and immunoreactive protein

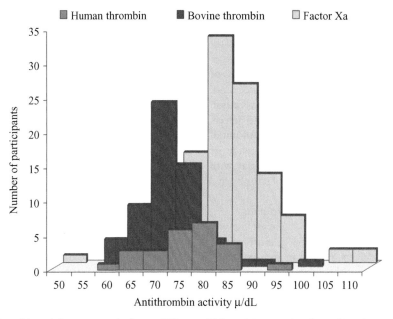

Figure 19.1 Antithrombin activity assay results from a UK National External Quality Assessment Scheme exercise in which participants were asked to test a sample from a donor heterozygous for antithrombin Cambridge II (Ala384Ser). The median antithrombin activity reported by 105 participants using factor Xa substrate was 83 μ/dL (range 50–110 μ/dL); by 25 participants using human thrombin substrate was 76 μ/dL (range 60–95 μ/dL); and by 59 participants using bovine thrombin substrate was 71 μ/dL (range 60–100 μ/dL).

C. In type II, the functional protein C level is substantially lower than that of the antigen. Type II deficiencies may be subdivided into those with reduced function detectable in both coagulation and amidolytic assays (about 95% of type II protein C deficiencies) and those with reduced activity detectable only in coagulation-based assays. To detect both type I and type II defects, a functional assay is required. The underlying genetic variant and associated phenotype are not predictive of thrombotic risk. The classification of protein C deficiency into type I and type II serves no useful clinical purpose.

Heritable protein C deficiency is usually an autosomal dominant trait. Homozygous protein C deficiency is an autosomal recessive disorder manifesting as progressive hemorrhagic skin necrosis—purpura fulminans—usually in the neonate (sometimes present at birth) but occasionally in older children or adults in association with sepsis. Homozygotes with a milder phenotype have also been shown to be compound heterozygotes.

The complexity of early protein C activity assays was avoided with the discovery of snake venoms capable of direct activation of protein C. The most widely used venom, available under the trade name Protac® (American Diagnostica), is isolated and purified from Agkistrodon contortrix (the southern copperhead snake). It activates protein C without affecting other components of hemostasis and without hydrolyzing, to any significant extent, chromogenic substrates for protein C. The APC formed can be quantitated by clotting or chromogenic methods, the latter being more specific.

Protein C assays—problems and dilemmas
In patients on vitamin K antagonists, protein C antigen will be overestimated by Laurell Rocket electrophoresis unless EDTA is present in the gel and buffer to ensure equal migration of carboxylated and non-carboxylated protein C [10]. More recently, other immunologic assays have been developed including the ELISA (enzyme-linked immunosorbent assay) [11] and ELFA (enzyme-linked fluorescent assay).

There is a wide overlap in protein C activity between heterozygous carriers and their unaffected relatives in families with protein C deficiency [12]. For samples where clotting factor activation is suspected, for example, pediatric samples and samples from patients with disseminated intravascular coagulation,

a blank (water substituted for Protac®) tube should be included in chromogenic assays to avoid overestimation of protein C activity due to autohydrolysis of the chromogenic substrate [13].

Some type II protein C defects, including some defects that impair the binding of protein C to protein S and calcium [14], will not be detected by chromogenic assay but will be apparent only when a clot-based assay is performed. Early suggestions that 40% of type II protein C defects would be detectable only by clot-based assay [14] were an overestimate since they preceded knowledge of the effect of APC resistance on some clot-based assays and it is likely that some individuals with factor V Leiden were erroneously diagnosed as having type II protein C deficiency. More recent estimates suggest that around 5% of type II protein C defects (about 1% of all protein C defects) have normal amidolytic activity and are detectable only on clot-based assay [15].

In a UK NEQAS BC exercise in which a sample homozygous for factor V Leiden was distributed to participants, there was a significant difference in the median protein C activity reported by participants using chromogenic assays and those using a clotting-based assay (Figure 19.2a), and more than half of the participants using a clotting-based assay erroneously diagnosed the sample as protein C deficient (Figure 19.2b) [16]. The effect of factor V Leiden may be avoided by predilution of plasma in PC deficient plasma, or the use of a chromogenic assay. In addition to the misleadingly low protein C activity levels which may be obtained with clotting-based assays in the presence of factor V Leiden, clotting-based assays are subject to interference by a number of other variables including elevated plasma factor VIII levels [17] or the presence of a lupus inhibitor [18] or heparin [19] or hyperlipidemia.

Rarely, it may be necessary to perform both chromogenic and clotting functional assays in addition to an immunologic assay to fully characterize an individual's protein C status, but these cases are the territory of experts whose advice and help should be sought.

Protein S

Protein S is a vitamin K-dependent protein. Approximately, 65% of the total plasma protein S is complexed with C4b-binding protein (C4bBP). The remainder, designated free protein S, remains

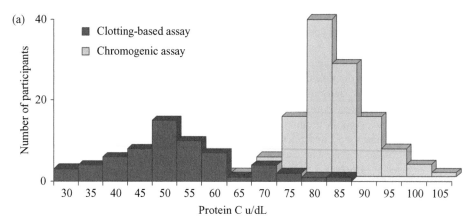

Figure 19.2a Protein C activity assay results from a UK National External Quality Assessment Scheme exercise in which participants were asked to test a sample from a donor with no protein C defect but homozygous for factor V Leiden. The median protein C activity for 116 participants using chromogenic assays was 82.0 μ/dL and for 62 participants using clotting based assays was 50 μ/dL.

uncomplexed and acts as a cofactor for APC in the degradation of factors Va and VIIIa. C4bBP-bound protein S also has APC-independent anticoagulant activity [20].

Heritable protein S deficiency is classified into three subtypes. Type I protein S deficiency is a quantitative defect caused by genetic abnormalities which result in the reduced production of structurally normal protein, with reduced plasma levels of both total and free protein S antigen and a decrease in functional protein S. Type II protein S deficiency has been characterized as a qualitative defect with reduced protein S activity

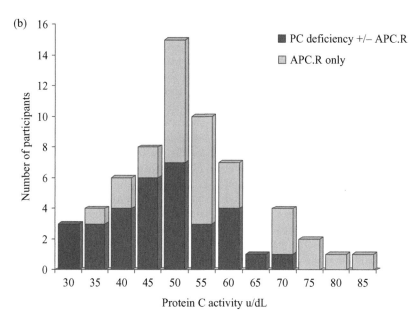

Figure 19.2b Thirty-two of the 62 participants using clotting-based assays erroneously reported that the donor was protein C (PC) deficient with or without evidence of increased resistance to activated protein C (APC.R). The remaining 30 reported the donor had only increased resistance to activated protein C.

but normal (or near normal) levels of both total and free protein S antigen. In type III deficiency, although free protein S antigen and functional protein S are reduced, the total protein S antigen level is normal. Evaluation of the relationship between protein S and C4bBP in families with protein S deficiency suggests that types I and III may be phenotypic variants of the same disorder [21].

Protein S assays—problems and dilemmas
Accurate diagnosis of protein S deficiency is widely accepted as problematic. An overlap of total protein S antigen levels occurs between normal and subjects with heritable protein S variants. Types II and III protein S deficiency are not detected by total protein S antigen assay. It has even been suggested that some total protein S antigen assays will fail to detect type I deficiency [22]. Free protein S antigen estimation is the preferred method for identifying protein S deficiency. Although free protein S antigen levels correlate well with protein S activity in subjects with types I and III protein S deficiency, they may not in patients with type II deficiency or an acquired deficiency.

Immunologic assays measure both fully carboxylated (active) and non-carboxylated (inactive) forms of free protein S and may overestimate the level of functional protein S. Free protein S antigen in a patient on warfarin will give higher values than those obtained using a functional assay. Total protein S antigen assays require conditions such that there is dissociation of the protein S-C4bBP complex, unless the antibodies used in the assay show equal affinity for bound and free protein S. Using ELISA methodology, high dilutions of plasma and long incubation times with primary antibody are required. If the dilution of the plasma or the incubation time is inadequate, total protein S levels may be underestimated. Measurement of free protein S antigen is required to distinguish type III protein S deficiency. Reduced free protein S antigen is the best indicator of a PROS1 genetic defect [22].

The original immunological assays for protein S antigen used polyclonal antibodies which could not distinguish between the free and C4bBp-bound protein S. Free protein S is measured in the supernatant fluid following precipitation of the C4bBP-bound complexes by polyethylene glycol (PEG). This method is very cumbersome and poorly reproducible because standardization of the PEG precipitation step is difficult. The extra sample processing step was perceived to contribute to poor precision for this assay, and encouraged the development of methods for direct measurement of free protein S. With increasing understanding of the interaction between protein S and C4bBP, it has become possible to prepare monoclonal antibodies against the protein S domain responsible for binding to C4bBP. These antibodies are relatively specific for free protein S and allow direct measurement of free protein S without the need for a precipitation stage. Latex immunoassays are now the most widely employed method for measuring free protein S antigen, using either two different monoclonal antibodies to free protein S or antibodies to free protein S and C4b BP. There are, however, also pitfalls related to the use of direct assays. It has been noted that when protein S levels are particularly reduced, monoclonal antibody-based assays may overestimate free protein S concentration relative to the PEG method. The incubation temperature for direct methods may be critical, and overestimation of free protein S in plasma from subjects with heritable protein S defects may occur [23].

Type II (qualitative) protein S defects may be missed if an immunologic assay only is used, and measuring protein S activity should, theoretically, be preferable to measurement of protein S antigen. Protein S activity may be measured by a number of prothrombin time or activated partial thromboplastin time-based assays. These assays measure the effect which degradation of factors Va and VIIIa by APC with free protein S as a cofactor has on a clotting time test. Commercial kits employ different methodologies. In some, activation is mediated by bovine thromboplastin and in others by factor Va or factor Xa. Ideally, these assays should reflect only free protein S activity but this is not always the case since separation of free protein S from C4bBP-complexed protein S is not performed in many of the available methods.

Although readily automated, protein S activity assays show considerable variation between methods, between laboratories, and even within laboratories. Cut-off values vary between laboratories, instruments, reagent handling, other preanalytical variables, and the use of calibrant or reference plasmas from different sources may contribute to differences in results observed between methods. Some individuals with protein S deficiency will not be detected with some of the commercial kits for measuring protein S

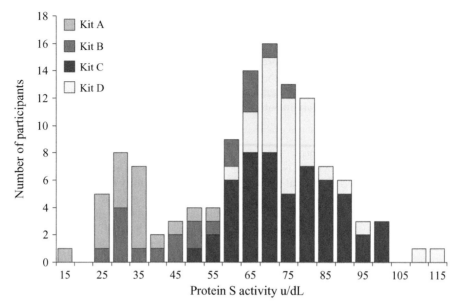

Figure 19.3 Protein S activity assay results from a UK National External Quality Assessment Scheme exercise in which participants were asked to test a sample from a donor with no protein S defect (median free protein S antigen 90.0 µ/dL, $n = 90$), but homozygous for factor V Leiden. The median protein S activity reported by 19 participants using kit A was 33.0 µ/dL; by 19 participants using kit B was 50.5 µ/dL; by 53 participants using kit C was 74.0 µ/dL; and by 28 participants using kit D was 75.4 µ/dL.

activity if the users employ the manufacturers' suggested reference ranges [24].

Protein S activity assays may be sensitive to the inherited APC resistance associated with factor V Leiden (Figure 19.3) and the acquired APC resistance observed in some patients with antiphospholipid antibodies. Protein S levels may be influenced by *in vitro* activation of factor VII, for example, as a consequence of repeated freeze–thawing of samples. Without careful consideration of confounding factors, protein S activity assay use can lead to erroneous diagnosis of protein S deficiency. Where a functional protein S assay is used as an initial screening test for protein S deficiency, low results should always be further investigated with an immunoreactive assay of free protein S [25].

Activated protein C resistance and factor V Leiden

APC resistance is defined as an impaired plasma anticoagulant response to APC added *in vitro*. APC with its cofactor protein S inactivates factors Va and VIIIa. APC cleaves factor Va at amino acid position Arg506 and subsequently at Arg306 and Arg679. The majority of patients with familial APC resistance have factor V Leiden [26], a point mutation in the gene for factor V which involves the 506 cleavage site.

Testing for APC resistance—problems and dilemmas

Many factors including age, gender, pregnancy, and estrogen use influence sensitivity to APC. The most commonly employed test system is aPTT-based. The aPTT is measured before and after the addition of exogenous APC and calcium to the test plasma. The resultant clotting times are expressed as a ratio, the so-called APC sensitivity ratio (APC.R). The original aPTT test has a wide range of reported sensitivities and specificities. Methodological variability can be reduced by "normalizing" the results by dividing the patient's APC.R by the APC.R of pooled normal plasma. If this system is adopted, it is important to establish that the normal plasma pool does not include a contribution from an individual who carries the factor V Leiden mutation since even a single affected donation is sufficient to affect the APC.R of the pool.

Although normalizing the result may reduce intralaboratory and interlaboratory variability, it does not significantly improve the diagnostic efficiency for APC resistance.

The originally described aPTT-based APC resistance test is not diagnostic of factor V Leiden since it is affected by plasma levels of factor VIII and protein S, and by the presence of antiphospholipid antibodies. It is also inaccurate if the patient has an elevated baseline aPTT due to the deficiency of clotting factors or the presence of heparin. Predilution of the test plasma one in five in factor V deficient plasma reduces the number of confounding factors and increases the specificity of the aPTT-based APC.R as a screen for factor V Leiden [27]. This modification makes the test close to 100% specific and sensitive to factor V Leiden [28]. It may be expected that the factor V deficient plasma into which the test plasma is diluted would supply adequate levels of protein S to counteract the effect of protein S deficiency in the test plasma. It has however been reported that protein S may become inactivated during the commercial preparation of factor V deficient plasma with the result that a test plasma may be erroneously classified as factor V Leiden positive [29].

Since the modified test is also aPTT based, it is subject to interference from the lupus anticoagulant in the test plasma. Diluting the patient plasma 1 in 40 in factor V deficient plasma [30] or adding phospholipid to the test sample to neutralize the lupus anticoagulant activity [31] may overcome the antiphospholipid interference. Prothrombin time or Russell viper venom-based tests have been described and are reported to be insensitive to lupus anticoagulants [32]. In practice, however, it is probably simpler to proceed directly to a genetic test for factor V Leiden in patients with antiphospholipid antibodies.

There is evidence that the APC.R determined with the original unmodified test correlates with venous thrombosis risk irrespective of whether or not factor V Leiden is present. The specificity of the modified APC.R test means that individuals who have increased APC resistance for reasons other than the possession of the factor V Leiden mutation will be overlooked if the original APC.R test is omitted from the screening procedure.

Detection of the factor V Leiden mutation
Factor V Leiden is a point mutation at nucleotide position 1691 that results in the elimination of an *Mnl*I restriction site. Detection of the factor V Leiden mutation relies on amplification of the mutation site from either genomic DNA or from mRNA followed by digestion of the product with *Mnl*I [33]. The presence of the factor V Leiden mutation is indicated by the absence of an *Mnl*I site at position 1691. Testing by polymerase chain reaction (PCR) allows clear distinction of heterozygotes and homozygotes. Many other DNA-based assays for factor V Leiden have been described, including ELISA, melting curve analysis, and fluorescence allele-specific discrimination methods [34].

Prothrombin G20210A mutation

The G–A transition at nucleotide 20210 in the 3′ untranslated region of the prothrombin gene is associated with elevated plasma prothrombin levels and an increased risk of venous thrombosis [35]. In the absence of a specific phenotypic test for the presence of the variant 20210A allele, DNA-based procedures are required. The 20210A transition is not associated with the introduction or loss of a specific restriction enzyme recognition site and detection methods that do not require the use of restriction enzyme digestion of the amplified PCR product have been devised.

For both factor V Leiden and prothrombin G20210A investigations, studies have demonstrated that errors are made by laboratories performing these complex tests, and it is important that robust assays with careful procedures and reporting systems are employed. Errors occur even in genetic testing and genetic tests are rarely repeated. Repeat testing should be considered at least for homozygous or doubly heterozygous patients where the thrombotic risk may be significantly increased.

Other tests

Homocysteine may be measured by a number of methods including fluorescence polarization immunoassay (FPIA) and HPLC. Between-centre agreement in UK NEQAS BC exercises is generally very good. The fibrinogen activity may be assessed by clotting-based methods and an immunological assay may be used to confirm dysfibrinogenemia. Although some studies in which raised levels of factors VIII, IX, or XI have been associated with thrombophilia were performed using immunological methods; others have employed clotting methods to demonstrate an association.

Global tests of the protein C anticoagulant pathway have been developed. These fulfill the requirements for identifying individuals with heritable protein C deficiency or APC resistance associated with factor V Leiden but do not reliably identify subjects with protein S defects [36].

What samples and when?

Sample quality is paramount. Although the thrombin time, antithrombin activity, aPTT, and APC resistance test have been shown not to be influenced by sample collection into plastic tubes, statistically significant but clinically irrelevant differences were noted in the levels of protein S activity and chromogenic protein C activity between samples collected into glass and into plastic [37]. The choice of anticoagulant can also affect some tests, notably the APC.R test [38].

Storage for 24 hours at either room temperature or 4°C has no significant effect on APC.R or assays of natural anticoagulants but artifactually increased APC resistance is seen in samples left for more than 24 hours post venipunctures [39]. Protein C and protein S levels may be reduced after 48 hours storage at either room temperature or 4°C so that the subjects with borderline low normal levels may be misclassified as thrombophilic. In contrast, antithrombin levels may rise after storage at either room temperature or 4°C, so that subjects with a mutation associated with borderline antithrombin activity may be misclassified as normal [39].

In general, antigen assays are unaffected by freeze–thawing of samples prior to analysis but functional assay results vary after freeze–thawing [39]. Platelet contamination or activation also results in artifactually increased resistance to APC [40]. Double centrifugation and freezing of samples into multiple aliquots and storage at 40°C or below before testing is recommended.

There is rarely any point in striving to obtain samples for tests for heritable thrombophilia when the patient presents with deep vein thrombosis or pulmonary embolism since the treatment of an acute venous thromboembolic event should not be influenced by the test results. Furthermore, consumption of the natural anticoagulants during the acute event may give misleading results. Testing, if it is considered desirable, is usually best delayed until at least a month after discontinuation of anticoagulation. Before testing, the patient should be carefully counseled about the implications and limitations of thrombophilia testing. Pregnancy and estrogen use reduce protein S levels significantly and increase resistance to APC. If possible, testing for heritable thrombophilia should be avoided during intercurrent illness, pregnancy, and the use of a combined oral contraceptive or hormone replacement therapy. PCR-based tests for factor V Leiden and the prothrombin 20210A allele are unaffected by the above factors.

Effective use of internal quality assurance and participation in accredited external quality assessment schemes is essential. Internal quality control can ensure between-run precision but it is important to include both normal and borderline abnormal samples to control the assay at different levels of measurement. External quality assessment programs not only identify errors in individual laboratory performance but may also highlight methodological errors and dilemmas in result interpretation.

Interpreting the results

Physiological and pathological variability

Many factors may affect the levels of the natural anticoagulants and other components of hemostasis. In adults, age- and sex-related variations in antithrombin activity and antigen levels are minor so the reference ranges in healthy populations are narrow. Compared with adults and even older children, neonates have significantly different levels of many hemostasis components. Andrew et al. in a number of seminal publications detailed reference ranges for many clotting factors and natural anticoagulants in both healthy full-term neonates [41] and in premature neonates [42]. Although still very useful as a guide, some of the ranges quoted would not necessarily transfer directly to currently used methods.

In general, thrombophilia testing in children should be discouraged. Routine testing for heritable thrombophilia in unselected children presenting with a first episode of VTE is not indicated; however, neonates and children with purpura fulminans should be tested for protein C and S deficiency [43].

Healthy newborns have about one-half the normal adult antithrombin concentration and gradually reach the adult level by 6 months of age. Protein C activity levels appear to be related to age and sex but this is explained by blood lipid levels. It is not necessary to use gender-specific reference ranges when testing for antithrombin or protein C deficiency. Protein S levels are higher in males than in females and premenopausal women have lower levels than postmenopausal women. Overdiagnosis of protein S deficiency is therefore a risk in women unless gender-specific protein S reference ranges are used. Because protein C and protein S are vitamin K dependent, their concentrations are reduced in neonates. APC resistance is greater in females than in males.

Significant decreases in antithrombin activity are observed in patients on heparin treatment and in those with current thrombosis. Profound decreases in plasma antithrombin are seen in disseminated intravascular coagulation, liver disease, and the nephrotic syndrome. Protein C activity is reduced by coumarins, in disseminated intravascular coagulation in severe liver disease, and in patients with sepsis. Measuring other vitamin K-dependent factors is often helpful in distinguishing heritable from acquired deficiency of protein C. Elevated levels of protein C have been reported in diabetic patients, in late pregnancy, during the puerperium, and in patients using oral contraceptives or anabolic steroids. Protein S levels fall progressively during pregnancy, are reduced to a lesser extent in women using estrogen-containing oral contraceptives or hormone replacement therapy, and decrease during treatment with oral anticoagulants. Acquired protein S deficiency is seen in some patients with antiphospholipid antibodies and in disseminated intravascular coagulation and liver disease.

Reference ranges

Attention to the validity of reference ranges for local methods and for the patient or population being studied is vital. Since so many preanalytical and analytical factors influence results, laboratories should determine their own local reference ranges for the tests which they offer—or at least validate the manufacturer's stated reference range(s). For reference ranges for tests on adults, at least 120 "normal" healthy subjects should be included. Forty individuals is the absolute minimum needed to allow a reasonable estimate

of the reference limits. The mean $+/-2$ standard deviations may be employed for normal Gaussian distributions. As far as possible, the sampling conditions applied to participants in the reference group should be applicable to the test population. Reference ranges must be constructed from samples handled in the same fashion as test samples. Reference ranges are applicable only to specific machine and reagent combinations and if any component of the "system" is changed, new reference ranges should be established. In some circumstances, the use of separate age- and/or gender-specific reference ranges is necessary, for example, in the neonate and during pregnancy.

It is appreciated that many laboratories find it increasingly difficult to recruit sufficient numbers of "normal" individuals to establish in-house reference ranges. Laboratories unable to establish a local reference range or at least validate the manufacturer's quoted range, should consider whether they should be offering a thrombophilia testing service. The importance of locally determined reference ranges was seen in a retrospective survey of protein S assay results in 19 UK NEQAS exercises sent to participants between May 1998 and November 2002. In each of the groups of sample types, protein S deficient ($n = 4$), factor V Leiden ($n = 5$), and other defects ($n = 10$), protein S activity results varied between assay methods (Table 19.3). In this survey, adoption of reference ranges provided from the literature or the manufacturer's data (without local validation) was shown to lead to errors in diagnosis [24].

Patient-specific interpretive comment

Accurate and meaningful interpretation of individual test results is crucial. Typically, thrombophilia test results are reported without patient-specific interpretive comment. Unfortunately, many requesting clinicians have little understanding of the vast number of factors which influence thrombophilia test results and may interpret the results inappropriately—giving the patient possibly false reassurance if the tests are negative or overstating the risk associated with one of the more prevalent defects (e.g., factor V Leiden). In one large US academic medical center, physicians responded positively to the introduction of interpretive comments saying that they improved the diagnostic process and helped prevent misdiagnosis. In

Table 19.3 Intermethod variability for protein S activity assays

Sample type		Protein S antigen μ/dL		Protein S activity μ/dL			
		Total PS	Free PS	All methods	Xa-based assay	Thromboplastin-based assay	Va-based assay
Protein S defect n = 4		47.8	18.4	27.6	39.6	29.2	21.5
No protein S defect	FV Leiden n = 5	81.9	86.9	65.2	45.0	67.9	69.2
	Other defect n = 10	88.2	80.0	87.0	79.1	83.5	82.3

Source: Data from UK National External Quality Assessment Scheme for Blood Coagulation, May 1998–November 2002.

addition, interpretations appeared to improve ordering practices [44].

Who should be tested?

A lengthy treatise on who should be tested and why is beyond the remit of this chapter. Suffice to say, where thrombophilia testing has been performed in the context of careful scientific studies it has led to greater understanding of the role of heritable thrombophilic defects in clinical disease, but it is often unclear what, if any, benefit accrues from testing individual patients in the clinical setting [43].

Within the past 4 or 5 years, it has become more widely appreciated that screening of unselected patients in the hope of preventing venous thrombosis or pregnancy vascular complications is of unproven clinical benefit and is not cost effective. Identifying a thrombophilia will not alter the management of an acute thrombotic event. Published results of the Multiple Environmental and Genetic Assessment (MEGA) study indicate that the incidence of recurrent venous thromboembolism is not reduced by thrombophilia testing [45]. Although finding a heritable thrombophilic defect usually has few implications for the patient with an acute venous thrombosis, it may be information viewed as useful to other family member. Investigating asymptomatic relatives, however, should be considered only in families which appear to be particularly prone to venous thrombosis (although it is impossible to define particularly prone to venous thrombosis) and limited to testing for high-risk thrombophilias such as deficiencies of antithrombin, protein C, or protein S [43]. Affected women in

symptomatic families may choose to avoid estrogen use for contraception or hormone replacement and may want to alert their antenatal care team to a potentially increased risk of a complicated pregnancy. Clinicians and their patients should, however, be aware that, although there is much published advice on the management of pregnant women with thrombophilia, with the exception of women with antiphospholipid syndrome, there is a lack of good evidence on which to base this advice.

Given the lack of evidence of clear benefit of thrombophilia testing in directing clinical management in most of the patients currently being tested and the potential for causing distress and possibly harm, clinicians should be advised that they should exercise restraint in ordering these tests and should consider carefully their reasons for testing individual patients. Venous thrombosis has a multicausal basis—the result of interaction of environmental factors with underlying genetic predisposition. Traditional laboratory tests have proven to be a blunt tool in assessing individual risk of venous thrombosis. Analysis of vast arrays of genes, although interesting, is not clinically applicable and will only explain part of the thrombotic risk. Proteomic analysis may help in characterizing biological pathways and pathophysiological interactions and in future may improve our ability to identify individuals at risk of venous thrombosis.

References

1. Lippi G, Salvagno GL, Ippolito L, Franchini M, Favaloro EJ. Shortened activated partial thromboplastin time: causes and management. *Blood Coagul Fibrinolysis.* 2010;21:459–463.

2. Harper PL, Daly M, Price J, Edgar PF, Carrell RW. Screening for heparin binding variants of antithrombin. *J Clin Pathol.* 1991;44:477–479.

3. Tollefsen DM, Majerus DW, Blank MK. Heparin cofactor II. Purification and properties of a heparin-dependent inhibitor of thrombin in human plasma. *J Biol Chem.* 1982;257:2162–2169.

4. Corral J, Hernandez-Espinosa D, Soria JM, et al. Antithrombin Cambridge II (A384S): an underestimated genetic risk factor for venous thrombosis. *Blood.* 2007;109:4258–4263.

5. Tait RC, Walker ID, Perry DJ, et al. Prevalence of antithrombin deficiency in the healthy population. *Br J Haematol.* 1994;87:106–112.

6. Harper PL, Luddington RJ, Daly M, et al. The incidence of dysfunctional antithrombin variants: four cases in 210 patients with thromboembolic disease. *Br J Haematol.* 1991;77:360–364.

7. Sanchez C, Alessi MC, Saut N, Aillaud MF, Morange PE. Relation between the antithrombin Cambridge II mutation, the risk of venous thrombosis, and the endogenous thrombin generation. *J Thromb Haemost.* 2008;6:1975–1977.

8. Perry DJ, Daly ME, Tait RC, et al. Antithrombin Cambridge II (Ala384Ser): clinical, functional, and haplotype analysis of 18 families. *Thromb Haemost.* 1998;79:249–253.

9. Jennings I, Kitchen S, Woods TA, Preston FE. Multi-laboratory testing in thrombophilia through the United Kingdom National External Quality Assessment Scheme (Blood Coagulation) Quality Assurance Program. *Semin Thromb Hemost.* 2005;31:66–72.

10. Mikami S, Tuddenham EG. Studies on immunological assay of vitamin K dependent factors. II. Comparison of four immunoassay methods with functional activity of protein C in human plasma. *Br J Haematol.* 1986;62:183–193.

11. Boyer C, Rothschild C, Wolf M, Amiral J, Meyer D, Larrieu MJ. A new method for the estimation of protein C by ELISA. *Thromb Res.* 1984;36:579–589.

12. Allaart CF, Poort SR, Rosendaal FR, Reitsma PH, Bertina RM, Briët E. Increased risk of venous thrombosis in carriers of hereditary protein C deficiency defect. *Lancet.* 1993;341:134–138.

13. Marlar RA, Mastovich S. Hereditary protein C deficiency: a review of the genetics, clinical presentation, diagnosis and treatment. *Blood Coagul Fibrinolysis.* 1990;1:319–330.

14. Marlar RA, Adcock DM, Madden RM. Hereditary dysfunctional protein C molecules (type II): assay characterization and proposed classification. *Thromb Haemost.* 1990;63:375–379.

15. Faioni EM, Franchi F, Asti D, Mannucci PM. Resistance to activated protein C mimicking dysfunctional protein C: diagnostic approach. *Blood Coagul Fibrinolysis.* 1996;7:349–352.

16. Jennings I, Kitchen S, Cooper PC, Rimmer JE, Woods TA, Preston FE. Further evidence that activated protein C resistance affects protein C coagulant activity assays. *Thromb Haemost.* 2000;83;171–172.

17. de Moerloose P, Reber G, Bouvier CA. Spuriously low levels of protein C with a Protac activation clotting assay. *Thromb Haemost.* 1988;59:543.

18. Simioni P, Lazzaro A, Zanardi S, Girolami A. Spurious protein C deficiency due to antiphospholipid antibodies. *Am J Hematol.* 1991;36:299–301.

19. Sturk A, Morrien-Salomons WM, Huisman MV, Borm JJ, Büller HR, ten Cate JW. Analytical and clinical evaluation of commercial protein C assays. *Clin Chim Acta.* 1987;165:263–270.

20. van de Poel RH, Meijers JC, Bouma BN. C4b-binding protein inhibits the factor V-dependent but not the factor V-independent cofactor activity of protein S in the activated protein C-mediated inactivation of factor VIIIa. *Thromb Haemost.* 2001;85:761–765.

21. Simmonds RE, Zoller B, Ireland H, et al. Genetic and phenotypic analysis of a large (122-member) protein S-deficient kindred provides an explanation for the familial coexistence of type I and type III plasma phenotypes. *Blood.* 1997;89:4364–4370.

22. Makris M, Leach M, Beauchamp NJ, et al. Genetic analysis, phenotypic diagnosis, and risk of venous thrombosis in families with inherited deficiencies of protein S. *Blood.* 2000;95:1935–1941.

23. Tsuda T, Tsuda H, Yoshimura H, Hamasaki N. Dynamic equilibrium between protein S and C4b binding protein is important for accurate determination of free protein S antigen. *Clin Chem Lab Med.* 2002;40:563–567.

24. Jennings I, Kitchen S, Cooper P, Makris M, Preston FE. Sensitivity of functional protein S assays to protein S deficiency: a comparative study of three commercial kits. *J Thromb Haemost.* 2003;1:1112–1114.

25. Haemostasis and Thrombosis Task Force, British Committee for Standards in Haematology. Investigation and management of heritable thrombophilia. *Br J Haematol.* 2001;114:512–528.

26. Bertina RM, Koeleman BPC, Koster T, et al. Mutation in blood coagulation factor V associated with resistance to activated protein C. *Nature.* 1994;369:64–67.

27. Jorquera JI, Montoro JM, Fernandez MA, Aznar JA, Aznar J. Modified test for activated protein C resistance. *Lancet.* 1994;344:1162–1163.

28. De Ronde H, Bertina RM. Careful selection of sample dilution and factor-V-deficient plasma makes the

modified activated protein C resistance test highly specific for the factor V Leiden mutation. *Blood Coagul Fibrinolysis*. 1999;10:7–17.

29. Samama MS, Gouin-Thibault I, Trossaert M, et al. Low levels of protein S activity in factor V depleted plasma used in APC resistance test. *Thromb Haemost*. 1998;80:715–716.

30. Benattar N, Schved JF, Biron-Andreani C. A new dilution for the modified APTT-based assay for activated protein C resistance: improvement of the reliability in patients with a lupus anticoagulant. *Thromb Haemost*. 2000;83:967–968.

31. Martorell JR, Munoz-Castillo A, Gil JL. False positive activated protein C resistance test due to antiphospholipid antibodies is corrected by platelet extract. *Thromb Haemost*. 1995;74:796–797.

32. Akhtar MS, Blair AJ, King TC, et al. Whole blood screening test for factor V Leiden using a Russell viper venom time-based assay. *Am J Clin Pathol*. 1998;109:387–391.

33. Bertina RM, Koeleman BP, Koster T, Sweeney JD. Mutation in blood coagulation factor V associated with resistance to activated protein C. *Nature*. 1994;369:64–67.

34. Ledford M, Friedman KD, Hessner MJ, Moehlenkamp C, Williams TM, Larson RS. A multi-site study for detection of the factor V (Leiden) mutation from genomic DNA using a homogeneous invader microtiter plate fluorescence resonance energy transfer (FRET) assay. *J Mole Diagn*. 2000;2:97–104.

35. Poort SR, Rosendaal FR, Reitsma PH, Bertina RM. A common genetic variation in the 3'-untranslated region of the prothrombin gene is associated with elevated plasma prothrombin levels and an increase in venous thrombosis. *Blood*. 1996;88:3698–3703.

36. Tripodi A, Akhavan S, Asti D, Faioni EM, Mannucci PM. Laboratory screening of thrombophilia. Evaluation of the diagnostic efficacy of a global test to detect congenital deficiencies of the protein C anticoagulant pathway. *Blood Coagul Fibrinolysis*. 1998;9:485–489.

37. Kratz A, Stanganelli N, Van Cott EM. A comparison of glass and plastic blood collection tubes for routine and specialized coagulation assays: a comprehensive study. *Arch Path Lab Med*. 2006;130:39–44.

38. De Ronde H, Bertina RM. Laboratory diagnosis of APC-resistance: a critical evaluation of the test and the development of diagnostic criteria. *Thromb Haemost*. 1994;72:880–886.

39. Luddington R, Peters J, Baker P, Baglin T. The effect of delayed analysis or freeze-thawing on the measurement of natural anticoagulants, resistance to activated protein C and markers of activation of the haemostatic system. *Thromb Res*. 1997;87:577–581.

40. Luddington R, Brown K, Baglin T. Effect of platelet phospholipid exposure on activated protein C resistance: implications for thrombophilia screening. *Br J Haematol*. 1996;92:744–746.

41. Andrew M, Paes B, Milner R, et al. Development of the human coagulation system in the full-term infant. *Blood*. 1987;70:165–172.

42. Andrew M, Paes B, Milner R, et al. Development of the human coagulation system in the healthy premature infant. *Blood*. 1988;72:1651–1657.

43. Baglin T, Gray E, Greaves M, et al. Clinical guidelines for testing for heritable thrombophilia. *Br J Haematol*. 2010;149:209–220.

44. Laposata ME, Laposata M, Van Cott EM, Buchner DS, Kashalo MS, Dighe AS. Physician survey of a laboratory medicine interpretive service and evaluation of the influence of interpretations on laboratory test ordering. *Arch Pathol Lab Med*. 2004;128:1424–1427.

45. Coppens M, Reijnders JH, Middeldorp S, Doggen CJ, Rosendaal FR. Testing for inherited thrombophilia does not reduce the recurrence of venous thrombosis. *J Thromb Haemost*. 2008;6:1474–1477.

20 Evaluation of antiphospholipid antibodies

Michael Greaves

Aberdeen Royal Infirmary, Head of College of Life Sciences and Medicine, University of Aberdeen, Scotland, UK

Antiphospholipid syndrome

Antiphospholipid syndrome is an important cause of thrombosis and pregnancy failure. Both are common from other causes in clinical practice and accurate diagnosis is essential to inform rational treatment decisions. The diagnosis is dependent upon recognition of the constellation of relevant clinical manifestations and confirmatory laboratory tests for antiphospholipid antibodies. Unfortunately, despite their widespread use, tests for antiphospholipid antibodies are not robust: there is no agreement on the most effective constellation of tests, standardization of methods is incomplete and reproducibility is poor. Because of these limitations the need for attention to quality assurance of tests for antiphospholipid antibodies and an awareness of their limitations are paramount if clinical management is to be optimal.

In this chapter, the features of antiphospholipid syndrome are first reviewed, and the nature of antiphospholipid antibodies described, in order to set the context for a discussion of the important issues around the laboratory evaluation of antiphospholipid antibodies.

The definition of antiphospholipid syndrome

Antiphospholipid syndrome is an acquired thrombophilia with an immune pathogenesis. Diagnosis requires the coexistence of clinical manifestations, thrombosis or pregnancy complications, and the presence of antiphospholipid antibodies. These include anticardiolipin antibodies, anti-beta2 glycoprotein I and lupus anticoagulant, which are described below. Internationally agreed diagnostic criteria for the syndrome have been established in order to improve diagnostic accuracy [1]. They are summarized in Table 20.1.

Antiphospholipid antibodies

The nomenclature of antiphospholipid antibodies can appear confusing as it is based on historical understanding which has been superceded without revision of the terminology. Antibodies which are apparently reactive with phospholipid have been recognized for many decades, in association with disease. The "serological false positive test for syphilis" is the earliest example. It was identified in some subjects with systemic lupus erythematosus (SLE) and was demonstrated to be due to antibodies in serum which bind to negatively charged phospholipid. Subsequently cardiolipin, a phospholipid component of the mitochondrial membrane, was used routinely as the antigen in diagnostic assays in SLE and some other systemic autoimmune diseases. Eventually it was noted that tests for these anticardiolipin antibodies could identify patients with a prothrombotic state: antiphospholipid syndrome.

It was observed independently that the plasma of some subjects with SLE has a prolonged clotting time, especially in the activated partial thromboplastin time

Quality in Laboratory Hemostasis and Thrombosis, Second Edition. Edited by Steve Kitchen, John D. Olson and F. Eric Preston.
© 2013 John Wiley & Sons, Ltd. Published 2013 by Blackwell Publishing Ltd.

Table 20.1 Clinical and laboratory criteria of antiphospholipid syndrome

Clinical criteria	Laboratory criteria
Thrombosis Arterial, venous, or microvascular thrombosis in any tissue or organ	IgG and/or IgM anticardiolipin antibodies at moderate or high concentration and/or: IgG and/or IgM anti-beta2 glycoprotein I at moderate or high concentration and/or

Pregnancy complications
 	
  Unexplained death of a morphologically normal fetus at or after 10 weeks
 	
  Three or more unexplained consecutive abortions before 10 weeks
 	
  Premature birth before 34 weeks due to severe pre-eclampsia or placental insufficiency
	Lupus anticoagulant

There must be at least one clinical and at least one laboratory criterion present.

The laboratory test must be consistently positive on at least two occasions 12 weeks apart as transient antibodies may occur, for example in infection, and such antibodies are not usually associated with clinical events.

The titer of anticardiolipin/anti-beta2 glycoprotein I antibody must be moderate or high, as low titer antibodies are common and may not be clinically significant.

The syndrome may occur against a background of systemic autoimmune disease, especially systemic lupus erythematosus (secondary antiphospholipid syndrome) or in isolation (primary antiphospholipid syndrome).

The common thrombotic events are venous thromboembolism and ischemic stroke but thrombosis in any vascular territory may occur. Some other clinical associations with antiphospholipid antibodies have been identified. These include thrombocytopenia, skin lesions including ulceration and livedo reticularis/recemosa, and non-stroke neurological conditions including transverse myelopathy.

Some other supposed associations between clinical events and antiphospholipid antibodies are less convincing and may represent chance findings of no clinical significance, for example, infertility [2].

(APTT) or kaolin clotting time (KCT), in the absence of any clinical bleeding tendency. This was shown to be due to the presence of an *in vitro* inhibitor of coagulation; the term lupus anticoagulant was coined. This lupus anticoagulant coagulation inhibitor is an immunoglobulin. In SLE, both anticardiolipin antibodies and lupus anticoagulant may be present and, paradoxically, the presence of antiphospholipid antibodies, including lupus anticoagulant, is not only unaccompanied by clinical bleeding but is associated with an increased risk of thrombosis: antiphospholipid syndrome. Subsequently the link was made to recurrent pregnancy failure and other pregnancy complications.

In addition to the paradox of the association between lupus anticoagulant and thrombosis rather than bleeding there is an additional complication in relation to terminology: it has been demonstrated clearly that, in relation to antiphospholipid antibodies, the relevant antigenic sites do not reside on phospholipids. In the early 1990's it was demonstrated that at least some antiphospholipid antibodies bind to a protein, beta2 glycoprotein I. This protein is present in high concentration in plasma. Beta2 glycoprotein I is a member of the family of complement control proteins (CCP). It binds avidly to anionic phospholipids and has a weak anticoagulant effect. Some other plasma proteins can also serve as target antigens for antiphospholipid antibodies. These include prothrombin, protein C, and annexin V. They all have a propensity to bind to anionic phospholipid. The apparent binding of antiphospholipid antibodies to phospholipid is through the clustering of antigenic sites on the target phospholipid-binding protein when the latter binds to a negatively charged phospholipid surface facilitating bivalent antibody binding to epitopes on the bound protein. In the diagnostic laboratory this phenomenon is exploited for the detection of antiphospholipid antibodies by coating of plastic wells with phospholipid, beta2 glycoprotein I, prothrombin, or other relevant protein in enzyme-linked immunosorbent assays (ELISA).

Lupus anticoagulants

Lupus anticoagulants are heterogeneous, an observation of some importance in relation to the need for the development of improved assays designed to detect clinically important lupus anticoagulant antibodies. Both antiprothrombin- and anti-beta2 glycoprotein I-type antiphospholipid antibodies may have lupus anticoagulant activity. The likely explanation is that binding of such antibodies to their phospholipid-binding protein target interferes with the assembly of the prothrombinase complex on the template provided by anionic phospholipids. For example, antibodies to beta2 glycoprotein I enhance the binding of beta2 glycoprotein I to phospholipid *in vitro*. As a result thrombin generation is slowed resulting in a prolonged time to clot formation in phospholipid-dependent coagulation tests, especially when available phospholipid is rate limiting such as in the KCT and the dilute Russell's viper venom time (DRVVT).

The pivotal role of beta2 glycoprotein I

Increased knowledge of the structure and properties of beta2 glycoprotein I has assisted in the understanding of the nature and pathogenicity of antiphospholipid antibodies. Beta2 glycoprotein I has five domains characterized by CCP repeats. The first four are similar, but the fifth is larger and includes a cluster of positively charged amino acids. This explains the anionic phospholipid-binding property. Antibodies may be directed against epitopes on any of the five domains. However, recent data indicate that it is only those which react with a specific epitope on domain I which have lupus anticoagulant activity. Furthermore, it is domain I antibodies which associate strongly with thrombotic manifestations [3].

Observational studies suggest that positivity in tests for lupus anticoagulant is more strongly associated with thrombosis [4] and recurrent late fetal loss [5] than is the presence of anticardiolipin antibodies.

There is potential to increase assay specificity still further by focusing on antibodies to domain I of beta2 glycoprotein I.

Lupus anticoagulant assays

All current tests for lupus anticoagulant are coagulation-based assays performed on citrated plasma. As such they are indirect tests and are not completely specific. For example, prolongation of clotting time can be obtained in the presence of other coagulation inhibitors or due to coagulation factor deficiency. However the specificity can be improved through the selection of reagents and conditions which increase sensitivity to lupus anticoagulant, by mixing studies to confirm inhibitory activity rather than factor deficiency, and by inclusion of additional steps to demonstrate the phospholipid-dependent nature of any inhibitor. There are numerous publications on the selection and performance of lupus anticoagulant assays, for example, the guidelines on this topic prepared by the British Committee for Standards in Haematology [6]. The coagulation tests which are generally regarded to be most useful in the diagnostic laboratory are the APTT, the KCT, and the DRVVT. There is no test which is completely sensitive to, and specific for, lupus anticoagulant and it is recommended that two tests of different types are used together to improve sensitivity. Furthermore, the presence of anionic phospholipid in test plasma can potentially reduce assay sensitivity. The most likely source is blood cell membrane. To minimize this possibility, plasma should be prepared as soon as possible after venepuncture, preferably within 1 hour, and subjected to further centrifugation to minimize phospholipid contamination.

The APTT

APTT reagents vary markedly in the composition and concentrations of phospholipid. This results in considerable heterogeneity in terms of sensitivity to lupus anticoagulant. Furthermore, the coagulation time in the APTT is influenced by the concentrations of all coagulation factors in the intrinsic and common pathways and this impacts on both sensitivity and specificity. For example, the shortening of the APTT which is associated with an increased concentration of factor VIII, a common phenomenon in systemic disease, may mask any prolongation of the APTT by a lupus inhibitor. The poor specificity caused by sensitivity to factor deficiency can be improved, however, by the use of mixing tests with normal plasma to confirm the presence of an inhibitor. Some other modifications to the APTT designed to improve specificity/sensitivity for lupus anticoagulant are the performance of the test in duplicate using lupus anticoagulant sensitive and insensitive reagents and the use of sensitive reagents in higher than usual dilution. In summary, when the APTT is employed as a screening test for lupus anticoagulant, it is essential that attention is paid to the limitations of the test for this purpose, optimal choice of reagents for maximum sensitivity and the pitfalls in interpretation of results.

The KCT

In the KCT there is no added phospholipid, clotting being dependent upon the low residual concentration of phospholipids in centrifuged plasma. This should render the test sensitive to lupus anticoagulant but the test suffers from the same problems as the APTT in relation to sensitivity and specificity because of the influence of factor deficiencies and other coagulation factor inhibitors on the clotting time. Specificity is improved through nullifying the effect of any factor deficiency by performing the test on a dilute mixture of test and normal plasma: a 1:4 mixture is recommended as this should guarantee the correction of any factor deficiency whilst sensitivity to lupus anticoagulant is generally retained.

The DRVVT

Russell's viper venom initiates clotting through the activation of factor X. Because fewer coagulation factors are required for clotting to occur, the use of the venom should result in a more specific test for lupus anticoagulant in comparison to the APTT and KCT. In addition, sensitivity is increased by the use of a high dilution of phospholipid. Specificity may be enhanced by demonstration of shortening of the clotting time of test plasma in a "platelet neutralization procedure." In this correction procedure anionic phospholipid is exposed on washed normal platelets by activation with calcium ionophore or through cell-lysis-induced repeated freezing and thawing. The

principle employed is that when such a preparation is added to the lupus anticoagulant plasma, the prolonged clotting time is corrected, but not if the prolongation is due to factor deficiency. Alternative reagents have been employed to demonstrate phospholipid dependence, including platelet-derived microvesicles and a preparation containing hexagonal phase phospholipids. Numerous commercial assay kits based on the DRVVT are available. Several methods for the calculation of the level of correction of prolonged DRVVT have been proposed. Unfortunately there is no consensus on the most appropriate method and nor is there conformity in relation to the degree of correction which most reliably indicates positivity for lupus anticoagulant, despite evidence that this would improve reproducibility between DRVVT assays [7].

In a survey carried out by the National External Quality Assurance Scheme (NEQAS) for blood coagulation in the United Kingdom [8], it was found that 98% of diagnostic laboratories employ the DRVVT for testing for lupus anticoagulant, 85% the APTT, and 34% the KCT. In addition, a small number of laboratories reported use of the tissue thromboplastin inhibition test/dilute prothrombin time. The principle of the test is that although thromboplastin contains very high concentrations of phospholipid, rendering the prothrombin time generally insensitive to lupus anticoagulant, when the thromboplastin reagent is diluted, the phospholipid concentration is the rate limiting factor, and inhibition of prothrombinase by lupus anticoagulant prolongs the clotting time. Thus, a progressive increase in clotting time with thromboplastin dilution is suggestive of lupus anticoagulant. Although the assay was found to be less sensitive than the KCT [9], Arnout et al. demonstrated subsequently that the sensitivity and specificity for lupus anticoagulant could be improved markedly when a recombinant tissue thromboplastin (Innovin) was used in the assay, compared with results with a rabbit brain thromboplastin (Simplastin)[10].

Numerous variations of the above assays have been recommended, and some other approaches for the identification of lupus anticoagulant positive plasmas. This reflects the lack of a completely satisfactory test. For example, snake venom enzymes which activate prothrombin directly have been used, in an attempt to improve specificity. Taipan venom and the venom of Pseudonaja textilis (Textarin) both activate prothrombin in a phospholipid- and calcium-dependent manner, Textarin requiring the presence of factor V in addition. Tests employing these venoms are sensitive to lupus anticoagulant if the concentration of the phospholipid employed is low. A modification of the Textarin-based assay which improves specificity employs a second venom-derived enzyme, Ecarin. Ecarin activates prothrombin in a phospholipid-independent manner and is, therefore, not sensitive to lupus anticoagulant. The Textarin/Ecarin ratio appears to have high sensitivity for lupus anticoagulant in some hands [11].

The British Committee for Standards in Haematology recommend the use of at least two coagulation assays with different principles for lupus anticoagulant detection—typically an APTT using a sensitive reagent and a mixing test to detect an inhibitor, and, based on its association with thrombosis in cohort studies, a DRVVT with a correction procedure. Updated international guidelines for lupus anticoagulant detection recommend against the use of the KCT due to its relatively poor reproducibility [12, 13].

Lupus anticoagulant assay performance

Because the tests for lupus anticoagulant are essentially indirect tests which may be influenced by the quality of the plasma sample, the presence of other inhibitors including anticoagulant drugs, coagulation factor deficiencies, and the choice of test, reagents, and the method of end-point detection, it is unsurprising that accuracy and reproducibility are not optimal. This has been revealed through external quality assurance programs. For example, in 1997 [8], Jennings et al. reported on the performance of lupus anticoagulant testing by 220 laboratories in the UK NEQAS for blood coagulation. Fewer than half of the laboratories identified a sample considered to be weakly positive for lupus anticoagulant correctly and around a quarter of laboratories misinterpreted a sample mildly deficient in factor IX as lupus anticoagulant positive. In a follow-up study reported in 2002 [14], there may have been some improvement but accurate identification of a weak lupus anticoagulant remained problematic for around a third of participating laboratories. Unsurprisingly, similar results have been obtained in other countries [15]. Furthermore, Pengo et al. [16] demonstrated that when a comprehensive range of assays was applied by a reference laboratory, around 25%

of plasmas considered to be positive for lupus anticoagulant by participating specialized laboratories represented false positive results. Because lupus anticoagulant is the most informative marker of thrombosis risk in antiphospholipid syndrome, false negative and false positive results are likely to adversely affect therapeutic decisions resulting in poor clinical outcomes.

In recognition of the limitations of current assays for lupus anticoagulant, recommendations have been made in an attempt to improve assay performance. Attention to pre-analytical variables has been referred to already. This applies to control plasmas also. In addition, local reference ranges using a minimum of 20 normal plasma samples should be established for each method and coagulometer. This applies equally to in-house methods and commercial kits. Pooled plasmas for calculation of clotting time ratios should be prepared from at least 12 individual normal plasma donations. In addition, when in-house assays are used, care must be taken to optimize assay conditions. For example, for the DRVVT, it is essential to titrate the venom reagent to determine the optimal clotting time for the coagulometer in use and to select the optimal dilution of phospholipid for maximal sensitivity and specificity.

Despite the recognition of these important variables and attention to them in many diagnostic laboratories there remains a lack of conformity in lupus anticoagulant testing. This is reflected in variations in assay selection and the number of individual assays used to test each sample. Even the degree of correction required for maximal specificity in confirmatory tests has not been agreed. These are obvious areas for improvement.

Some other approaches to improvement in the accuracy of lupus anticoagulant tests have been suggested. These include the development of widely available reference materials and standards, and new assays which better identify clinically important lupus anticoagulants. In relation to reference materials the ideal would be well characterized lupus anticoagulant positive plasmas from subjects with a firm diagnosis of antiphospholipid syndrome. However, a sufficient and regular supply of such materials for global use is not feasible. Alternative solutions have been sought, including the use of normal pooled plasma spiked with monoclonal antibodies to beta2 glycoprotein I or prothrombin. Although this approach appears to have some utility in assay standardization [17] an obvious drawback is that the spiked plasmas may not adequately reflect the characteristics of clinically important antiphospholipid antibodies.

Whether the introduction of more specific tests for subtypes of lupus anticoagulants which are most closely linked to thrombosis and pregnancy failure might improve diagnostic accuracy is of interest but remains speculative. Research in this area has been led by the group of de Groot. As described above, lupus anticoagulant activity is a feature of some antiprothrombin and some anti-beta2 glycoprotein I antibodies. They may occur alone or in combination in lupus anticoagulant positive plasmas [18]. Lupus anticoagulants which are prothrombin-dependent can be distinguished from the beta2 glycoprotein-I dependent antibodies by modified coagulation tests. Importantly, it appears that it is the latter antibodies which associate with thrombotic events in patients. Furthermore, in a landmark paper, de Laat and colleagues [3] demonstrated, in elegant experiments employing deletion mutants of beta2 glycoprotein I, that among anti-beta2 glycoprotein I antibodies it is the IgG antibodies which recognize the sequence Gly40-Arg43 of domain I which have lupus anticoagulant activity. This raises the possibility of the development of new, more specific tests for clinically important antibodies. One such APTT-based lupus anticoagulant assay which employs cardiolipin vesicles as a confirmatory reagent is deserving of further assessment [19]. Addition of cardiolipin vesicles shortened the prolonged clotting time caused by anti-beta2 glycoprotein I antibodies with lupus anticoagulant activity, but further prolonged the clotting time in plasma with antiprothrombin antibodies with lupus anticoagulant activity. Pengo et al. used a different approach [20]. They found that a reduction in the final calcium concentration in a DRVVT and a dilute prothrombin time assay further prolonged the clotting time in the presence of beta2 glycoprotein I-dependent lupus anticoagulants whereas there was a shortening of clotting time in lupus anticoagulant positive, anti-beta2 glycoprotein I negative plasmas. Such approaches could significantly improve the specificity of lupus anticoagulant assays for antiphospholipid syndrome. However, for now, there should be concerted efforts to standardize approaches to the use of coagulation assays for the diagnosis of antiphospholipid syndrome. Also, it is essential that diagnostic and research laboratories engaged in the identification of lupus anticoagulant

positive plasmas use robust internal quality assurance measures and take part in external quality assurance programs in order to provide some reassurance on performance in this difficult area.

Assay of lupus anticoagulant in subjects treated with coumarin

The accurate identification of lupus anticoagulant in a patient with reduced concentrations of gamma-carboxylated coagulation factors due to treatment with coumarin is particularly challenging. Perhaps the simplest approach is to perform a lupus anticoagulant assay on a mixture of test and normal plasma on the assumption that the concentrations of vitamin K-dependent coagulation factors are increased to within the normal range in the plasma mix. However, inevitably this results in a dilution of the lupus anticoagulant immunoglobulin also, with consequential reduced assay sensitivity. Indeed, this dilution effect on the antibody has been demonstrated to significantly impair the detection of lupus anticoagulant, confirming the limitations of this method [21]. Alternative approaches include the use of the Taipan snake venom time with a platelet neutralization procedure [22] and the Taipan snake venom time combined with the Ecarin time [23]. However, when one considers the poor performance of lupus anticoagulant assays performed without the added complication of reduced levels of vitamin K-dependent coagulation factors it seems unlikely there can be confidence in the diagnosis of the presence of lupus anticoagulant in a subject under treatment with coumarin. As such, and in view of the implications of a diagnosis of antiphospholipid syndrome for duration of anticoagulant therapy, it would seem to be preferable to briefly interrupt anticoagulant treatment in order to perform lupus anticoagulant assays in those cases where a confident diagnosis is paramount.

There has been concern over the prolongation of the prothrombin time/INR due to lupus anticoagulant and the possibility that this may result in insufficiently intensive anticoagulation in subjects with antiphospholipid syndrome who are treated with coumarin. However, in one large series only around 4% of lupus anticoagulant plasmas from non-anticoagulated patients had prolonged prothrombin time using a recombinant thromboplastin (Innovin) [24]. In general there appears to be little interference by lupus anticoagulants in the prothrombin time/INR if insensitive thromboplastin is employed with instrument-specific international sensitivity index (ISI) [25]. (For further discussion of INR use in the presence of antiphospholipid antibodies, see Chapter 18, Monitoring Oral Anticoagulant Therapy).

Anticardiolipin assays

The solid phase assays employed for detection and quantitation of anticardiolipin antibodies have been refined over two decades. Commercial kits for the quantitation of IgG and IgM anticardiolipin antibodies are readily available. They carry theoretical advantages over lupus anticoagulant assays: testing in bulk is achievable, standards are readily available, coagulation factor deficiencies are irrelevant, immunoglobulin inhibitors of specific clotting factors do not interfere in the assay, and therapeutic anticoagulants have no impact on assay results. Unfortunately, however anticardiolipin ELISAs cannot substitute for lupus anticoagulant assays for diagnostic purposes because in some subjects with antiphospholipid syndrome who are lupus anticoagulant positive, tests for anticardiolipin are negative and the sensitivity of the tests for thrombosis differs, lupus anticoagulant being more specific.

The use of affinity purified standards is essential. They allow expression of IgG and IgM anticardiolipin antibodies in widely accepted antiphospholipid units: GPLU and MPLU respectively. This is of great practical importance as the consensus guidelines for the firm diagnosis of antiphospholipid syndrome specify that as a diagnostic criterion, anticardiolipin antibody must be present in medium or high titer, defined as >40 GPLU or MPLU or >99th percentile. This reflects the observation that low titer anticardiolipin antibodies are a frequent incidental finding. They are detected in up to 5% of tests and are often transient. Any relationship to thrombosis or pregnancy complications is weak or absent.

Although IgM anticardiolipin is included as a criterion in the consensus guideline, observational studies have generally suggested that the IgM isotype is only weakly associated with clinical events, if at all. Tests for IgA anticardiolipin are available but do not seem to be of diagnostic value and, as antibodies of IgA

isotype do not form part of the consensus criteria for diagnosis, the use of IgA anticardiolipin ELISAs in the diagnostic laboratory cannot be recommended. There have been numerous descriptions of ELISAs employing alternative anionic phospholipids, for example, phosphatidylserine. In general, such assays behave in a similar manner to anticardiolipin assays and their employment does not aid diagnosis of antiphospholipid syndrome.

Anticardiolipin assay performance

Despite the advantages of solid phase assays for the detection of antiphospholipid antibodies, not least the ready availability of standards, assay performance is disappointing. For example, in 1995 Reber et al. compared the values obtained for six anticardiolipin standards in nine commercial anticardiolipin assay kits and an in-house method [26]. Concordance was extremely poor, to the extent that the highest standard employed would not have been deemed even moderately positive in some assays according to the current consensus guideline for the diagnosis of antiphospholipid syndrome. This implies that the attribution of a diagnosis of antiphospholipid syndrome in a particular patient may reflect the choice of anticardiolipin assay kit rather than the truth. A more recent report indicates that this unacceptable situation had not been resolved. In their analysis, in 2002, of results from 56 laboratories testing 12 samples for IgG and IgM anticardiolipin as part of an external quality assurance scheme, Favaloro and Silvestrini reported an overall interlaboratory coefficient of variation of >50% in 74% of tests [27]. Remarkably, they were led to conclude that "In the majority of cases laboratories could not decide on whether a laboratory was cardiolipin positive or negative." Unacceptable coefficients of variation between assays even when plasmas spiked with lyophilized, affinity purified immunoglobulin are used as test samples has been reported also [14], highlighting the lack of uniformity of assay reagents and methods currently employed.

Variables which have been identified to influence anticardiolipin assay performance include the quality of the cardiolipin used and the technique employed for coating plates. The use of uncoated wells/plates as blanks is essential in order to allow for non-specific binding [28]. An expert group has recommended four requirements for antiphospholipid ELISAs which may reduce interlaboratory variability [29]. These are: performance of assays in duplicate; determination of the cut-off for positivity by analysis of at least 50 samples from normal subjects, preferably age- and sex-matched with the typical clinic population; calculation of the cut-off level in percentiles; and employment of stable standards. It seems unlikely that all of this advice is routinely followed by the majority of diagnostic laboratories at the present time.

Based on the nature of the putative pathogenic antibodies described above it is essential that anticardiolipin assays detect only those antibodies which are beta2 glycoprotein I-dependent. This can be provided in the fetal calf serum or adult bovine serum in the blocking agent which is used to reduce non-specific binding, or in the sample diluent. This requirement for diagnostic anticardiolipin assays to measure beta2 glycoprotein I-dependent antibodies and their generally poor performance has led to an ongoing debate regarding whether anticardiolipin assays should be replaced by anti-beta2 glycoprotein I ELISAs or whether they are complementary [30]. The emerging evidence from case series, that the number of different tests type positive provides important information regarding the likely clinical implications, suggests that the tests are indeed complimentary to some degree at least [31, 32].

Anti-beta2 glycoprotein I antibody assays

Improvements in our understanding of the nature of antiphospholipid antibodies led to the development of ELISAs for the determination of anti-beta2 glycoprotein I. Several commercial assay kits are routinely available for diagnostic use. In view of the observation that it is beta2 glycoprotein I-dependent lupus anticoagulants which are most strongly associated with clinical manifestations in antiphospholipid syndrome, and because the clinically relevant antibodies detected in anticardiolipin assays are beta2 glycoprotein I-dependent, it is reasonable to suppose that the assay of antibodies which bind specifically to beta2 glycoprotein I would provide improved diagnostic specificity. To some extent this may be true: Galli et al. undertook a systematic review of the literature and reached the conclusion that anti-beta2

glycoprotein I antibodies are more strongly associated with thrombosis than anticardiolipin antibodies [33]. Also, as indicated above, some anticardiolipin assays detect non-beta2 glycoprotein I-dependent antibodies. In some cases these antibodies are induced by infection and have no significance as far as risk of thrombosis is concerned. However, the situation is not completely straightforward. First, the anti-beta2 glycoprotein I assays are less well standardized at present, in comparison with the long-established anticardiolipin assays. A titer in excess of the 99th centile is regarded as significant according to the international consensus criteria [1]. Second, the work of de Groot and colleagues already referred to indicates that it is only a subset of anti-beta 2 glycoprotein I antibodies which have lupus anticoagulant activity (those recognizing Gly40-Arg43 on domain I) and it is lupus anticoagulant-type antibodies which associate most strongly with thrombosis. Third, anti-beta2 glycoprotein I antibodies have been reported to be present in association with infections: specifically syphilis, leptospirosis, visceral leishmaniasis, and leprosy [34]. However, in a group of subjects with leprosy, Arvieux et al. [35] demonstrated that the anti-beta2 glycoprotein I antibodies which were present in a high proportion of subjects were distinct from those in antiphospholipid syndrome with respect to IgG subclass, avidity, and epitope specificity. These observations provide further impetus to efforts to develop assays for antiphospholipid syndrome-specific anti-beta2 glycoprotein I antibodies.

Anti-beta2 glycoprotein I antibody assay performance

Disappointingly, anti-beta2 glycoprotein I assays appear to share the problem of poor interlaboratory reproducibility exhibited by anticardiolipin assays. For example, Reber and colleagues reported on 28 test samples analyzed across 21 European centers [36]. The proportion of results deemed to be positive ranged from 50% to 93% for IgG isotype and from 13% to 70% for IgM. Similarly, Favaloro et al. [37] reported poor performance of anti-beta2 glycoprotein I assays in an external quality assurance scheme. Interlaboratory coefficients of variation were more than 50% in 19 of 27 sera. The obvious implication, once again, is that whether a patient is deemed to have antiphospholipid syndrome varies depending upon the location of the diagnostic laboratory performing the assays. This is a highly unsatisfactory situation as the risk of recurrent thrombosis in antiphospholipid syndrome may be high and the principal treatment is anticoagulation with warfarin, an intervention which is associated with a significant rate of iatrogenic bleeding.

Antiprothrombin antibodies appear to be of low specificity for the diagnosis of antiphospholipid syndrome and assays for antiprothrombin antibodies are likely to suffer from the same issues of poor reproducibility as do anticardiolipin and anti-beta2 glycoprotein I assays. As such their use by diagnostic laboratories cannot be supported at the present.

The clinical implications of positive tests for antiphospholipid antibodies

It is recognized now that antiphospholipid antibodies are a quite frequent finding in apparently healthy people and even more frequent in some patient groups in which they may represent an epiphenomenon, such as in infertile women, migraineurs, and patients with multiple sclerosis [2, 38–42]. A lack of awareness of this is likely to lead to overdiagnosis of antiphospholipid syndrome. Therefore, in reaching diagnostic and therapeutic decisions in the clinic, it is essential to consider the specific and individual clinical circumstances, the range of positive tests, and the immunoglobulin isotype and titer. Patients with true antiphospholipid syndrome are likely to have the relevant history of (frequently unprovoked) thrombosis and/or unexplained pregnancy failure together with both lupus anticoagulant and high titer IgG antibodies in the solid phase assays.

Summary and conclusion

Although the features of antiphospholipid syndrome and the diagnostic criteria are well defined, the serious deficiencies in the quality of the available laboratory tests for the condition have not been given adequate consideration in clinical practice. Assays for lupus anticoagulant, anticardiolipin, and anti-beta2 glycoprotein I all perform poorly in quality assurance exercises. There is a need for consensus among laboratory scientists, clinicians, and manufacturers of laboratory reagents and equipment on the most effective combination of assays and choice of reagents and methods for optimal sensitivity and specificity. At the same time, research should concentrate on the development of assays for disease-specific antiphospholipid antibodies.

References

1. Miyakis S, Lockshin MD, Atsumi T, et al. International consensus statement on an update of the classification criteria for definite antiphospholipid syndrome (APS). *J Thromb Haemost.* 2006;4(2):295–306.
2. Buckingham KL, Chamley LW. A critical assessment of the role of antiphospholipid antibodies in infertility. *J Reprod Immunol.* 2009;80(1–2):132–145.
3. de Laat B, Derksen RH, Urbanus RT, de Groot PG. IgG antibodies that recognize epitope Gly40-Arg43 in domain I of beta 2-glycoprotein I cause LAC, and their presence correlates strongly with thrombosis. *Blood.* 2005;105(4):1540–1545.
4. Galli M, Luciani D, Bertolini G, Barbui T. Lupus anticoagulants are stronger risk factors for thrombosis than anticardiolipin antibodies in the antiphospholipid syndrome: a systematic review of the literature. *Blood.* 2003;101(5):1827–1832.
5. Opatrny L, David M, Kahn SR, Shrier I, Rey E. Association between antiphospholipid antibodies and recurrent fetal loss in women without autoimmune disease: a metaanalysis. *J Rheumatol.* 2006;33(11):2214–2221.
6. Greaves M, Cohen H, MacHin SJ, Mackie I. Guidelines on the investigation and management of the antiphospholipid syndrome. *Br J Haematol.* 2000;109(4):704–715.
7. Gardiner C, MacKie IJ, Malia RG, et al. The importance of locally derived reference ranges and standardized calculation of dilute russell's viper venom time results in screening for lupus anticoagulant. *Br J Haematol.* 2000;111(4):1230–1235.
8. Jennings I, Kitchen S, Woods TA, Preston FE, Greaves M. Potentially clinically important inaccuracies in testing for the lupus anticoagulant: an analysis of results from three surveys of the UK national external quality assessment scheme (NEQAS) for blood coagulation. *Thromb Haemost.* 1997;77(5):934–937.
9. Exner T. Comparison of two simple tests for the lupus anticoagulant. *Am J Clin Pathol.* 1985;83(2):215–218.
10. Arnout J, Vanrusselt M, Huybrechts E, Vermylen J. Optimization of the dilute prothrombin time for the detection of the lupus anticoagulant by use of a recombinant tissue thromboplastin. *Br J Haematol.* 1994;87(1):94–99.

11. Forastiero RR, Cerrato GS, Carreras LO. Evaluation of recently described tests for detection of the lupus anticoagulant. *Thromb Haemost.* 1994;72(5):728–733.

12. Keeling D, Mackie I, Moore GW, Greer IA, Greaves M. Guidelines on the investigation and management of antiphospholipid syndrome. *Br J Haematol.* 2012 Feb 8. doi: 10.1111/j.1365-2141.2012.09037.x.[Epub ahead of print].

13. Pengo V, Tripodi A, Reber G, et al. Update on the guidelines for LA detection. *J Thromb Haemost.* 2009;7:1737–1740.

14. Jennings I, Greaves M, Mackie IJ, Kitchen S, Woods TA, Preston FE. UK National External Quality Assessment Scheme for Blood Coagulation. Lupus anticoagulant testing: improvements in performance in a UK NEQAS proficiency testing exercise after dissemination of national guidelines on laboratory methods. *Br J Haematol.* 2002;119(2):364–369.

15. Tripodi A, Biasiolo A, Chantarangkul V, Pengo V. Lupus anticoagulant (LA) testing: performance of clinical laboratories assessed by a national survey using lyophilized affinity-purified immunoglobulin with LA activity. *Clin Chem.* 2003;49(10):1608–1614.

16. Pengo V, Biasiolo A, Bison E, Chantarangkul V, Tripodi A. Italian Federation of Anticoagulation Clinics (FCSA). Antiphospholipid antibody ELISAs: survey on the performance of clinical laboratories assessed by using lyophilized affinity-purified IgG with anticardiolipin and anti-beta2-glycoprotein I activity. *Thromb Res.* 2007;120(1):127–133.

17. Jennings I, Mackie I, Arnout J, Preston FE. UK National External Quality Assessment Scheme for Blood Coagulation. Lupus anticoagulant testing using plasma spiked with monoclonal antibodies: performance in the UK NEQAS proficiency testing programme. *J Thromb Haemost.* 2004;2(12):2178–2184.

18. Horbach DA, van Oort E, Derksen RH, de Groot PG. The contribution of anti-prothrombin-antibodies to lupus anticoagulant activity–discrimination between functional and non-functional anti-prothrombin-antibodies. *Thromb Haemost.* 1998;79(4):790–795.

19. de Laat HB, Derksen RH, Urbanus RT, Roest M, de Groot PG. Beta2-glycoprotein I-dependent lupus anticoagulant highly correlates with thrombosis in the antiphospholipid syndrome. *Blood.* 2004;104(12):3598–3602.

20. Pengo V, Biasiolo A, Pegoraro C, Iliceto S. A two-step coagulation test to identify antibeta-glycoprotein I lupus anticoagulants. *J Thromb Haemost.* 2004;2(5):702–707.

21. Moore GW, Savidge GF. The dilution effect of equal volume mixing studies compromises confirmation of inhibition by lupus anticoagulants even when mixture specific reference ranges are applied. *Thromb Res.* 2006;118(4):523–528.

22. Rooney AM, McNally T, Mackie IJ, Machin SJ. The taipan snake venom time: a new test for lupus anticoagulant. *J Clin Pathol.* 1994;47(6):497–501.

23. Moore GW, Smith MP, Savidge GF. The ecarin time is an improved confirmatory test for the taipan snake venom time in warfarinized patients with lupus anticoagulants. *Blood Coagul Fibrinolysis.* 2003;14(3):307–312.

24. Moore GW, Rangarajan S, Holland LJ, Henley A, Savidge GF. Low frequency of elevated prothrombin times in patients with lupus anticoagulants when using a recombinant thromboplastin reagent: implications for dosing and monitoring of oral anticoagulant therapy. *Br J Biomed Sci.* 2005;62(1):15–18; quiz 47.

25. Tripodi A, Chantarangkul V, Clerici M, Negri B, Galli M, Mannucci PM. Laboratory control of oral anticoagulant treatment by the INR system in patients with the antiphospholipid syndrome and lupus anticoagulant. results of a collaborative study involving nine commercial thromboplastins. *Br J Haematol.* 2001;115(3):672–678.

26. Reber G, Arvieux J, Comby E, et al. Multicenter evaluation of nine commercial kits for the quantitation of anticardiolipin antibodies. The Working Group on Methodologies in Haemostasis from the GEHT (groupe d'etudes sur l'hemostase et la thrombose). *Thromb Haemost.* 1995;73(3):444–452.

27. Favaloro EJ, Silvestrini R. Assessing the usefulness of anticardiolipin antibody assays: a cautious approach is suggested by high variation and limited consensus in multilaboratory testing. *Am J Clin Pathol.* 2002;118(4):548–545

28. De Moerloose P, Reber G, Vogel JJ. Anticardiolipin antibody determination: comparison of three ELISA assays. *Clin Exp Rheumatol.* 1990;8(6):575–577.

29. Tincani A, Allegri F, Balestrieri G, et al. Minimal requirements for antiphospholipid antibodies ELISAs proposed by the European forum on antiphospholipid antibodies. *Thromb Res.* 2004;114(5–6):553–558.

30. de Moerloose P, Reber G. Antiphospholipid antibodies: do we still need to perform anticardiolipin ELISA assays? *J Thromb Haemost.* 2004;2(7):1071–1073.

31. Pengo V, Ruffatti A, Legnani C, et al. Incidence of a first thromboembolic event in asymptomatic carriers of high-risk antiphospholipid antibody profile: a multicenter prospective study. *Blood.* 2011;118(17):4714–4718.

32. Pengo V, Ruffatti A, Legnani C, et al. Clinical course of high-risk patients diagnosed with antiphospholipid syndrome. *J Thromb Haemost.* 2010;8(2):237–242.

33. Galli M, Luciani D, Bertolini G, Barbui T. Anti-beta 2-glycoprotein I, antiprothrombin antibodies, and the risk

of thrombosis in the antiphospholipid syndrome. *Blood.* 2003;102(8):2717–2723.

34. Santiago M, Martinelli R, Ko A, et al. Anti-beta2 glycoprotein I and anticardiolipin antibodies in leptospirosis, syphilis and kala-azar. *Clin Exp Rheumatol.* 2001;19(4):425–430.

35. Arvieux J, Renaudineau Y, Mane I, Perraut R, Krilis SA, Youinou P. Distinguishing features of anti-beta2 glycoprotein I antibodies between patients with leprosy and the antiphospholipid syndrome. *Thromb Haemost.* 2002;87(4):599–605.

36. Reber G, Tincani A, Sanmarco M, de Moerloose P, Boffa MC. Standardization group of the European Forum on Antiphospholipid Antibodies. *J Thromb Haemost.* 2004;2(10):1860–1862.

37. Favaloro EJ, Wong RC, Jovanovich S, Roberts-Thomson P. A review of beta2-glycoprotein-l antibody testing results from a peer-driven multilaboratory quality assurance program. *Am J Clin Pathol.* 2007;127(3):441–448.

38. Hughes GR. Migraine, memory loss, and "multiple sclerosis". Neurological features of the antiphospholipid (Hughes') syndrome. *Postgrad Med J.* 2003;79(928):81–83.

39. Avcin T, Markelj G, Niksic V, et al. Estimation of antiphospholipid antibodies in a prospective longitudinal study of children with migraine. *Cephalalgia.* 2004;24(10):831–837.

40. Williams FM, Cherkas LF, Bertolaccini ML, et al. Migraine and antiphospholipid antibodies: no association found in migraine-discordant monozygotic twins. *Cephalalgia.* 2008;28(10):1048–1052.

41. Heinzlef O, Weill B, Johanet C, et al. Anticardiolipin antibodies in patients with multiple sclerosis do not represent a subgroup of patients according to clinical, familial, and biological characteristics. *J Neurol Neurosurg Psychiatry.* 2002;72(5):647–649.

42. Liedorp M, Sanchez E, van Hoogstraten IM, et al. No evidence of misdiagnosis in patients with multiple sclerosis and repeated positive anticardiolipin antibody testing based on magnetic resonance imaging and long term follow-up. *J Neurol Neurosurg Psychiatry.* 2007;78(10):1146–1148.

21 Monitoring heparin therapy

Marilyn Johnston
Consultant, Hemostasis Reference Laboratory Hamilton, ON, Canada

Heparin

The discovery of heparin dates back to 1916. In that year, Jay McLean, a medical student at Johns Hopkins University, was searching for substances that caused clotting. Experimenting with homogenized dog liver, instead of finding a clotting material, McLean found a substance that prevented clotting. He named it heparin, from the Latin word for liver, hepar [1]. Heparin was first used in humans around 1940. It was prepared from extractions from porcine mucosa, and the procedure today is basically the same. Heparin, a sulfated glycosaminoglycan, has a mean size of 15,000 Daltons with a range of 3000 to 30,000 Daltons and is highly negatively charged.

This material is called unfractionated heparin (UFH), referring to the wide range of molecular weight products of which only a third have anticoagulant properties.

Mechanism of action

The determination of the mechanism of action for heparin developed through studies carried out over several years by a variety of researchers. In 1939, Brinkhous et al. [2] reported that heparin required a plasma cofactor in order for it to act as an anticoagulant. Abildgaard later identified this cofactor as antithrombin (AT) [3]. The mechanism for heparin–AT interaction was further studied by both Lindahl [4] and Rosenberg [5], showing that heparin binds to AT

through lysine residues. This produces a conformational change at the arginine reactive centre, converting AT from a slow progressive inhibitor to a rapid-acting one. The AT linked to heparin forms a covalent bond to the serine proteases of the coagulation pathway, irreversibly inhibiting their activity.

Subsequent work has shown that heparin binds to AT through a unique pentasaccharide sequence present in about one-third of UFH molecules [6]. Once bound, the heparin–AT complex can irreversibly inhibit the serine proteases of the coagulation pathway, but the strongest inhibition is against thrombin (IIa) and factor Xa (Xa). Thrombin is more readily inhibited than Xa by the heparin–AT complex (Figure 21.1). Over years of *in vitro* experimentation with UFH, clinical use, and clinical trials, heparin has been found to have a number of limitations.

Limitations of heparin

Pharmacokinetic

Heparin has been shown to bind nonspecifically to proteins, endothelial cells, and macrophages, thereby reducing its anticoagulant activity in a variable manner. Being negatively charged, heparin binds independent of the pentasaccharide to a variety of plasma proteins. These include histidine-rich glycoprotein, vitronectin, lipoproteins, fibronectin, and fibrinogen. Many of these proteins are acute phase reactants, and, when treating patients with

Quality in Laboratory Hemostasis and Thrombosis, Second Edition. Edited by Steve Kitchen, John D. Olson and F. Eric Preston.
© 2013 John Wiley & Sons, Ltd. Published 2013 by Blackwell Publishing Ltd.

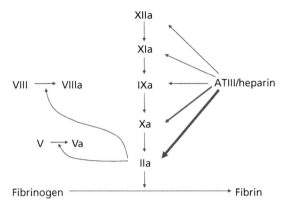

Figure 21.1 Heparin/antithrombin irreversibly inactivates the serine proteases of the coagulation pathway with the strongest inhibition against factor Xa (Xa), and thrombin (IIa). After Hirsh [7], with permission from PMPH-USA, Ltd.

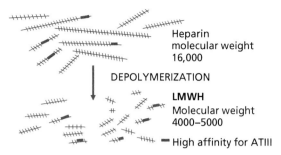

Figure 21.2 Commercial-grade heparin is chemically or enzymatically depolymerized to create LMWH that contains the high-affinity pentasaccharide. After Hirsh [7], with permission from PMPH-USA, Ltd.

venous thromboembolism, post surgery, and post myocardial infarction (MI), the variable levels of these proteins can lead to under-dosing heparin [8] as well as to a variable response of heparin from patient to patient. Heparin will also bind to platelet factor 4 (PF4) [9] and high molecular weight von Willebrand factor (vWF) secreted from the activated platelet or endothelium [10].

Clinical

Heparin can cause thrombocytopenia and osteoporosis.

Heparin-induced thrombocytopenia (HIT) is a result of heparin's high affinity for PF4. This binding results in a structural change in the PF4 so that it is recognized as a foreign protein and antibodies can therefore be produced [11]. These IgG antibodies form complexes with PF4 and heparin on the platelet surface, triggering platelet activation through the Fc receptors on the platelet membrane (Chapter 16).

Osteoporosis is a complication in approximately 2–3% of patients after 3 months of continuous heparin use. The mechanisms are well described in a paper by Shaughnessy and colleagues [12].

Low molecular weight heparins

In the early 1970s researchers began experimenting with techniques to reduce the wide molecular weight

range of heparin with a view to limiting the negative aspects of heparin treatment.

Johnson and Anderson [13] used gel filtration to separate heparin into four molecular weight groups. They found that as the molecular weight size decreased, the activated partial thromboplastin time (aPTT) became progressively shorter while the fractions still retained the ability to inhibit activated factor X. This observation has resulted in a plethora of research, the goal being finding an anticoagulant that provides protection from clot formation without the side effects of excessive bleeding.

Low molecular weight heparins (LMWHs) are prepared from UFH by chemical or enzymatic depolymerization and are, on average, one-third the molecular weight of the parent compound [7] (see Figure 21.2). Ultralow molecular weight heparins (U-LMWH) have been developed where the molecular weights are defined between 2000 and 3000 Daltons. Semuloparin, an U-LMWH, has also been enriched with AT-binding sites allowing anticoagulant activity to be directed toward Xa with little effect on IIa [14].

Because different methods of preparation are used, LMWHs are not equal, both when used clinically for a specific indication and in the laboratory, where the Xa:IIa ratios vary (Table 21.1). The LMWH preparations with the lower Xa:IIa ratios will have a greater effect on the activity assays of coagulation.

Inactivation of IIa by LMWH requires the simultaneous binding to the pentasaccharide and a minimum of an additional 13 saccharide units. Inactivation of Xa requires only the pentasaccharide unit [7] (Figure 21.3).

245

	Anti-Xa to anti-IIa ratio	MW range
Dalteparin	2.7:1	2000–9000
Enoxaparin	3.8:1	3000–8000
Tinzaparin	1.9:1	3000–6000
Reviparin	3.5:1	Mean MW 4000
Nadroparin	3.6:1	Median MW 4500
Ardeparin	1.9:1	Mean MW 6000

MW, Molecular weight

Current techniques used to measure heparin in plasma

aPTT
Protamine sulfate (PS) neutralization
Xa inhibition, chromogenic and clotting
IIa inhibition, chromogenic and clotting

Of these, the Xa inhibition chromogenic method is the most widely used for LMWH, fondaparinux, and the newer direct inhibitors of Xa including rivaroxaban (Chapter 24).

The aPTT still remains the procedure of choice for monitoring UFH. It is a simple, rapid, and inexpensive assay providing results within 30 minutes of blood collection. However, the method is difficult to standardize. The aPTT requires the entire cascade of coagulation proteins to be intact for the accurate measurement of heparin levels. Patients with lupus anticoagulant or antiphospholipid syndrome generally have prolonged aPTTs and must be monitored using heparin assays.

Besides levels of the various coagulation factors, reagents and instrumentation will affect the sensitivity to heparin and can result in a fourfold difference in results between reagents, making the results from one laboratory to another difficult to correlate [15]. A study by Bates et al. assayed six different aPTT reagents on five instrument platforms and compared the results to the anti-Xa heparin levels [15]. The conclusion was that, for the reagents studied and presuming the therapeutic interval to be 0.3–0.7 IU/mL of heparin, using a ratio of 2.0:3.5 more closely represented the therapeutic heparin level than the reported 1.5:2.5 times control plasma.

Studies have been carried out by the ISTH/SSC in an attempt to standardize the aPTT method by applying a correction factor similar to the use of an international sensitivity index (ISI) for prothrombin time testing [16]. Because of the wide variety of phospholipids, activators, and instruments, there was limited success and further work has not been initiated. It is recommended that each aPTT method be calibrated against anti-Xa heparin assays. The following is an accepted method for standardization [17].

Recommended protocol

1 Blood is collected from patients (ideally 50 patients) being treated with continuous intravenous heparin.

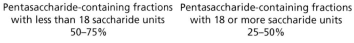

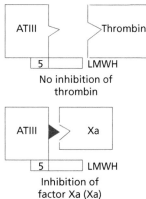

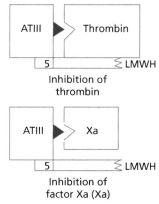

Figure 21.3 Low molecular weight activity. Approximately 25–50% of the LMWH molecules of different commercial preparations contain at least 18 saccharide units; these molecules inhibit both thrombin and Xa. The remaining 50–75% of LMWH molecules contain fewer than 18 saccharide units and only inhibit Xa. After Hirsh [7], with permission from PMPH-USA, Ltd.

These samples are taken at least 4–6 hours after a heparin bolus but less than 24 hours after the first dose of warfarin.

2 Blood samples are centrifuged at a minimum of 1700 G for 15 minutes. The plasma is transferred to a clean tube and recentrifuged for 5 minutes at 1700 G. The plasma is carefully transferred to a storage tube and frozen at −35°C or colder until testing is performed.

3 The plasma is thawed to 37°C for 5 minutes and the aPTT and heparin levels measured.

4 The relationship between aPTT and heparin level is plotted using linear regression analysis. The heparin level is plotted on the x axis and the aPTT values on the y axis. The line of best fit is calculated from the regression equation.

An alternate procedure and one that is less onerous is to freeze platelet-poor plasma from heparinized patients with known anti-Xa heparin levels at −70°C. Before retiring one lot number of aPTT reagent, aPTT measurements with the current reagent lot number and the new reagent lot number are performed side by side. If the values are within the tolerance of the assay, no further work is required. If the aPTT results are different, a regression analysis is performed using the anti-Xa values previously established, or the full procedure as described above is repeated.

Split samples may also be used. Once the laboratory has narrowed down the possible replacement of an aPTT reagent, then split samples may be measured with the new and old reagents. The comparison data are plotted with the old reagent on the x axis and the new on the y axis. Regression analysis or simply visual analysis is performed to check for discrepant results. A difference of 5 seconds between pairs is considered acceptable. The means and standard deviations for each set of data are calculated and recorded for use in charting the cumulative summation of difference over time [18]. By doing this, the cumulative shift in the reagent performance in the presence of heparin can be determined. A cumulative change of 5–7 seconds is reason for concern while a cumulative change of more than 7 seconds requires action. This may require looking at different reagents to choose one with a similar pattern as the previous reagent with an acceptable level of variation, or performing the aPTT, Xa heparin levels as in the full protocol for establishing a therapeutic range or informing the physicians of the change in the aPTT therapeutic range. Spiking heparin

into normal pooled plasma is not an acceptable procedure for determining the aPTT therapeutic range for heparin. The *in vitro* spiked plasma invariably gives a much steeper aPTT heparin response curve than *ex vivo* samples. This is due, in part, to the normal levels of coagulation proteins in the spiked normal plasma.

The therapeutic range for UFH levels is 0.2–0.4 IU/mL using protamine sulfate neutralization assay method [19] or 0.30–0.70 IU/mL using anti-Xa assays [20].

PS neutralization assay

The assay is based on the neutralization of UFH, a highly negatively charged molecule, by PS, a positively charged protein. A series of concentrations of PS are prepared and added to plasma. Thrombin is added and the clotting times measured. The concentration of PS to normalize the IIa clotting time of the test plasma is considered the heparin concentration. This procedure can only be used for UFH [21].

Chromogenic Xa inhibition heparin assays

The chromogenic assay was introduced in the late 1970s and still remains the assay of choice for monitoring LMWH and other Xa inhibitors. LMWH does not require constant monitoring. The drug is provided as weight-adjusted doses and monitoring is generally not required except for the following: patients who are very obese, very thin patients, patients with renal disease, patients with malignancy, women in the third trimester pregnancy, pediatric patients [22]. The clinical condition of the patient dictates the frequency of testing in these groups. Patients with renal disease should be monitored closely at the beginning of their treatment and then less often.

There are a number of different assays available to the laboratory; these include one-stage, and two-stage chromogenic or clotting inhibition assays. The chromogenic assays are all based on the original description by Teine et al. [23].

A generic two-stage chromogenic factor Xa heparin assay

The principle of all chromogenic heparin assays is the same: heparin in the sample binds with AT forming heparin–AT complexes. The heparin–AT complex inhibits Xa which has been added in excess. The residual Xa activity is measured by its action on a specific substrate, sensitive, and highly specific for Xa. The resulting release of paranitroaniline (pNA) is measured at 405 nM, and the reaction is inversely proportional to the concentration of heparin in the plasma.

Heparin + AT(plasma and exogenous) → [Hep-AT]
[Hep-AT] + [FXa (excess)] → [FXa-AT-Hep.]
   + [residual FXa]
[residual FXa] + Substrate → Peptide + pNA

The differences among assays are the incubation time of the reaction, the buffer used to dilute the plasma, the substrate, and the addition of exogenous AT. The presence of dextran sulfate (DXS) in the buffer reduces the influence of PF4 [24]. The assays may be one- or two-stage procedures and may be used for measurement of LMWH or UFH with the appropriate calibration line. Single calibration lines incorporating both LMWH and UFH (hybrid lines) have been validated and are commercially available. Studies have been encouraging using a single calibration line [25].

Interfering substances

One should be aware of the limitations of concentrations of interfering substances. The manufacturer for each assay provides maximum allowable levels of bilirubin, hemoglobin, and triglycerides.

One-stage chromogenic assays

One-stage methods for measuring heparin have been developed to simplify the assay and improve turnaround time. These assays do not add exogenous AT.

The assay is based on the principle of competitive inhibition. Xa is added to a plasma substrate mix resulting in two simultaneous reactions: hydrolysis of substrate by Xa and inhibition of Xa by the heparin–AT complex. Once the reaction reaches equilibrium, the quantity of PNA released from the substrate is inversely proportional to the concentration of heparin in the test plasma.

Heparin + AT (plasma) + Substrate + Xa → pNA

There are differing opinions on whether exogenous AT should be added to a heparin assay. One opinion is that the AT should not be added so one would rely on the level of AT in the patient's plasma. This would represent the functional response within the patient. Others believe AT should not be a rate-limiting protein and should be added to the test procedure to ensure 100% levels are present. This allows for the absolute drug concentration within the patient.

In patients with AT levels between 35% and 130%, the addition of exogenous AT has no effect on the resulting heparin concentration [26].

Xa inhibition clotting assays

Assays are commercially available that are based on the principle of the ability of heparin to complex with AT resulting in the inhibition of Xa.

An example of such an assay [27] uses undiluted plasma mixed with an equal volume of Xa and is incubated for a fixed period of time. This mix is then recalcified by the addition of a Recalmix consisting of calcium chloride, brain cephalin (phospholipid), factor V, and fibrinogen. The clotting time is measured and interpolated from a previously constructed calibration curve. Exogenous AT is not added in this assay, and the manufacturer recommends diluting the test plasma in normal pooled plasma if the patient is known to be AT deficient, or a newborn. Patients treated with warfarin should have their plasma diluted in normal plasma to correct for the low factor II levels in their plasma.

Another example of such an assay incorporates bovine AT into the procedure. In this assay, the patient plasma is diluted with 1:3 (UFH) and 1:5 (LMWH) in saline and an equal volume of AT is added. The concentration of AT is not given. The mix is allowed to incubate, followed by the addition of an excess of bovine Xa. The mix is further incubated followed by the addition of specially treated substrate plasma. Details are not given. After a short incubation, 0.025 M CaCl$_2$ is added and the clotting time measured.

In these assays, calibration curves can be prepared using the heparin preparation used for treatment, or a commercial secondary standard referenced against the World Health Organization (WHO) second International LMWH standard or the WHO sixth International UFH standard. The concentrations of heparin are plotted on the x axis of semi-log or log–log graph paper and the time in seconds for each respective point plotted on the y axis.

As with the chromogenic assays, the question of the calibration material and control plasmas is an issue and will be described below.

IIa inhibition assays

Available assays use bovine IIa and human AT. The inhibition of IIa by LMWH is variable and the assay is not recommended for LMWH determination. The assay can be used for UFH and is one of the assays used by manufacturers to assign potency to UFH.

The assay principles are the same as for the Xa inhibition assays except IIa replaces the Xa in the assay.

Heparin + AT → [Hep-AT]
[Hep-AT] + [excess IIa] → [FIIa-Hep-AT]
    + [residual IIa]
[IIa (residual)] + IIa-Substrate → Peptide + pNA

Quality control and assurance

Preanalytical variables

Specimen collection
Careful venipuncture technique must be used when collecting blood for all coagulation testing, including heparin assays.

The tourniquet should be applied for a minimal period of time and the venipuncture must be clean with a good flow of blood into the collection tube. Difficult venipunctures may result in platelet activation and subsequent release of PF4. PF4 readily binds UFH, resulting in an underestimation of the drug. The affinity for LMWH to PF4 is less, but still careful venipuncture is essential. The needle gauge also will contribute to platelet activation and a 21 gauge needle or less is recommended.

The blood (9 volumes) is collected into 0.109 M (3.2%) buffered citrate anticoagulant (1 volume). Other concentrations of citrate are not recommended for coagulation assays. There are special tubes available to minimize platelet activation: citrate, theophylline, adenosine and dipyridamole (CTAD) are available from Becton Dickinson.

Blood processing
Blood should be processed within 1 hour of collection. Centrifugation at a minimum of 1700 G for 15 minutes at 22°C (room temperature) is recommended. Following centrifugation, the plasma is carefully removed from the collection tube using a plastic pipette and placed in a plastic tube or container and capped.

To ensure minimal platelets, essentially platelet-free plasma, a double centrifugation technique is recommended. After the first centrifugation, the plasma is removed from the tube as above and the plasma centrifuged again for 5 minutes at the same speed. The plasma from this tube is carefully removed and placed in a clean plastic tube ready for freezing or assay. It is strongly advised that one of these procedures be used if the plasma is to be frozen [28].

Heparin calibration curves

The WHO provides biological reference preparation for a number of coagulation proteins including heparin. The current primary heparin standards available are:

sixth International Standard for UFH, 07/328, 2009, is available in lyophilized form at a concentration 2145 IU/ampoule,

second International standard for LMWH, 01/608, 2008, for LMWH is available in lyophilized form at a concentration of 1097 IU/mL anti-Xa units and 326 IU anti-IIa per ampoule.

Most manufacturers of heparin assay kits have available UFH and LMWH calibration material. This material is a secondary standard and should always be referenced by the manufacturer against the primary WHO standard. The type of LMWH used to spike the secondary plasma standard should also be made available to the laboratory by the manufacturer.

In a 2004 College of American Pathologists (CAP) survey, an UFH heparin sample was sent to 82 laboratories. The results among laboratories and among methodologies when read off a calibration curve prepared with UFH demonstrated reasonable correlation among methods, but still a wide range among laboratories, 0.2 to 0.64 anti-Xa units/mL. The imprecision was marked among methodologies and laboratories when the sample values were read off a LMWH calibration curve. In both instances the one-stage assay measured lower levels of heparin. These findings demonstrate the need for two calibrators, one for UFH and one for LMWH. Hybrid calibration curves have been introduced and it remains to be seen if the assays incorporating the two heparins into a single calibration curve will result in improved precision.

It has also been recommended that a calibration line specific for the type of LMWH being used in patient treatment be established. Two publications, both in abstract form, have demonstrated that this may not be required [29, 30]. The slopes and intercepts of plasma spiked with different LMWHs showed similar slopes and intercepts and although different, the differences would not be clinically significant. This is reassuring and adds confidence in using a commercially prepared calibration material even though it may be a different LMWH from that being used in the hospital.

Control plasmas

Control plasmas may be purchased from the kit manufacturer; however, it is preferable, at least at the validation stage of the assay, to prepare in-house controls. This is especially true if a laboratory is using a commercial calibration material to establish the calibration line. At least two levels of heparin controls are necessary, with one level just at the lower part of the reference line and one level close to the upper end.

This may be done by preparing a pool of normal plasma that has been rendered platelet-free (see sample preparation). A commercial plasma may be used but it must be plasma that has been prepared for this specific use, that is, it MUST be free of platelets before freezing and lyophilization. Any residual PF4 resulting from inadequate preparation will produce falsely low heparin levels.

The heparin used to spike the plasma when possible should be the same heparin used for patient treatment.

Results from quality assurance programs

In 2011, two quality assurance programs, ECAT Foundation and Thrombosis and Quality Manage-

ment Program – Laboratory Services (QMP-LS), each undertook a heparin survey. Lyophilized samples spiked with UFH and LMWH were distributed to 130 and 14 laboratories respectively, and each laboratory was asked to assay the sample using an anti-Xa heparin assay. The results were similar in both programs: anti-Xa heparin assay kits containing DXS recovered higher levels of UFH than those kits that did not contain DXS.

However, when the LMWH samples were tested, only a slight difference in results was seen between the two types of assay kits. In the ECAT survey, the between-laboratory variation was better for the LMWH than for UFH, 14% CV for the LMWH compared to a CV of 37–63% depending on the amount of heparin spiked into the plasma (Dr. Piet Meijer, Director ECAT foundation, Leiden, The Netherlands, personal communication). To determine if these differences were seen in samples from patients receiving therapeutic UFH, QMP-LS compared six frozen patient samples, using two kits with DXS and one kit without DXS. The samples were run at different hospitals and no bias was seen using the assay kits containing DXS [31]. A second study was performed in which 20 clinical samples were distributed to five hospital laboratories, two laboratories using a kit without DXS and three laboratories each using a different heparin kit containing DXS. No differences were seen in these sets of patient samples with only the expected scatter seen between the laboratories. The clinical sample values measured using kits with DXS were not higher than the values obtained using kits without DXS (Dr. W. Brien and Vanessa Chan, Hospital for Sick Children, Toronto, Canada, personal communication).Overestimation of heparin activity using assay kits with DXS has been described in cardiopulmonary bypass patients as well as postheparin reversal by protamine [32]. These results would be consistent with high levels of PF4 found in postcardiopulmonary bypass patients with heparin binding to PF4 making the heparin unavailable for assay. DXS could dissociate the heparin and higher levels of heparin would be measured.

The plasma used for spiking quality assurance samples may have higher levels of PF4 or other heparin-binding proteins. Lyophilization may also cause some changes in protein binding resulting in higher levels of heparin measured with assays containing DXS. Additional studies are ongoing.

Summary

Monitoring UFH

The aPTT remains the most commonly used method for monitoring UFH in spite of all its known standardization issues. Although it is a functional assay, it has many limitations, variable levels of clotting factors for one, masking the heparin anticoagulant effect. Anti-IIa and anti-Xa chromogenic heparin assays could be used but because of the costs, these assays have not become mainstream for monitoring UFH. Rosborough [33] addressed the question of cost by monitoring 268 patients treated with UFH with both aPTT and anti-Xa assays. He found that those patients monitored with the anti-Xa assay had fewer dose adjustments and fewer tests in a 24-hour period, and that in a 96-hour period, the anti-Xa assay cost $4.37 more than the aPTT assay.

Anti-IIa clotting assays have in the past been more difficult to standardize and were not widely used. This is changing with commercial kits being available and the need to assay direct thrombin inhibitors. Anti-II assays are now used by manufacturers of heparin to assign the potency replacing the method of timing the clotting of sheep's blood. Heparin potency is now labeled as International Standard, IS units replacing the US Pharmacopeia (USP) unit.

Monitoring LMWH

The aPTT and anti-IIa assays cannot be used for monitoring LMWH. The anti-Xa chromogenic or clotting is the method of choice. Standardization for both these assays is possible through the use of international standards and all commercial reference plasmas should be traceable to these standards. This will lead to better precision and accuracy between laboratories. Evidence of this has been demonstrated in recent CAP and ECAT surveys and in the 2003 collaborative study to calibrate the WHO Second International Standard where the coefficients of variation between laboratories were approximately 5% despite different kits and methods being used [34].

The Future

The current assays for measuring heparin have been criticized for not adequately measuring the biological effect of the drug. The endogenous thrombin potential (ETP) assay has the possibility of fulfilling this requirement but at present, it still remains primarily a research test.

References

1. Mclean J. The thromboplastic action of cehalin. *Am J Physiol*. 1916;41:250–257.
2. Brinkhous KM, Smith HP, Warner ED, Seegers WH. The inhibition of blood clotting: an unidentified substance which acts in conjunction with heparin to prevent the conversion of prothrombin into thrombin. *Am J Physiol*. 1939;125:683–687.
3. Abildgaard U. Highly purified antithrombin III with heparin cofactor activity prepared by disc electrophoresis. *Scan J Clin Lab Invest*. 1968;21:89–91.
4. Lindahl U, Bäckström G, Höök M, Thunberg L, Fransson LA, Linker A. Structure of the antithrombin-binding site of heparin. *Proc Natl Acad Sci USA*. 1979;6:3198–3202.
5. Rosenberg RD, Lam L. Correlation between structure and function of heparin. *Proc Natl Acad Sci USA*. 1979;76:1218–1222.
6. Casu B, Oreste P, Torri G, et al. The structure of heparin oligosaccharide fragments with high anti- (factor Xa) activity containing the minimal antithrombin III-binding sequence. *Biochem J*. 1981;97:599–609.
7. Hirsh J. *Low Molecular Weight Heparins*. 4th ed. Shelton, CT: PMPH-USA, Ltd.; 1999.
8. Hirsh J, van Aken WG, Gallus AS, et al. Heparin kinetics in venous thrombosis and pulmonary embolism. *Circulation*. 1976;53:691–695.
9. Amiral J, Bridey F, Dreyfus M, et al. Platelet factor 4 complexed to heparin is the target for antibodies generated in heparin-induced thrombocytopenia. *Thromb Haemost*. 1992;68:95–96.
10. Sobel M, McNeill PM, Carlson PL, et al. Heparin inhibition of von Willebrand factor-dependent platelet function in vitro and in vivo. *J Clin Invest*. 1991;87:1787–1793.
11. Kelton JG, Smith JW, Warkenting TE, Hayward CP, Denomme GA, Horsewood P. Immunoglobulin G from patients with heparin-induced thrombocytopenia binds to a complex of heparin and platelet factor 4. *Blood*. 1994;83:3232–3239.

12. Shaughnessy SG, Young E, Deschamps P, Hirsh J. The effects of low molecular weight and standard heparin on calcium loss from fetal rat calvaris. *Blood*. 1995;86(4):1368–1373.

13. Johnson EA, Kirkwood TB, Stirling Y, et al. Four heparin preparations: anti-Xa potentiating effect of heparin after subcutaneous injection. *Thromb Haemost*. 1976;35:586–591.

14. Kakkar A, Agnelli G, Fisher W, et al. The ultra-low-molecular-weight heparin semuloparin for prevention of venous thromboembolism in patients undergoing major abdominal surgery. *Blood (ASH Annual Meeting Abstracts)*. 2010;116:188.

15. Bates SM, Weitz JI, Johnston M, Hirsh J, Ginsberg JS. Use of a fixed activated partial thromboplastin time ratio to establish a therapeutic range for unfractionated heparin. *Arch Intern Med*. 2001;161:385–391.

16. Van der Veld EA, Poller L. The aPTT monitoring of heparin–the ISTH/ICSH collaborative study. *Thrombo Haemost*. 1995;73(1):73–81.

17. Brill-Edwards P, Ginsberg JS, Johnston M, Hirsh J. Establishing a therapeutic range for heparin therapy. *Ann Intern Med*. 1993;119:104–109.

18. Olson JD, Arkin CH, Brandt JT, et al. Laboratory monitoring of unfractionated heparin therapy. *Arch Pathol & Lab Med*. 1998;122(9):782–798.

19. Chiu HM, Hirsh J, Yung WL, Regoeczi E, Gent M. Relationship between anticoagulant and antithrombotic effects of heparin in experimental venous thrombosis. *Blood*. 1977;49:171–184.

20. Hirsh J, Fruster V. Guide to anticoagulant therapy. I: heparin. *Circulation*. 1994;89:1449–1468.

21. Refn I, Vestergaad L. The titration of heparin with protamine. *Scand J Clin Lab Invest*. 1954;6:284.

22. Laposata M, Green D, van Cott ENM, Barrowcliffe TW, Goodnight SH, Sosolik RC. The clinical use and laboratory monitoring of low molecular weight heparin, danaparoid, hirudin and related compounds, and argatroban. College of American Pathologist Conference XXXI on Laboratory Monitoring of Anticoagulant Therapy. *Arch Pathol Lab Med*. 1998;122:799–807.

23. Teien AN, Lie M. Evaluation of an amidolytic heparin assay method: increased sensitivity by adding purified antithrombin III. *Thromb Res*. 1977;10:399–410.

24. Lyons SG, Lasser EC, Stein R. Modification of an amidolytic heparin assay to express protein-bound heparin and to correct for the effect of antithrombin III concentration. *Thromb Haemost*. 1987;58:884–887.

25. McGlasson D, Fritsma GA. Comparison of two anti-Xa assays using a single calibration curve for monitoring heparin anticoagulation. *J Throm Haemost*. 2007;Supplement, P-S- 092.

26. Diapharma website: www.diapharma.com Chromogenix Heparin Monograph.

27. Yin ET, Wessler S, Butler JV. Plasma heparin: a unique, practical submicrogram sensitive assay. *J Clin Lab Med*. 1973;81:298–310.

28. NCCLS (CLSI) document H21-A3. (1998) *Collection, Transport and Processing of Blood S for Coagulation Testing and General Performance of Coagulation Assays*. Approved Guideline, Third Edition.

29. Chan AKC, Black L, Ing C, Williams S, Brandao L. Do we need different standard curves for measuring different low molecular weight heparins? *J Throm Haemost*. 2007;5(suppl 2):P-S-128.

30. McGrath J, Johnston M, Angeloni F, Ginsberg J. Does monitoring patients on low molecular weight heparin (LMWH) require type specific reference lines for antifactor Xa heparin assays? *J Throm Haemost*. 2001;Supplement, P-S-2239.

31. QMP-LS Coagulation committee comments page 5, 2011;05–25.

32. Mouton C, Calderon J, Janvier G, Vergnes MC. Dextran sulphate included in factor Xa assay reagent overestimates heparin activity after heparin reversal by protamine. *Thromb Res*. 2003;111:273–279.

33. Rosborough TK. Monitoring unfractionated heparin therapy with antifactor Xa activity results in few monitoring tests and dosage changes the monitoring with the activated partial thromboplastin time. *Pharmacotherapy*. 1999;19(6):760–766.

34. Barrowcliffe TW. Laboratory monitoring of low molecular-weight heparin therapy—part II. *J Thromb Haemost*. 2005;3:575–576.

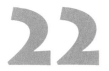

22 Monitoring oral anticoagulant therapy with vitamin K antagonists

Armando Tripodi

University School of Medicine and IRCCS Cà Granda Maggiore Hospital Foundation, Milan, Italy

Introduction

Vitamin K antagonists (VKA) are widely used as oral anticoagulants for the treatment of venous thromboembolism and for the prevention of systemic embolism in patients with atrial fibrillation or prosthetic heart valves [1]. VKA exert their anticoagulant effect by interfering with the cyclic conversion of vitamin K, thus inhibiting the carboxylation of glutamate residues to gamma-carboxyglutamate at the N-terminal domains of the procoagulant factors IX, VII, X, and II, and of the naturally occurring anticoagulants protein C, protein S, and protein Z [1]. The process of gamma-carboxylation which takes place in the hepatocytes is mediated by the enzyme carboxylase with vitamin K acting as a cofactor. As a consequence of the antagonizing effect of oral anticoagulants, vitamin K-dependent coagulation factors are synthesized as a-carboxylated or partially carboxylated forms that do not bind phospholipid surfaces, thus leading to defective coagulation *in vivo* and *in vitro* [1]. The dose–response effect of VKA is variable and their dosage must be monitored closely to prevent undesirable over- or under-anticoagulation. Assessing the effect directly through the measurement of their plasmatic concentration (although feasible [2]) would be of little value and difficult in practice [1]. Interaction of VKA with other drugs, dependency from diet, seasonal variation, and age suggest that assessing plasma coagulability by means of laboratory tests may be the most appropriate method for drug dosage [1].

The establishment of therapeutic intervals (i.e., optimal level of anticoagulation to prevent thrombosis, but still sufficient to minimizing the hemorrhagic risk) has in fact been achieved by dosing VKA through a coagulation test [1].

The prothrombin time (PT) was the logical choice because it is a global test sensitive to most of the coagulation factors depressed by VKA intake, it is also easy to perform and relatively inexpensive. However, an important limitation of the PT soon became evident. Thromboplastin preparations extracted from different tissues showed different responsiveness to the coagulation defect induced by VKA intake, thus making PT results obtained with different thromboplastins in different laboratories not comparable [3]. As a consequence, patients had to refer to the same laboratory for monitoring and the adoption of *"universal"* therapeutic intervals established by clinical trials was not possible. This situation has limited for many years the use of oral anticoagulants, despite the fact that early clinical trials of treatment and prophylaxis showed promising results.

During the last decades of the twentieth century many attempts have been made to make PT results comparable (see reference 3 for review) which culminated in the adoption of the system elaborated by Kirkwood [4] and later endorsed by the World Health Organization (WHO) [5, 6].

This system is based on the expression of PT results by means of a common scale called international normalized ratio (INR) [6]. Commercial

Quality in Laboratory Hemostasis and Thrombosis, Second Edition. Edited by Steve Kitchen, John D. Olson and F. Eric Preston.
© 2013 John Wiley & Sons, Ltd. Published 2013 by Blackwell Publishing Ltd.

thromboplastins are calibrated against an international reference preparation (IRP) for thromboplastin held by WHO by measuring paired PTs with both reagents for plasmas from healthy individuals and from patients stabilized on VKA [6]. The procedure allows the determination of the international sensitivity index (ISI), which is an index of the responsiveness of the reagent to be calibrated (working thromboplastin) to the coagulation defect induced by VKA, relatively to the IRP [6]. By definition, an ISI equal to 1.00 means the same responsiveness as the IRP, whereas an ISI greater or smaller than 1.00 means lesser or greater responsiveness, respectively [6]. Knowledge of the ISI value permits the conversion of PT results obtained with any given working reagent into the INR [6]. The following paragraphs will be devoted to discussing how the system works, what its limits are, and future directions.

Thromboplastin calibration

There are two models of calibration: full calibration, according to the WHO, and local calibration. The two models are interrelated and the second is a simplification of the first. The relative merits and shortcomings of the two models will be discussed below. For more details the reader may refer to the references 6 and 7.

WHO calibration

The ISI value is determined by parallel testing for PT of the plasmas from 20 healthy subjects and 60 patients stabilized on VKA treatment with an IRP and with the thromboplastin to be calibrated [6]. Patients must be chosen from among those who are in good health and those on long-term treatment (at least 6 months) [6]. Additionally, they must not be on heparin therapy and should not have undergone major dose changes during the last two visits [6]. Healthy individuals must be chosen among those who do not have personal or family history of hemorrhagic or thrombotic diseases, or other diseases known to alter hemostasis [6]. The calibration procedure may be conveniently performed over ten working sessions (not necessarily consecutive) each including two healthy individuals and six patients [6]. In principle the plasmas should be fresh, but frozen plasmas can also be used,

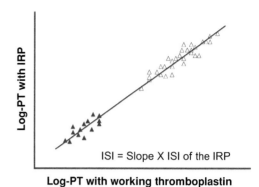

Figure 22.1 Calibration of prothrombin time (PT) measuring systems according to the World Health Organization (WHO) model. IRP: international reference preparation for thromboplastin. ISI: international sensitivity index. Closed and open symbols: PT values from healthy individuals and patients on VKA treatment, respectively.

especially for batch-to-batch calibration of the same thromboplastin [6]. Plasmas are intended as single donations, but pooled plasmas may also be suitable [6]. Testing is usually performed as single determinations by using the manual (tilt tube) technique or automated coagulometers for clot detection [6]. The manual technique for clot detection is mandatory for testing with the IRP [6].

As shown in Figure 22.1, paired PT values are plotted as coagulation times (seconds) on a double-log scale (IRP on the vertical axis), and the best-fit orthogonal regression line is drawn through the data points [6]. The slope of the line represents the responsiveness of the working reagent to the defect induced by VKA relatively to that of the IRP [6]. The ISI is calculated as the product of the slope times the ISI value of the IRP [6]. The final ISI will be assigned after identification and removal of data points whose INR as determined with both the IRP and the working thromboplastin is outside the interval 1.5–4.5 [6]. Likewise, data points lying at a perpendicular distance of three or more standard deviations from the line must also be identified and discarded before the final calculation of the ISI [6].

The precision of the calibration is acceptable if the coefficient of variation (CV) of the slope is 3% or less [6]. The CV depends not only on the precision of the measurements obtained with the IRP and the working thromboplastin, but also on the numbers and distribution of plasmas from the normal donors and patients on VKA used for calibration [6]. Another important requisite to judge the calibration is to test whether or not the orthogonal regression line drawn through the patient-only data points passes through the mean of the data points obtained for the healthy subjects [6]. Statistical analyses specifically designed for this requirement are available [8], but in practice it may suffice to test whether the values of the INR determined with the ISI calculated for the patient-only line deviates from the INR determined with the ISI calculated for the normal-plus-patients line [6]. If this difference is greater than 10%, alternative calculation of the INR may be required [8], but this does not occur very frequently.

Hierarchy of WHO international reference preparations

IRPs are crucial for the model of WHO calibration. As shown in Figure 22.2, two different IRPs are presently available from WHO and an additional one from the Institute for Reference Materials and Measurements (IRMM) of the European Commission. rTF/09 is a human recombinant relipidated tissue factor [9]; RBT/05 [10] and CRM 149 S [11] are from rabbit brain. All of them have been indirectly calibrated against the primary IRP coded 67/40 to which an arbitrary ISI equal to 1.00 had been assigned. Between the present IRPs and 67/40 there have been other

preparations (see Figure 22.2) whose stocks are now exhausted. All of them have been directly or indirectly calibrated against 67/40, so that continuity of the system is ensured. The reason to maintain at least two IRPs is twofold.

The *first* rests on the assumption that the calibration is more precise when performed against an IRP of the same species of the working thromboplastin. This would require an additional IRP of bovine origin, which was in fact available until recently [12], but it was dismissed on the ground that very few commercial thromboplastins of bovine origin are available [13]. Furthermore, evidence has been provided that bovine thromboplastins can be reliably calibrated by using IRPs from rabbit origin [13].

The *second* reason to maintain more than one IRP rests on the fact that these preparations although stable may deteriorate over time. The presence of at least two IRPs permits occasional checking of their relative stability by cross-calibrations [14]. When stocks of any of the IRPs is close to exhaustion or shows signs of deterioration, a replacement preparation is selected and calibrated by large international collaborative studies against all the existing IRPs. The assigned ISI is the average of all the individual values obtained with each IRP [6, 15]. Established IRPs are distributed upon request to manufacturers and national control laboratories along with protocols to be used for calibration of commercial thromboplastins and national secondary standards.

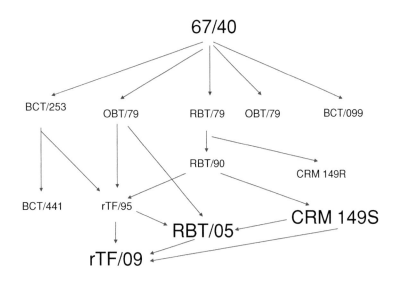

Figure 22.2 Hierarchy of international reference preparation (IRP) for thromboplastin. IRPs coded as small font have already been dismissed.

Local calibration

The responsibility to determine the ISI usually rests on the manufacturer as the above full calibration according to WHO recommendations would be beyond the expertise of most clinical laboratories. However, in recent years it has become evident that the ISI of commercial thromboplastins depends not only on reagents but also on coagulometers used for testing [16–18]. The effect of the coagulometer on the ISI may be minimized by two alternative procedures.

The *first* is to calibrate commercial thromboplastins on specific coagulometers. This can be achieved by testing plasmas with the IRP by the manual technique and with the working thromboplastin by the coagulometer. This gives an instrument-specific ISI value. It is the best solution, but difficult to put in practice because of the many possible thromboplastin/coagulometer combinations.

The *second* option requires that the calibration is performed locally by the user. Two different systems of local calibration have been devised over the last 15 years and are now available.

Local ISI determination

This system requires a set of lyophilized plasmas certified in terms of PT by using an IRP and the manual technique [19]. These calibration plasmas can then be tested locally by means of the thromboplastin/coagulometer combination and the value plotted against the certified PT value with the IRP [19]. The slope of the best-fit orthogonal regression line can eventually be used to calculate the local ISI in a manner analogous to that of the WHO-recommended procedure (Figure 22.3).

'Direct' INR determination

The second system suitable for local calibration requires a set of lyophilized calibration plasmas certified directly in terms of the INR by means of an IRP [20]. These calibration plasmas are then tested locally, and their coagulation times plotted against the certified INR values to draw a local calibration curve that may ultimately serve to convert patient coagulation times into INR (Figure 22.4).

Pros and cons of local calibration

The pros of these procedures are that they do not require expertise with the manual technique to record

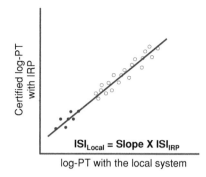

Figure 22.3 Local calibration of prothrombin time (PT) measuring system by means of lyophilized plasmas certified in terms of PT with an international reference preparation (IRP) for thromboplastin. ISI: international sensitivity index. Closed and open symbols: PT values from healthy individuals and patients on VKA treatment, respectively.

coagulation times and need neither the IRP nor the availability of considerable numbers of fresh plasmas from healthy individuals and patients on VKA treatment. Furthermore, the *"direct"* INR determination does not require knowledge of the ISI nor that of the mean normal PT (see later).

The cons are that they use lyophilized plasmas that do not necessarily mimic their fresh counterparts. Numerous surveys carried out over the last 15 years have shown light and shadows associated with the use of these simplified procedures for local calibration [21–24].

In general, the two procedures proved effective in improving the interlaboratory agreement of the INR

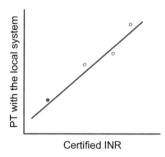

Figure 22.4 Local calibration of prothrombin time (PT) measuring system by means of lyophilized plasmas certified in terms of INR with an international reference preparation (IRP) for thromboplastin. Closed and open symbols: PT values from healthy individuals and patients on VKA treatment, respectively.

[21, 22], although doubts may remain about the efficacy to maintain the accuracy of the INR measurement [25]. The most important shortcoming associated with these procedures is that the INR determined for the calibration plasmas is often dependent on the type of thromboplastin or IRP used for testing [26]. The abovementioned differences, which vary with different sets of plasmas, are often greater than those recorded for fresh plasmas [26]; this probably means that the process of lyophilization (protein denaturation, addition of preservatives, buffers, and stabilizers) make those plasmas somewhat different from their fresh counterparts, with which they are supposed to be compared. Furthermore, the source of those plasmas may also play a role [26].

In this respect, artificially depleted plasmas obtained by selective absorption of vitamin K-dependent coagulation factors mimic the prolongation of the coagulation times recorded for plasmas from patients on VKA, but their composition is different for obvious reasons.

Plasmas from patients on VKA (coumarin plasmas) would be more suitable, but are more difficult to obtain in large amounts and with the range of INR required to cover the whole spectrum of anticoagulation.

The working party of the International Society on Thrombosis and Haemostasis has issued guidelines on how to prepare and use calibration plasmas [7], to which the reader may refer for more details. The most important recommendation stemming from the guidelines is that each set of calibration plasmas must be validated before it can be used for local calibration [7]. The validation requires that ten or more fresh plasmas from patients on VKA be tested for the INR by using the local combination of thromboplastin/coagulometer previously calibrated by the set of calibration plasmas [7]. The INR for the same plasmas will then be determined by the same combination of thromboplastin/coagulometer calibrated as recommended by the WHO (fresh plasmas and the IRP). If the mean values of the two determinations do not differ for more than 10%, the set of plasmas may be used for local calibration of subsequent lots of the same thromboplastin when used in combination with the same coagulometer [7]. Practical experience made with several sets of lyophilized calibration plasmas showed that generalization on the use of these plasmas for all types of thromboplastins may prove unfeasible

[23]. The reasons are presently unknown and probably rest on the interaction between thromboplastins and lyophilized plasmas. The (theoretical) argument that coumarin plasmas work better than artificially depleted plasmas in the above respect has been disputed [27], and this emphasizes the need to validate calibration plasmas before use with a particular combination of thromboplastin/coagulometer. Procedures for validation of INR and local calibration of PT/INR systems have also been issued by the Clinical and Laboratory Standards Institute (CLSI) [28].

Conversion of PT into INR and issues affecting results

Conversion of PT into INR

Once a combination of thromboplastin/coagulometer has been calibrated, the conversion of the coagulation time (seconds) into INR is straightforward. If the ISI of the thromboplastin/coagulometer is known the patient coagulation time is converted into ratio (patient-to-normal coagulation time), and this is raised to a power equal to the ISI of thromboplastin/coagulometer combination according to the equation [6]:

$$INR = (PT_{patient}/MNPT)^{ISI}$$

where the MNPT is the geometrical mean normal PT obtained by testing plasmas from 20 or more healthy individuals.

If the system ISI is not known, the patient coagulation time may be converted into INR by "*direct*" interpolation by means of a locally determined calibration curve relating coagulation times for the calibration plasmas versus the respective certified INR values [7].

By definition, the INR value for any given patient is the PT ratio that would have been obtained had the patient's plasma been tested with the IRP instead of the working thromboplastin [6].

Issues affecting results

Looking at equation that define the INR one can easily realize how and to what extent any of the parameters needed for its calculation may affect the final result.

Patient PT

The variables that may influence this parameter are pre-analytical and analytical. Among the first, the most important are the quality of venipuncture, the effect brought about by the blood collection system, the type and concentration of the anticoagulant, the centrifugation, and the type and time of storage before analysis. The analytical variables are concerned with the type of thromboplastin and coagulometers and the concentration of calcium chloride.

As for any other coagulation test, blood for the PT test should be obtained by clean venipuncture with minimum stasis to avoid undesirable activation of blood coagulation. Blood must be transferred rapidly into the tube containing the appropriate proportion of anticoagulant and mixed gently by repeated inversion to prevent the onset of coagulation activation. The use of evacuated tubes for blood collection is recommended, as it ensures a more standardized procedure of blood drawing than the syringe technique. The anticoagulant of choice for blood coagulation testing is trisodium citrate at a concentration of 109 mM (corresponding to 3.2%) [6], although concentrations ranging from 105 mM to 109 mM may be acceptable [29]. In many countries the concentration of 129 mM (or 3.8%) is still used, but this should be urgently replaced as the concentration of citrate may considerably influence the determination of the ISI and therefore of the INR. Evidence has been provided that the low concentration of the anticoagulant (in the face of a standard concentration of calcium chloride) results in shorter coagulation times. This shortening, however, does not affect normal and anticoagulated plasmas to the same extent and has, therefore, considerable effect on the ISI of any thromboplastin/coagulometer combination [30].

The correct proportion of blood to anticoagulant is 9:1. In evacuated tubes, this proportion is ensured by the vacuum, if sufficient time is allowed for the blood to flow. Visual inspection of the correct level of the blood in the tube is, however, highly recommended. Citrate does not cross cell membranes; therefore its concentration is higher in plasmas from patients with high hematocrit and lower in plasma from patients with low hematocrit. This translates in longer or shorter coagulation times, respectively. However, correction for the proportion of blood to anticoagulant is not strictly needed unless the patient's hematocrit is very low (<0.20) or very high (>0.60). Whenever needed, a correction chart proposed by Ingram & Hills [31] can be used to determine the appropriate amounts of citrate to be used in combination with the abnormal hematocrit.

Tubes for blood collection may considerably influence the PT, especially for patients on VKA. This holds true even when the concentration of the anticoagulant is maintained constant [29, 32]. The main reasons for those differences rest on the type of plastic (or siliconized glass) and the effect of buffers or contaminants [33]. Users should be aware of those differences and should check new brands of tubes to ascertain whether they are comparable to the old brands [34]. Whenever needed new values for the ISI and mean normal PT must be established and applied to the calculation of the INR.

Centrifugation should be carried out at a speed sufficient to get platelet-poor plasma. Residual platelets do not affect the PT very much; therefore, centrifugation for 15 minutes at 2000 g is adequate. To avoid deterioration of coagulation factors, it is advised that the centrifugation be carried out at (controlled) room temperature. Prior to the analyses, plasma samples must be stored at room temperature (20–24°C) to avoid cold activation of factor VII, which might considerably shorten the PT especially for patients on VKA. Although storage times up to 24 hours have been advocated as safe [35], occasional changes may occur in individual patients, and it is therefore strongly recommended that the analyses be complete not later than 4 hours from blood collection. This may prove increasingly challenging owing to laboratory consolidation, whereby blood samples must travel long distances prior to reaching the centralized laboratory. Frozen plasmas may be used provided that they have been stored in capped plastic tubes, rapidly frozen (liquid nitrogen) and stored at temperature lower than −30°C. Thawing before analysis should be performed rapidly (immersion of tubes in a water bath at 37°C for 1–2 minutes) to avoid the formation of cryoprecipitate.

Mean normal PT (MNPT)

The guidelines issued by WHO state that the value to be used as denominator in the equation to calculate the INR should be the geometric mean of the PT values for 20 or more healthy individuals [6]. This value must be determined locally with the combination of thromboplastin/coagulometer used for testing patient plasmas. The value is valid for that particular batch of thromboplastin, and must be recalculated whenever changes of thromboplastin and/or coagulometer do occur.

As an alternative to the MNPT, the PT value of pooled normal plasma, stored frozen and tested along with the patient plasmas may be also appropriate, provided that the material has been prepared by pooling a sufficient number of individual donations to ensure an average value close to the MNPT. Likewise, commercial lyophilized normal pooled plasmas may also be suitable if they have been prepared as above and their clotting times are close to the MNPT [36].

ISI

Being exponential, the effect of the ISI on the INR calculation may be considerable, especially with relatively unresponsive thromboplastins (ISI >1.00). The WHO guidelines recommend the use of thromboplastins with ISI values close to 1.00, although ISI ranging from 0.90 to 1.70 (determined with manual technique) may be acceptable [6].

Limits of the INR

General limits

It should be realized that the INR is an average approximate scale and therefore occasional between-system differences may occur even in the face of well-calibrated thromboplastin/coagulometer combinations. The PT test, which forms the basis for the INR scale, is a global test responsive to many coagulation factors (VII, X, V, II, and fibrinogen). Some of these factors are vitamin K-dependent (VII, X, and II), and therefore they are taken into consideration by the calibration procedure. However, the relative responsiveness of different thromboplastins to the activity of individual vitamin K-dependent coagulation factors may vary. Furthermore, other coagulation factors to which the PT is responsive (V and fibrinogen) are vitamin K-independent and therefore escape the calibration procedure [37]. It is therefore not surprising that small variations in the above coagulation factors may give rise to variation in the INR value measured with different thromboplastins even when they are accurately calibrated. The above differences are, however, not great enough to hamper the use of the INR in the clinical practice of dose prescription of VKA treatment as demonstrated by the relatively low rate of adverse events recorded in a large field inception cohort study carried out in oral anticoagulation clinics using the INR [38].

Specific limits

In addition to the above general limitations, clinicians using the INR scale for dose prescription should be aware of other specific limitations of this scale.

Patients not yet stabilized on VKA treatment
Strictly speaking the scale is valid only for patients stabilized on VKA. In fact, the ISI is determined by using plasmas from patients who are in the stable phase of VKA treatment [6]. This has two important implications.

First, the responsiveness of the thromboplastin to the defect induced by VKA intake is calculated when vitamin K-dependent coagulation factors are stably depressed. During the induction phase, the coagulation factors are depressed at a different rate depending on the relative half-life of the individual factors with factor VII being the first and factor II the last to be reduced. Obviously, those thromboplastins that are more responsive to factor VII will give INR values greater than those that are less responsive. Notwithstanding this limit, the INR scale can be safely used even during the induction phase [39].

The *second* implication is that the scale is (at least in principle) not valid for patients other than those treated with VKA. For instance, recent evidence highlighted this fact showing that the INR is unable to harmonize results obtained for patients with cirrhosis [40]. The most likely explanation is that the defect induced by VKA intake (similar though it may seem) is qualitatively different from that induced by cirrhosis. The lack of harmonization of the INR in the setting of cirrhosis is disturbing as the PT–INR has long been (and is still) used as a parameter to assess survival in patients with chronic liver disease [41] and ultimately to calculate the "*model for end stage liver disease (MELD)*" score which is ostensibly used to prioritize patients for liver transplantation [42]. If one considers that the INRs for patients with cirrhosis are not harmonized in different laboratories, the practical implication is that there is no parity of organ allocation, as it depends on the responsiveness of the thromboplastin used for testing by a particular laboratory. This translates into the undesirable situation where those patients who refer for INR measurement to laboratories using relatively more responsive thromboplastins may achieve priority for liver transplantation. The possible solution would be to calibrate the INR measuring system by determining the ISI for patients with chronic liver disease in a manner analogous to that for patients on VKA, whereby plasmas from the latter are replaced with plasmas from the former [40]. This system of alternative calibration proved feasible [40, 43], but implies that manufacturers should provide two different ISI (i.e., the ISI_{vka} and the ISI_{liver}) for each of their reagents. Recommendations on how to deal with this issue have been provided by the working group of the Scientific and Standardization Committee of the International Society on Thrombosis and Haemostasis [44].

INR values outside the interval of anticoagulation corresponding to 1.5–4.5

Strictly speaking, the INR is valid within the interval of anticoagulation corresponding to 1.5–4.5. This is because plasmas from patients selected for calibration lay within this interval, therefore the linearity of relationship and the ensuing validity of the ISI cannot be checked outside this interval. This implies that INR values greater than 4.5 are not very accurate and should be interpreted with caution.

Heparin

The treatment of acute venous thromboembolism requires embrication of heparin with VKA at least until the patient INR is within the therapeutic interval [1]. During this phase the PT is prolonged as a function of VKA intake, but (although to a lesser extent) also as a function of heparin. Therefore, the prescribing physician might be induced to withdraw heparin before the INR has reached the real therapeutic interval. Most of the commercial thromboplastins contain in their formulation antiheparin substances (polybrene or heparinases) which are able to quench heparin up to 1 U/mL activity. It is recommended to look at the package insert of the thromboplastin for more details.

Lupus anticoagulant (LA)

Patients with LA may occasionally present with prolonged PT. This means that when they are treated with VKA because of a thrombotic event their INR reflect the combined effects of anticoagulation and LA and this may make the assessment of the degree of anticoagulation uncertain. Numerous studies addressed this issue and although results are somewhat contrasting the conclusion is that there is no massive influence of LA on the INR [45–47]. There are, however, thromboplastins and patients for whom an effect has been shown [46, 47]. Whenever possible the PT should be measured before starting treatment with VKA. In case of prolongation there is an indication to switch to an insensitive thromboplastin.

Alternatively, other methods of laboratory control less sensitive or insensitive may be used. For instance, combined thromboplastins (brain extracts added with optimal amounts of factor V and fibrinogen) require plasma/thromboplastin ratios lower than that of conventional thromboplastins. Such thromboplastins are apparently less sensitive to the LA because the effect of the anticoagulant would be diluted out [48]. Another option would be monitoring the treatment through the measurement of an individual coagulation factor. The preferred candidate would be factor X, for which there are methods based on amidolytic measurement not influenced by LA [47]. It should, however, be realized that no validated therapeutic intervals based on such measurements are available.

Implementation of the INR

The full implementation of the INR requires combined efforts and partnership from the industry, national control laboratories, laboratory workers, and clinicians.

According to WHO recommendations, manufactures of commercial thromboplastins should determine the ISI of their reagents and state the value together with the coagulometer(s) for which they are valid on the package insert. Batch-to-batch consistency cannot be given for granted and the ISI should be checked for each production lot. Manufacturers should also state clearly the IRP (or secondary standard) and the procedure adopted for calibration.

The WHO strongly encourages health authorities to establish one or more National Control

Laboratories [6]. These laboratories should supervise the correct implementation of the INR, monitor the performance of clinical laboratories through the organization of regular external quality control surveys specifically designed for the INR, check of the validity of the ISI of commercial thromboplastins, establish national secondary standards where required, and provide assistance/advice to manufacturers for calibration of thromboplastins.

Laboratory workers are instrumental for the implementation of the INR. Besides being responsible for the correct measurement, they also play a key role in disseminating the relevant information to clinicians to whom the system of calibration and its limit should be explained.

Conclusions and future directions

The PT test was described nearly 80 years ago to investigate the coagulability of plasmas from patients with liver disease [49]. Since then it has been extensively used as a laboratory tool to investigate congenital and acquired coagulopathies, and for the laboratory control of oral anticoagulant therapy. Because of the increasing numbers of patients who benefit from oral anticoagulation, the PT is probably the most frequently asked coagulation test.

Attempts have been made to replace the PT with other tests such as single-factor measurements [50] or biochemical markers of coagulation activation [51, 52], but these attempts did not go beyond the publication of reports in scientific journals.

It may be predicted that the PT will stay in place at least until new direct antithrombin or anti-factor Xa drugs [53], which (allegedly) do not require laboratory monitoring, will enter the scene of treatment and prophylaxis of venous and arterial thromboembolism.

However, in spite of its popularity, when used to monitor patients on VKA, PT has many shortcomings, some of them not entirely resolved. Among them an adequate and robust system of local calibration is the most urgent to be tackled and resolved. Certified calibration plasmas are the way to go, but their quality should be improved to make them more similar to fresh plasmas. Preliminary experience showed that fresh frozen plasmas may be more suitable than lyophilized plasmas for local calibration [26], but their shipment to distant locations (although

possible) is problematic. There is, therefore, an urgent need to explore new venues for lyophilization with the aim of maintaining unaltered the properties of fresh coumarin plasmas.

References

1. Ansell J, Hirsh J, Poller L, Bussey H, Jacobson A, Hylek E. The pharmacology and management of the vitamin K antagonists: the Seventh ACCP Conference on Antithrombotic and Thrombolytic Therapy. *Chest.* 2004;126(suppl 3):204S–233S. Erratum in: *Chest.* 2005;127:415–416. Dosage error in text.
2. Lombardi R, Chantarangkul V, Cattaneo M, Tripodi A. Measurement of warfarin in plasma by high performance liquid chromatography (HPLC) and its correlation with the international normalized ratio. *Thromb Res.* 2003;111:281–284.
3. Poller L. International normalized ratios (INR): the first 20 years. *J Thromb Haemost.* 2004;2:849–860.
4. Kirkwood TB. Calibration of reference thromboplastins and standardisation of the prothrombin time ratio. *Thromb Haemost.* 1983;49:238–244.
5. WHO Expert Committee on Biological Standardization. Thirty-third report. *World Health Organ Tech Rep Ser.* 1983;687:81–105.
6. van den Besselaar AMHP, Poller L, Tripodi A. WHO Expert Committee on Biological Standardization. Forty-eighth report. Guidelines for thromboplastins and plasma used to control oral anticoagulant therapy. WHO Technical Report Series. 1999;889:64–93.
7. van den Besselaar AMHP, Barrowcliffe TW, Houbouyan-Réveillard LL, et al. On behalf of the Subcommittee on Control of Anticoagulation of the Scientific and Standardization Committee of the ISTH. Guidelines on preparation, certification and use of certified plasmas for ISI calibration and INR determination. *J Thromb Haemost.* 2004;2:1946–1953.
8. Tomenson JA. A statistician's independent evaluation. In: van den Besselaar AMHP, Lewis SM, Gralnick HR, eds. *Thromboplastin calibration and oral anticoagulant control.* Boston: Martinus Nijhoff; 1984:87–108.
9. Tripodi A, Chantarangkul V, van den Besselaar AMHP, Witteveen E, Hubbard AR. On behalf of the Subcommittee on Control of Anticoagulation of the Scientific and Standardisation Committee of the International Society on Thrombosis and Haemostasis. International collaborative study for the calibration of a proposed international standard for thromboplastin, human, plain. *J Thromb Haemost.* 2010;8:2066–2068.
10. Chantarangkul V, van den Besselaar AMHP, Witteveen E, Tripodi A. International collaborative study for

the calibration of a proposed international standard for thromboplastin, rabbit, plain. *J Thromb Haemost.* 2006;4:1339–1345.

11. van den Besselaar AMHP. Multi-center calibration of the third BCR reference material for thromboplastin, rabbit, plain, coded CRM 149S. Long-term stability of previous BCR reference materials. *Thromb Haemost.* 1995;74:1465–1467.

12. Hermans J, van den Besselaar AM, Loeliger EA, van der Velde EA. A collaborative calibration study of reference materials for thromboplastins. *Thromb Haemost.* 1983;50:712–717.

13. van den Besselaar AM, Tripodi A. Is there a need for replacement of the International Reference Preparation for Thromboplastin, Bovine, Combined (OBT/79)? *J Thromb Haemost.* 2005;3:2365–2366.

14. Linsinger TP, van den Besselaar AMHP, Tripodi A. Long-term stability of relationships between reference materials for thromboplastins. *Thromb Haemost.* 2006;96:210–214.

15. Tripodi A, Poller L, van den Besselaar AMHP, Mannucci PM. A proposed scheme for calibration of international reference preparations of thromboplastin for the prothrombin time. On behalf of the Subcommittee on Control of Anticoagulation. *Thromb Haemost.* 1995;74:1368–1369.

16. Poggio M, van den Besselaar AMHP, van der Velde EA, Bertina RM. The effect of some instruments for prothrombin time testing on the International Sensitivity Index (ISI) of two rabbit tissue thromboplastin reagents. *Thromb Haemost.* 1989;62:868–874.

17. Chantarangkul V, Tripodi A, Mannucci PM. The effect of instrumentation on thromboplastin calibration. *Thromb Haemost.* 1992;67:588–589.

18. van den Besselaar AMHP, Houbouyan LL, Aillaud MF, et al. Influence of three types of automated coagulometers on the international sensitivity index (ISI) of rabbit, human, and recombinant human tissue factor preparations–a multicenter study. *Thromb Haemost.* 1999;81:66–70.

19. Poller L, Triplett DA, Hirsh J, Carroll J, Clarke K. A comparison of lyophilized artificially depleted plasmas and lyophilized plasmas from patients receiving warfarin in correcting for coagulometer effects on international normalized ratios. *Am J Clin Pathol.* 1995;103:366–371.

20. Houbouyan LL, Goguel AF. Long-term French experience in INR standardization by a procedure using plasma calibrants. *Am J Clin Pathol.* 1997;108:83–89.

21. Chantarangkul V, Tripodi A, Cesana BM, Mannucci PM. Calibration of local systems with lyophilized calibrant plasmas improves the interlaboratory variability of the INR in the Italian external quality assessment scheme. *Thromb Haemost.* 1999;82:1621–1626. Erratum in: *Thromb Haemost.* 2000;83:VIII.

22. Kitchen S, Jennings I, Woods TA, Preston FE. Local calibration of international normalised ratio improves between laboratory agreement: results from the UK National External Quality Assessment Scheme. UK NEQAS (Blood Coagulation) Steering Committee. *Thromb Haemost.* 1999;81:60–65.

23. van den Besselaar AMHP, Houbouyan-Reveillard LL. Field study of lyophilized calibrant plasmas for fresh plasma INR determination. *Thromb Haemost.* 2002;87:277–281.

24. Poller L, Keown M, Ibrahim S, et al. European Concerted Action on Anticoagulation. Comparison of local International Sensitivity Index calibration and 'Direct INR' methods in correction of locally reported International Normalized Ratios: an international study. *J Thromb Haemost.* 2007;5:1002–1009.

25. van den Besselaar AMHP. International normalized ratio: towards improved accuracy. *Thromb Haemost.* 1999;82:1562–1563.

26. van den Besselaar AMHP, Houbouyan-Reveillard LL, Aillaud MF, et al. Multicenter evaluation of lyophilized and deep-frozen plasmas for assignment of the International Normalized Ratio. *Thromb Haemost.* 1999;82:1451–1455.

27. Poller L, van den Besselaar AMHP, Jespersen J, Tripodi A, Houghton D. A comparison of artificially-depleted, lyophilized coumarin and fresh coumarin plasmas in thromboplastin calibration. European Concerted Action on Anticoagulation. *Br J Haematol.* 1998;101:462–467.

28. Procedures for Validation of INR and Local Calibration of PT/INR Systems; Approved Guideline. CLSI document H54-A [ISBN 1-56238-000-0]. Clinical and Laboratory Standards Institute, 940 West Valley Road, Suite 1400, Wayne, PA 19087-1898 USA, 2005.

29. van den Besselaar AMHP, Chantarangkul V, Tripodi A. A comparison of two sodium citrate concentrations in two evacuated blood collection systems for prothrombin time and ISI determination. *Thromb Haemost.* 2000;84:664–667.

30. Chantarangkul V, Tripodi A, Clerici M, Negri B, Mannucci PM. Assessment of the influence of citrate concentration on the International Normalized Ratio (INR) determined with twelve reagent-instrument combinations. *Thromb Haemost.* 1998;80:258–262.

31. Ingram GI, Hills M. The prothrombin time test: effect of varying citrate concentration. *Thromb Haemost.* 1976;36:230–236.

32. van den Besselaar AMHP, Bertina RM, van der Meer FJ, den Hartigh J. Different sensitivities of various

thromboplastins to two blood collection systems for monitoring oral anticoagulant therapy. *Thromb Haemost*. 1999;82:153–154.

33. van den Besselaar AMHP, Witteveen E, Meeuwisse-Braun J, van der Meer FJ. The influence of exogenous magnesium chloride on the apparent INR determined with human, rabbit, and bovine thromboplastin reagents. *Thromb Haemost*. 2003;89:43–47.

34. Tripodi A, Chantarangkul V, Bressi C, Mannucci PM. How to evaluate the influence of blood collection systems on the international sensitivity index. Protocol applied to two new evacuated tubes and eight coagulometer/thromboplastin combinations. *Thromb Res*. 2002;108:85–89.

35. Rao LV, Okorodudu AO, Petersen JR, Elghetany MT. Stability of prothrombin time and activated partial thromboplastin time tests under different storage conditions. *Clin Chim Acta*. 2000;300:13–21.

36. Peters RH, van den Besselaar AM, Olthuis FM. Determination of the mean normal prothrombin time for assessment of international normalized ratios. Usefulness of lyophilized plasma. *Thromb Haemost*. 1991;66:442–445.

37. Tripodi A, Chantarangkul V, Akkawat B, Clerici M, Mannucci PM. A partial factor V deficiency in anticoagulated lyophilized plasmas has been identified as a cause of the international normalized ratio discrepancy in the external quality assessment scheme. *Thromb Res*. 1995;78:283–292.

38. Palareti G, Leali N, Coccheri S, et al. Bleeding complications of oral anticoagulant treatment: an inception-cohort, prospective collaborative study (ISCOAT). Italian Study on Complications of Oral Anticoagulant Therapy. *Lancet*. 1996;348:423–428.

39. Johnston M, Harrison L, Moffat K, Willan A, Hirsh J. Reliability of the international normalized ratio for monitoring the induction phase of warfarin: comparison with the prothrombin time ratio. *J Lab Clin Med*. 1996;128:214–217.

40. Tripodi A, Chantarangkul V, Primignani M, et al. The International Normalized Ratio Calibrated for Cirrhosis (INR$_{liver}$) Normalizes PT Results for MELD Calculation. *Hepatology*. 2007;46:520–527.

41. Malinchoc M, Kamath PS, Gordon FD, Peine CJ, Rank J, ter Borg PC. A model to predict poor survival in patients undergoing transjugular intrahepatic portosystemic shunts. *Hepatology* 2000; 31:864–71.

42. Wiesner R, Edwards E, Freeman R, Harper A, Kim R, Kamath P, Kremers W, Lake J, Howard T, Merion RM, Wolfe RA, Krom R. United Network for Organ Sharing Liver Disease Severity Score Committee. Model for end-stage liver disease (MELD) and allocation of donor liver. *Gastroenterology* 2003; 124: 91–6.

43. Bellest L, Eschwege V, Poupon R, Chazoullieres O, Robert A. A modified international normalized ratio as an effective way of prothrombin time standardization in hepatology. *Hepatology*. 2007;46:528–534.

44. Tripodi A, Baglin T, Robert A, Kitchen S, Lisman T, Trotter JF. On behalf of the Subcommittee on Control of Anticoagulation of the Scientific and Standardisation Committee of the International Society on Thrombosis and Haemostasis. Reporting Prothrombin Time Results as International Normalised Ratios for Patients with Chronic Liver Disease. *J Thromb Haemost*. 2010;8:1410–1412.

45. Moll S, Ortel TL. Monitoring warfarin therapy in patients with lupus anticoagulants. *Ann Intern Med*. 1997;127:177–185.

46. Robert A, Le Querrec A, Delahousse B, et al. Control of oral anticoagulation in patients with the antiphospholipid syndrome–influence of the lupus anticoagulant on International Normalized Ratio. Groupe Methodologie en Hemostase du Groupe d'Etudes sur l'Hemostases et la Thrombose. *Thromb Haemost*. 1998;80:99–103.

47. Tripodi A, Chantarangkul V, Clerici M, Negri B, Galli M, Mannucci PM. Laboratory control of oral anticoagulant treatment by the INR system in patients with the antiphospholipid syndrome and lupus anticoagulant. Results of a collaborative study involving nine commercial thromboplastins. *Br J Haematol*. 2001;115:672–678.

48. Rapaport SI, Le DT. Thrombosis in the antiphospholipid antibody syndrome. *New Eng J Med*. 1995;333, 665.

49. Quick AJ. The prothrombin time in hemophilia and obstructive jaundice. *J Biol Chem*. 1935;109:73–74.

50. Furie B, Diuguid CF, Jacobs M, Diuguid DL, Furie BC. Randomized prospective trial comparing the native prothrombin antigen with the prothrombin time for monitoring oral anticoagulant therapy. *Blood*. 1990;75:344–349.

51. Millenson MM, Bauer KA, Kistler JP, Barzegar S, Tulin L, Rosenberg RD. Monitoring "mini-intensity" anticoagulation with warfarin: comparison of the prothrombin time using a sensitive thromboplastin with prothrombin fragment F1+2 levels. *Blood*. 1992;79:2034–2038.

52. Tripodi A, Cattaneo M, Molteni A, Cesana BM, Mannucci PM. Changes of prothrombin fragment $1 + 2$ (F $1 + 2$) as a function of increasing intensity of oral anticoagulation—considerations on the suitability of F $1 + 2$ to monitor oral anticoagulant treatment. *Thromb Haemost*. 1998;79:571–573.

53. Franchini M, Mannucci PM. A new era of anticoagulants. *Eur J Intern Med*. 2009;20:562–568.

263

23 Monitoring new anticoagulants

Elaine Gray[1] & Trevor W. Barrowcliffe[2]

[1]National Institute for Biological Standards and Control, Potters Bar, UK.
[2]Formerly National Institute for Biological Standards and Control (NIBSC), Potters Bar, Hertfordshire, UK

Introduction

Unfractionated heparin (UFH) and warfarin have been in use as therapeutic anticoagulants since the 1930s and 1950s, respectively. While these two anticoagulants are effective in the prevention and treatment of thrombosis, there are drawbacks to their use. These include unpredictability in the dosage required for therapeutic effect, the need for continuous monitoring, and in the case of UFH, the development of antibodies that can lead to heparin-induced thrombocytopenia. Low-molecular-weight heparins (LMWHs), derivatives of UFH, were first described in 1976 [1] and have been in clinical use since the 1980s. The clinical advantages of LMWHs include greater predictability, dose-dependent plasma concentrations, a long half-life, and less bleeding for a given antithrombotic effect [2]. LMWHs are administered in fixed doses for prophylaxis and body weight adjusted doses for the treatment of thrombosis. Laboratory monitoring is not generally necessary [3]. However, dose-finding trials have not been carried out in specific populations, such as patients with renal failure or severe obesity. It has been suggested that monitoring should be considered in such patients [4–6]. Several laboratory assays have been proposed for this purpose, including the antifactor Xa assay, and more global clotting tests, such as the Heptest [6, 7]. Antifactor Xa chromogenic assay kits are now widely available, and the antifactor Xa assay is the test currently recommended by the American College of Chest physicians for monitoring of LMWHs [8].

New anticoagulants

In the past decade, development of new anticoagulants has focused on two major drug classes that have high specificity for either factor Xa or thrombin. These new generation anticoagulants are small molecules, produced either by chemical synthesis or recombinant technology. Their pharmacokinetics and pharmacodynamics are more predictable than warfarin, UFH, and LMWHs. Indirect FXa inhibitors such as fondaparinux and idraparinux bind specifically to antithrombin and are reported to have 100% bioavailability following subcutaneous injection. Coagulation monitoring has not been recommended for these therapeutics [9]. However, it is prudent to have appropriate and sensitive methods that will detect the concentration and activity of these therapeutics in case of overdose or for monitoring specific patient groups. Table 23.1 shows examples of these new anticoagulants. The indirect FXa inhibitors are antithrombin dependent and inhibit only free FXa, while the direct FXa inhibitors are antithrombin independent and inhibit both free FXa and FXa bound in the prothrombinase complex. While FXa inhibitors inhibit FXa that then leads to inhibition of the process of thrombin formation, the direct thrombin inhibitors

Quality in Laboratory Hemostasis and Thrombosis, Second Edition. Edited by Steve Kitchen, John D. Olson and F. Eric Preston.
© 2013 John Wiley & Sons, Ltd. Published 2013 by Blackwell Publishing Ltd.

Table 23.1 Indirect, direct FXa inhibitors and thrombin inhibitors that are in clinical use or in clinical trials

Indirect FXa inhibitors	Direct FXa inhibitors	FXa and thrombin inhibitors	Direct thrombin inhibitors
Fondaparinux	Otamixaban	BIBT 986	Dabigatran etexilate
Idraparinux	DX-9065a		Lepirudin
	Rivaroxaban		Bivalirudin
Biotinylated idraparinux	Apixaban		Argatroban
	LY517717		
	YM150		
	Edoxaban		
	PRT-054021		

(DTIs) target thrombin, the enzyme that converts fibrinogen to fibrin. Although the net effect of FXa and thrombin inhibitors is the suppression of coagulation, the mechanisms by which these inhibitors exert their action differ and therefore different laboratory monitoring methods will vary in their sensitivities to these inhibitors.

Calibration for accuracy of measurement

Unlike UFH and LMWHs, which are heterogeneous and polydisperse polysaccharides, these new anticoagulants are mostly chemically synthesized and homogeneous entities. However, their mechanisms of action are complex and therefore they behave more similarly to a biological than a chemically defined drug. The measurement of these anticoagulants should, therefore, follow the principle of bioassay that is, "like versus like" [10]. Regardless of assay methods used, each product should be used to construct calibration curves for the estimation of *ex vivo* plasma concentrations or activities of that product. The activity of these products should be expressed in either mass or molar concentrations rather than units. Figure 23.1 shows standard curves for two DTIs, argatroban and hirudin in an anti-IIa chromogenic assay. Although both anticoagulants inhibit thrombin, they yielded calibration curves with significantly different slopes and hence the standards are not interchangeable for the accurate estimation of plasma concentrations of either thrombin inhibitors.

Methods for monitoring indirect FXa inhibitors

Indirect FXa inhibitors such as fondaparinux and idraparinux potentiate the inactivation of free FXa

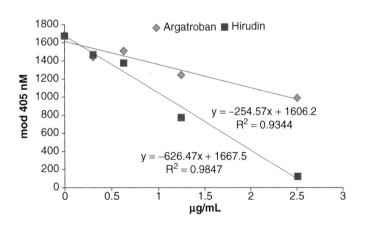

Figure 23.1 Anti-IIa chromogenic assay: standard curves for argatroban and hirudin.

by antithrombin. The routine prothrombin time (PT) and activated partial thromboplastin time (APTT) screening tests are not sensitive to this class of inhibitors. Walenga and Hoppensteadt [11] found that within the therapeutic range, APTT was insensitive to fondaparinux. The College of American Pathologists proficiency test results in 2006 showed that prophylactic or therapeutic concentrations of fondaparinux prolonged the PT by approximately 1 second and the APTT by 4–5 seconds [12]. The anti-Xa clot-based or chromogenic assays are the most sensitive method for monitoring this class of inhibitors. Heptest is the only commercially available clot-based anti-Xa assay, while there are a number of anti-Xa chromogenic kits, all of which are designed for LMWHs rather than for small synthetic indirect FXa inhibitors. The principle of the Heptest is based on the ability of heparin and similar compounds to catalyze the inhibition of exogenous FXa by antithrombin in plasma. The residual FXa is determined by the addition of phospholipid and calcium to the plasma and the end point of the assay is the measurement of clotting times. The resultant clotting times may also be influenced by inhibition of prothrombin activation and thrombin inhibition. Therefore the clot-based Heptest is less specific than the chromogenic methods. The chromogenic assays have the same principle as the Heptest, but residual FXa is estimated by the addition of a peptide substrate specific for FXa. Upon cleavage by FXa, the peptide substrate releases *p*-nitroaniline that can be monitored by OD at 405 nM. For fondaparinux, variability in results using different anti-Xa kits calibrated with different LMWHs indicated that there is a need to use a fondaparinux preparation as the reference standard and that the concentration of fondaparinux should be estimated in μg/mL [13, 14]. Concerns were also raised over the presence or absence of exogenous antithrombin in these kits. It has been suggested that at high doses, the monitoring anti-Xa assay may need to be supplemented with antithrombin to obtain the total amount of pentasaccharide in circulation [11]. However, results from a number of studies have shown that there were no significant differences between the amount of fondaparinux detected using anti-Xa methods with or without exogenous antithrombin [13–16].

Recently, a prothrombinase-induced clotting time (PiCT) assay has been introduced [17] and found to be useful for monitoring UFH, LMWH, indirect and direct FXa inhibitors, and DTIs. This is a two-step assay that appears to have a wide dynamic range, and is able to detect high concentrations of anticoagulants. In this test, the plasma sample containing the anticoagulant is mixed with a reagent containing a combination of a defined amount of FXa, phospholipids, and RVV-V, an enzyme from the venom of the snake *Daboia russelli* that directly activates FV. After 180-second incubation, the amount of prothrombinase complex formed is related to the residual FXa. The clotting time is recorded following the addition of calcium. Figure 23.2 shows an example of standard curves produced by an UFH, an LMWH and fondaparinux. The results from the PiCT assay correlate well with Heptest and chromogenic FXa assays [18, 19]. A one-step modification of this assay is also

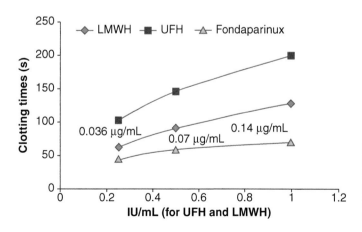

Figure 23.2 PiCT: calibration curves for UFH, LMWH, and fondaparinux. Concentrations of UFH and LMWH in IU/mL, were as stated on the axis, while the concentration of fondaparinux in μg/mL, is next to the datapoints.

available and has been found to be more sensitive to certain types of anticoagulants.

Methods for monitoring direct Xa inhibitors

The logical choice of monitoring methods for direct FXa inhibitors is anti-Xa based assays. Recent reports indicated that anti-Xa chromogenic methods and rivaroxaban calibrators are the assays of choice for quantification of rivaroxaban levels in plasma and that PT and APTT can be used as a screening test for the presence of the Xa inhibitor [20, 21]. Guidance from the British Committee for Standards in Haematology (BCSH) supports the use of the anti-Xa assays [22]. However, it has been noted that anti-Xa chromogenic assays with exogenous antithrombin could give an apparently higher concentration of rivaroxaban [23]. The pharmacokinetic and pharmacodynamic studies of direct Xa inhibitors such as otamixaban and DX 9065a indicated that clot-based assays can also be employed for monitoring this class of anticoagulants [24–30]. In these studies, increase in anti-Xa activity as assessed by anti-Xa chromogenic assay, prolongation of clotting times in the Heptest, APTT, PT, dilute prothrombin time (dPT), Russell's viper venom clotting time (RVVT), dilute Russell's viper venom clotting time (dRVVT) were found to correlate well with plasma concentrations of the Xa inhibitors as measured by liquid chromatography/tandem mass spectrometry (LC/MS/MS). APTT and PT reagents vary in their sensitivity to different FXa inhibitors and local validation of these methods is necessary before the use of these reagents for monitoring of therapy [30–32].

It should be noted that therapeutic APTT ratios and PT INR established for UFH, LMWHs, and warfarin should not be used as guidance for the safety and efficacy of these drugs. The PiCT test has also been investigated for monitoring of DX 9065a, but was only found to be sensitive to this inhibitor when the modified one-step method (omission of the 180s pre-incubation step) was used [33].

Methods for monitoring DTIs

DTIs are now used clinically for the prophylaxis and treatment of thrombosis and related cardiovascular diseases. Although all these inhibitors bind to thrombin and inhibit its activity, their chemical structures, binding affinities, and modes of action are different and, accordingly, their behavior in various monitoring tests are different. Routine anticoagulant monitoring tests such as the APTT have been used to estimate the activity of these inhibitors [8]. Other tests such as the ecarin clotting time (ECT), anti-IIa chromogenic assays, and point-of-care ECT have also been used for monitoring [34–36]. Gray and Harenberg [37] evaluated the robustness and the sensitivity of these different monitoring methods in an international collaborative study utilizing a panel of plasmas spiked with lepirudin and argatroban. This study found that the APTT (when expressed as a ratio to normal plasma) and the ECT tests gave the lowest interlaboratory variability. The APTT and anti-IIa chromogenic assays showed similar sensitivity to lepirudin and argatroban, but all three ECT kits (wet ECT, dry ECT, TIM) were more sensitive to argatroban than to lepirudin (Figures 23.3a and 23.3b).

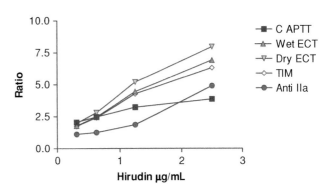

Figure 23.3a Geometric mean ratios of responses of lepirudin-spiked plasmas to normal plasma.

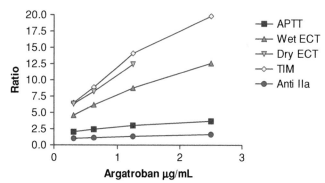

Figure 23.3b Geometric mean ratios of responses of argatroban-spiked plasmas to normal plasma.

These findings were confirmed by Gosselin et al. [38]. The two-step PiCT test was found to yield more reproducible results, but a linear dose–response relationship was not obtained within the therapeutic ranges of all of the thrombin inhibitors [39]. Several reports [40–43] on *in vitro* assays of dabigatran indicated that Hemoclot, a dilute thrombin time assay, was the most sensitive assay and showed a linear correlation with increase in clotting time and concentration of dabigatran; BCSH guidelines [22] supports the use of this test for the quantification of dabigatran. Commercially available dabigatran reference plasmas also aid accurate estimation of plasma concentration of the thrombin inhibitor. APTT and ECT were found to be useful in providing qualitative assessment of dabigatran, while the PT was found to be the least sensitive.

Methods for monitoring dual inhibitor of FXa and thrombin

BIBT 986 is the only synthetic anticoagulant that inhibits both FXa and thrombin. Theoretically, both FXa and thrombin-based assays would be suitable methods for monitoring this inhibitor. Pharmacokinetics and pharmacodynamics studies [44, 45] in humans have shown that there is a linear relationship between plasma concentrations of the drug and pharmacodynamic responses assessed by changes in clotting times of routine screening coagulation tests such as the APTT, thrombin time (TT), and ECT. Similar to other thrombin inhibitors, BIBT 986 is also able to lengthen the PT, but the sensitivity is poor by comparison to APTT, TT, and ECT.

Monitoring anticoagulants using global screening tests

Screening tests such as the APTT and the PT only provide a snapshot of the coagulation status and do not take into account the dynamics of the hemostatic pathways. Due to the recent availability of automated and semi-automated instruments for global methods such as the thrombin generation test and thromboelastography (TEG), there is now an increased interest in these informative but laborious tests for monitoring of procoagulant and anticoagulant therapies.

The thrombin generation test measures thrombin production over time and can be quantified by calculating the area under the thrombin generation curve. This area under the curve is commonly referred to as the endogenous thrombin potential (ETP). Other parameters such the lag time, peak thrombin, and the overall shape of the curves also provide useful information on the activity of the therapeutics. Anticoagulants that give similar prolongation of APTT and PT may have different behavior in the thrombin generation test. Figures 23.4a and 23.4b show thrombin generation curves of plasma spiked with hirudin or argatroban. With increasing concentration, hirudin delayed thrombin generation without decreasing the overall amount of thrombin generated, while argatroban delayed thrombin generation as well as reducing the amount of thrombin generated (Table 23.2). The interlaboratory reproducibility of thrombin generation test results is poor even when the same concentrations of tissue factor/phospholipid were used [46, 47]. Standardization of methods is required before a useful clinical correlation can be drawn.

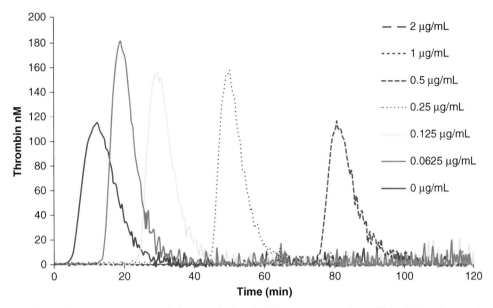

Figure 23.4a Thrombin generation curves of plasma spiked with different concentrations of hirudin. Results are obtained from the Thrombinoscope. Thrombin was not detected with plasmas spiked with 1 or 2 µg/mL of hirudin.

The point-of-care-based (TEG) or thromboelastometry (ROTEM) measures the mechanics of clot formation and lysis [48]. Preliminary studies on anticoagulants are being made by research laboratories [49, 50]. However, the interlaboratory reproducibility of these tests is difficult to assess as whole blood samples are normally used for testing. External quality assessment providers are recognizing the need for standardization of these tests and currently the United Kingdom National External Quality Assessment Scheme (NEQAS) is organizing proficiency tests for these techniques [51].

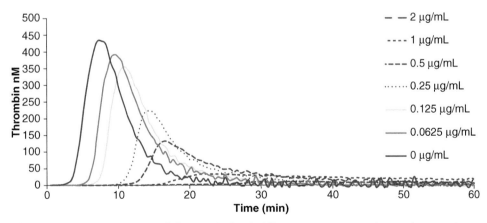

Figure 23.4b Thrombin generation curves of plasma spiked with different concentrations of argatroban. Results are obtained from the Thrombinoscope. Thrombin was not detected with plasma sample spiked with 2 µg/mL of argatroban.

269

Table 23.2 Inhibition of thrombin generation by hirudin and argatroban, measured by the Thrombinoscope, using 1 pM tissue factor/4 μM phospholipid in normal platelet poor plasma

	Thrombin inhibitors	Concentration μg/mL						
		0	0.0625	0.125	0.25	0.5	1	2
Lag time (min)	Hirudin	5.83	14.35	24.88	43.83	76.36	NC	NC
	Argatroban	3.89	6.22	7.67	11.44	12.89	16.22	25.11
ETP Min*nM	Hirudin	1303	1498	1399	1312	1132	NC	NC
	Argatroban	3084	3017	2698	1933	1737	NC	NC

NC, not calculated

Summary

The new anticoagulants can be broadly classified into FXa and thrombin inhibitors. The FXa inhibitors can be monitored by anti-Xa chromogenic or clot-based methods, while the APTT and ECT are useful for thrombin inhibitors. The PiCT tests appear to be sensitive to a wide range of anticoagulants. As these new therapeutics have different mechanisms to the traditional anticoagulants such as heparin and warfarin and since there are no international standards available, product-specific reference materials should be used to standardize the different methods used for monitoring.

References

1. Johnson EA, Kirkwood TB, Stirling Y, et al. Four heparin preparations: anti-Xa potentiating effect of heparin after subcutaneous injection. *Thromb Haemost*. 1976;35(3):586–591.
2. Warkentin TE, Levine MN, Hirsch J, et al. Heparin-induced thrombocytopenia in patients treated with low-molecular-weight heparin or unfractionated heparin. *N Engl J Med*. 1995;332:1330–1325.
3. Hirsh J, Raschke R. Heparin and low-molecular weight heparin. The seventh ACCP Conference on antithrombotic and thrombolytic therapy. *Chest*. 2004;126:188S–203S.
4. Kessler CM. Low molecular weight heparins: practical considerations. *Semin Hematol*. 1997;34:35–42.
5. Abbate R, Gori AM, Farsi A, Attanasio M, Pepe G. Monitoring of low-molecular- weight heparins. *Am J Cardiol*. 1998;82:33L–36L.
6. Samama MM. Contemporary laboratory monitoring of low molecular weight heparins. *Clin Lab Med*. 1995;15:119–123.
7. Kessler CM, Esparraguera IM, Jacobs HM, et al. Monitoring the anticoagulant effects of a low molecular weight heparin preparation. *Am J Clin Pathol*. 1995;103:642–648.
8. Garcia DA, Baglin TP, Weitz JI, Samama MM. Parenteral Anticoagulants: antithrombotic therapy and preventions thrombosis, 9th ed: American College of Chest Physicians Evidence-based Clinical Practice Guidelines. *Chest*. 2012;141(suppl):e24S–e43S.
9. Gross PL, Weitz JI. New anticoagulants for treatment of venous thromboembolism. *Arterioscler Thromb Vasc Biol*. 2008;28:380–386.
10. Barrowcliffe TW. Heparin assays and standardisation. In: Lane DA, Lindahl U, eds. *Heparin: Chemical and Biological Properties, Clinical Applications*. London: Edward Arnold; 1989;393–416.
11. Walenga JM, Hoppensteadt DA. Monitoring the new antithrombotic drugs. *Semin Thromb Hemost*. 2004;30(6):683–695.
12. Smogorzewska A, Brandt JT, Chandler WL, et al. Effect of fondaparinux on coagulation assays: results of College of American Pathologists proficiency testing. *Arch Pathol Lab Med*. 2006;130:1605–1611.
13. Depasse F, Gerotziafas GT, Busson J, van Dreden P, Samama MM. Assessment of three chromogenic and one clotting assays for the measurement of synthetic pentasaccharide fondaparinux (Arixtra®) anti-Xa activity. *J Thromb Haemost*. 2004;2:346–348.
14. Dämgen-von Brevern G, Kläffling C, Lindhoff-Last E. Monitoring anticoagulation by fondaparinux: determination of anti factor Xa-level. *Hamostaseologie*. 2005;25(3):281–285.
15. Klaeffling C, Piechottka G, Daemgen-von Brevern G, et al. Development and clinical evaluation of two chromogenic substrate methods for monitoring fondaparinux sodium. *Ther Drug Monit*. 2006;28(3):375–381.
16. Paolucci F, Frasa H, Van Aarle F, et al. Two sensitive and rapid chromogenic assays of fondaparinux sodium

(Arixtra) in human plasma and other biological matrices. *Clin Lab.* 2003;49(9–10):451–460.

17. Calatzis A, Spannagl M, Gempeler-Messina P, Kolde HJ, Schramm W, Haas S. The prothrombinase induced clotting test: A new technique for the monitoring of anticoagulants. *Haemostasis.* 2000;30(suppl 2):172–174.

18. Harenberg J, Giese C, Hagedorn A, Traeger I, Fenyvesi T. Determination of antithrombin-dependent factor Xa inhibitors by prothrombin-induced clotting time. *Semin Thromb Hemost.* 2007;33(5):503–507.

19. Graff J, Picard-Willems B, Harder S. Monitoring effects of direct FXa-inhibitors with a new one-step prothrombinase-induced clotting time (PiCT) assay: comparative in vitro investigation with heparin, enoxaparin, fondaparinux and DX 9065a. *Int J Clin Pharmacol Ther.* 2007;45(4):237–243.

20. Douxfils J, Mullier F, Loosen C, Chatelain C, Chatelain B, Dogné JM. Assessment of the impact of rivaroxaban on coagulation assays: Laboratory recommendations for the monitoring of rivaroxaban and review of the literature. *Thromb Res.* 2012;130(6):956–966.

21. Miyares MA, Davis K. Newer oral anticoagulants: A review of laboratory monitoring options and reversal agents in the hemorrhagic patient. *Am J Health Syst Pharm.* 2012;69(17):1473–1484.

22. Baglin T, Keeling D, Kitchen S. Effects on routine coagulation screens and assessment of anticoagulant intensity in patients taking oral dabigatran or rivaroxaban: Guidance from the British Committee for Standards in Haematology. *Br J Haematol.* 2012;159(4):427–429. doi: 10.1111/bjh.12052. [Epub ahead of print]

23. Mani H, Rohde G, Stratmann G, et al. Accurate determination of rivaroxaban levels requires different calibrator sets but not addition of antithrombin. *Thromb Haemost.* 2012;108(1):191–198.

24. Gerbutavicius R, Iqbal O, Messmore HL, et al. Differential effects of DX-9065a, argatroban, and synthetic pentasaccharide on tissue thromboplastin inhibition test and dilute Russell's viper venom test. *Clin Appl Thromb Hemost.* 2003;9(4):317–323.

25. Tobu M, Iqbal O, Ma Q, et al. Global anticoagulant effects of a synthetic anti-factor Xa inhibitor (DX-9065a): implications for interventional use. *Clin Appl Thromb Hemost.* 2003;9(1):1–17.

26. Rezaie AR. DX-9065a inhibition of factor Xa and the prothrombinase complex: mechanism of inhibition and comparison with therapeutic heparins. *Thromb Haemost.* 2003;89(1):112–121.

27. Paccaly A, Ozoux ML, Chu V, et al. Pharmacodynamic markers in the early clinical assessment of otamixaban, a direct factor Xa inhibitor. *Thromb Haemost.* 2005;94(6):1156–1163.

28. Paccaly A, Frick A, Ozoux ML, et al. Pharmacokinetic/pharmacodynamic relationships for otamixaban, a direct factor Xa inhibitor, in healthy subjects. *J Clin Pharmacol.* 2006;46(1):45–51.

29. Hinder M, Frick A, Jordaan P, et al. Direct and rapid inhibition of factor Xa by otamixaban: a pharmacokinetic and pharmacodynamic investigation in patients with coronary artery disease. *Clin Pharmacol Ther.* 2006;80(6):691–702.

30. Mueck W, Becka M, Kubitza D, Voith B, Zuehlsdorf M. Population model of the pharmacokinetics and pharmacodynamics of rivaroxaban—an oral, direct factor Xa inhibitor—in healthy subjects. *Int J Clin Pharmacol Ther.* 2007;45:335–344.

31. Tobu M, Iqbal O, Hoppensteadt DA, Shultz C, Jeske W, Fareed J. Effects of a synthetic factor Xa inhibitor (JTV-803) on various laboratory tests. *Clin Appl Thromb Hemost.* 2002;8(4):325–336.

32. Laux V, Perzborn E, Kubitza D, Misselwitz F. Preclinical and clinical characteristics of rivaroxaban: a novel, oral, direct factor Xa inhibitor. *Semin Thromb Hemost.* 2007;33(5):515–523.

33. Graff J, Picard-Willems B, Harder S. Monitoring effects of direct FXa-inhibitors with a new one-step prothrombinase-induced clotting time (PiCT) assay: comparative in vitro investigation with heparin, enoxaparin, fondaparinux and DX 9065a. *Int J Clin Pharmacol Ther.* 2007;45(4):237–243.

34. Nowak G, Bucha E. Quantitative determination of hirudin in blood and body fluids. *Semin Thromb Hemost.* 1996;22:197–202.

35. Hafner G, Fickenscher K, Friesen HJ, et al. Evaluation of an automated chromogenic substrate assay for the rapid determination of hirudin in plasma. *Thromb Res.* 1995;77:165–173.

36. Koster A, Hansen R, Grauhan O, et al. Hirudin monitoring using the TSA ecarin clotting time in patients with heparin-induced-thrombocytopenia type II. *J Cardiothorac Vasc Anesth.* 2000;14:249–252.

37. Gray E, Harenberg J, ISTH Control of Anticoagulation SSC Working Group on Thrombin Inhibitors. Collaborative study on monitoring methods to determine direct thrombin inhibitors lepirudin and argatroban. *J Thromb Haemost.* 2005;3(9):2096–2097.

38. Gosselin RC, King JH, Janatpour KA, Dager WE, Larkin EC, Owings JT. Comparing direct thrombin inhibitors using aPTT, ecarin clotting times, and thrombin inhibitor management testing. *Ann Pharmacother.* 2004;38(9):1383–1388.

39. Fenyvesi T, Jörg I, Harenberg J. Monitoring of anticoagulant effects of direct thrombin inhibitors. *Semin Thromb Hemost.* 2002;28(4):361–368.

40. van Ryn J, Stangier J, Haertter S, et al. Dabigatran etexilate—a novel, reversible, oral direct thrombin inhibitor: interpretation of coagulation assays and reversal of anticoagulant activity. *Thromb Haemost.* 2010;103(6):1116–1127.

41. Stangier J, Feuring M. Using the HEMOCLOT direct thrombin inhibitor assay to determine plasma concentrations of dabigatran. *Blood Coagul Fibrinolysis.* 2012;23(2):138–143.

42. Douxfils J, Mullier F, Robert S, Chatelain C, Chatelain B, Dogné JM. Impact of dabigatran on a large panel of routine or specific coagulation assays. Laboratory recommendations for monitoring of dabigatran etexilate. *Thromb Haemost.* 2012;107(5):985–997.

43. Curvers J, van de Kerkhof D, Stroobants AK, van den Dool EJ, Scharnhorst V. Measuring direct thrombin inhibitors with routine and dedicated coagulation assays: which assay is helpful? *Am J Clin Pathol.* 2012;138(4):551–558.

44. Leitner JM, Jilma B, Mayr FB, et al. Pharmacokinetics and pharmacodynamics of the dual FII/FX inhibitor BIBT 986 in endotoxin-induced coagulation. *Clin Pharmacol Ther.* 2007;81(6):858–866.

45. Graefe-Mody EU, Schühly U, Rathgen K, Stähle H, Leitner JM, Jilma B. Pharmacokinetics and pharmacodynamics of BIBT 986, a novel small molecule dual inhibitor of thrombin and factor Xa. *J Thromb Haemost.* 2006;4(7):1502–1509.

46. Lawrie AS, Gray E, Leeming D, et al. A multicentre assessment of the endogenous thrombin potential using a continuous monitoring amidolytic technique. *Br J Haematol.* 2003;123(2):335–341.

47. Dargaud Y, Luddington R, Gray E, et al. Effect of standardization and normalization on imprecision of calibrated automated thrombography: an international multicentre study. *Br J Haematol.* 2007;139(2):303–309.

48. Luddington RJ. Thromboelastography/thromboelastometry. *Clin Lab Haematol.* 2005;27:81–90.

49. Demir M, Iqbal O, Hoppensteadt DA, et al. Anticoagulant and antiprotease profiles of a novel natural heparinomimetic mannopentaose phosphate sulfate (PI-88). *Semin Thromb Hemost.* 2000;26(suppl 1):39–46.

50. Mousa SA. Comparative efficacy of different low-molecular-weight heparins (LMWHs) and drug interactions with LMWH: implications for management of vascular disorders. *Clin Appl Thromb Hemost.* 2001;7(2):131–140.

51. Jennings I, Kitchen DP, Woods TA, Kitchen S, Walker ID. Emerging technologies and quality assurance: the United Kingdom National External Quality Assessment Scheme perspective. *Semin Thromb Hemost.* 2007;33(3):243–249.

Index

Quality in Laboratory Hemostasis and Thrombosis, Second Edition. Edited by Steve Kitchen, John D. Olson and F. Eric Preston.
© 2013 John Wiley & Sons, Ltd. Published 2013 by Blackwell Publishing Ltd.

Printed and bound by CPI Group (UK) Ltd, Croydon, CR0 4YY

16/04/2025

14658503-0004